Diagnostic Imaging of Novel Coronavirus Pneumonia

Minming Zhang • Bin Lin
Editors

Diagnostic Imaging of Novel Coronavirus Pneumonia

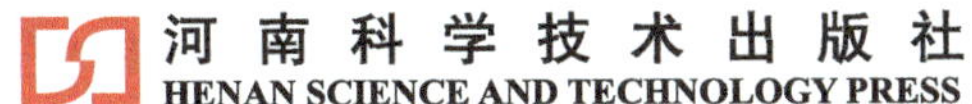

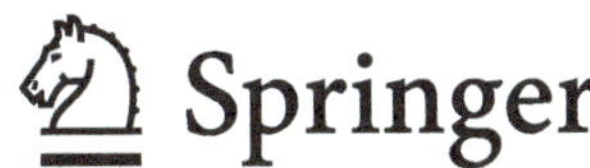

Editors
Minming Zhang
Department of Radiology
The Second Affiliated Hospital
Zhejiang University School of Medicine
Hangzhou
China

Bin Lin
Department of Radiology
The Second Affiliated Hospital
Zhejiang University School of Medicine
Hangzhou
China

ISBN 978-981-15-5994-5   ISBN 978-981-15-5992-1 (eBook)
https://doi.org/10.1007/978-981-15-5992-1

B&R Book Program
The printed edition is not for sale in China Mainland. Customers from China Mainland please order the print book from: Henan Science and Technology Press.
Jointly published with Henan Science and Technology Press

This Springer imprint is published by the registered company Springer Nature Singapore Pte Ltd.
The registered company address is: 152 Beach Road, #21-01/04 Gateway East, Singapore 189721, Singapore

Preface

Since December 2019, there has been an outbreak of Coronavirus disease 2019 (COVID-19) pandemic across the world, and now the number of people who have been infected with this disease has exceeded 10 million and more than 500 thousand of them have died. Chest CT examination may help to find pulmonary lesions, and the characteristic imaging manifestations of CT may give us an indication of the infectious agents of the pneumonia; therefore, chest CT examination plays a positive role in isolating the suspected patients as early as possible in the process of preventing and controlling the disease. In addition, chest CT examination has important effects in predicting the outcome of the disease, evaluating the therapeutic effect, and identifying the mixed infection and complications.

In the epidemic prevention and control, radiologists of China have played an important role and also have accumulated rich valuable experience. For this reason, we have written this book so as to share the experiences of our team with our counterparts in the world.

The editorial board members of this book are radiologists from several designated hospitals for the treatment of COVID-19, who are working at the frontline for China's prevention and control of COVID-19. In order to compile this book, the editorial board members read a lot of literature. They reviewed the clinical records, laboratory examination results, and imaging data of thousands of cases. Hundreds of the typical cases were selected and included in this book, and the comments of these cases were added.

It is hoped that this book can help radiologists and clinicians around the world to understand the typical imaging manifestations of the disease, and further provide valuable information for scientific research, diagnosis, treatment, and prevention of the disease. As the current epidemic situation is constantly changing, our understanding of the disease may not be comprehensive. Therefore, this book is likely to be insufficient. We sincerely invite colleagues and readers to correct us.

Hangzhou, Zhejiang, China — Minming Zhang
July 1, 2020

Contents

Editors and Contributors

Editors-in-Chief

Minming Zhang Department of Radiology, the Second Affiliated Hospital, Zhejiang University School of Medicine, Hangzhou, China

Bin Lin Department of Radiology, the Second Affiliated Hospital, Zhejiang University School of Medicine, Hangzhou, China

Associate Editors-in-Chief

Hui Mao Department of Radiology and Imaging Sciences, Emory University School of Medicine, Atlanta, GA, USA

Zongyu Xie Department of Radiology, the First Affiliated Hospital of Bengbu Medical College, Bengbu, China

Xiqi Zhu Department of Radiology, Nanxishan Hospital of Guangxi Zhuang Autonomous Region, Guilin, China

Yuantong Gao Department of Radiology, the Third Affiliated Hospital of Wenzhou Medical University, Ruian, China

Contributors

Lulu Gao Department of Radiology, Zhejiang Hospital, Hangzhou, China

Yuqing Gao Department of Radiology, the First Affiliated Hospital of Bengbu Medical College, Bengbu, China

Pingding Kuang Department of Radiology, the Second Affiliated Hospital, Zhejiang University School of Medicine, Hangzhou, China

Shuhua Li Department of Radiology, the First Affiliated Hospital of Bengbu Medical College, Bengbu, China

Yongchou Li Department of Radiology, the Third Affiliated Hospital of Wenzhou Medical University, Ruian, China

Nan Lu Department of Radiology, the Second Affiliated Hospital, Zhejiang University School of Medicine, Hangzhou, China

Jian Lv Department of Radiology, Nanxishan Hospital of Guangxi Zhuang Autonomous Region, Guilin, China

Zhujing Shen Department of Radiology, the Second Affiliated Hospital, Zhejiang University School of Medicine, Hangzhou, China

Chao Wang Department of Radiology, the Second Affiliated Hospital, Zhejiang University School of Medicine, Hangzhou, China

Jian Wang Department of Radiology, Tongde Hospital of Zhejiang Province, Hangzhou, China

Lihua Wang Department of Radiology, the Second Affiliated Hospital, Zhejiang University School of Medicine, Hangzhou, China

Liya Wang Southern Medical University Affiliated Longhua People's Hospital, Shenzhen, Guangdong, China

The Third School of Clinical Medicine Southern Medical University, Shenzhen, Guangdong, China

Qiyuan Wang Department of Radiology, the Second Affiliated Hospital, Zhejiang University School of Medicine, Hangzhou, China

Xiaopei Xu Department of Radiology, the Second Affiliated Hospital, Zhejiang University School of Medicine, Hangzhou, China

Fan Yang Department of Radiology, the Second Affiliated Hospital, Zhejiang University School of Medicine, Hangzhou, China

Xiaocheng Zhang Department of Radiology, the Second Affiliated Hospital, Zhejiang University School of Medicine, Hangzhou, China

Cancan Zhao Department of Radiology, the First Affiliated Hospital of Bengbu Medical College, Bengbu, China

Tongtong Zhao Department of Radiology, the Second People's Hospital of Fuyang City, Fuyang, China

Hanpeng Zheng Department of Radiology, YueQing People's Hospital, WenZhou, China

Haisheng Zhou Department of Radiology, YueQing People's Hospital, WenZhou, China

1 Overview of the COVID-19

Yuantong Gao, Liya Wang, Bin Lin, Hui Mao, and Minming Zhang

1.1 Identification and Nomenclature of COVID-19

The novel coronavirus that caused pandemic in 2020 started from a number of cases of unexplained pneumonia in the city of Wuhan, Hubei Province, China, in December of 2019. Unlike the other human coronavirus previously reported, this new strain of coronavirus is much more contagious and rapidly spread in the city of Wuhan and subsequently various regions of China from the epicenter of Wuhan. Within several weeks, many countries of Asia, Europe, North America, and Oceania reported the confirmed cases with the worldwide total number quickly rising to over 5.35 million and more than 343,000 deaths on May 24, 2020. The World Health Organization (WHO) initially named this novel coronavirus as "2019 Novel Coronavirus" (2019-nCoV) on January 12, 2020. National Health Commission of China named the pneumonia caused by 2019-nCoV as Novel Coronavirus Pneumonia (NCP) on January 20, 2020. In the meantime, National Health Commission of China issued an announcement to include this disease in the category B infectious diseases as stipulated in the Law of the People's Republic of China on the Prevention and Treatment of Infectious Diseases, but to manage this disease according to Class A infectious diseases. On February 11, 2020, Tedros Adhanom Ghebreyesus, director general of WHO, announced the revised name of the pneumonia caused by novel coronavirus as "Coronavirus Disease 2019" (COVID-19). At the same time, the International Committee for Virus Classification named the novel coronavirus "Severe Acute Respiratory Syndrome Coronavirus 2" (SARS-CoV-2). Given the high incidence of SARS-CoV-2 infection and the rapid increase of the cases globally, WHO officially declared on March 11, 2020 in Geneva that the COVID-19 caused by SARS-CoV-2

Y. Gao
Department of Radiology, the Third Affiliated Hospital of Wenzhou Medical University, Ruian, China

L. Wang
Department of Radiology, Southern Medical University Affiliated Longhua People's Hospital, Shenzhen, Guangdong, China

Department of Radiology, the Third School of Clinical Medicine Southern Medical University, Shenzhen, Guangdong, China

B. Lin · M. Zhang (✉)
Department of Radiology, the Second Affiliated Hospital, Zhejiang University School of Medicine, Hangzhou, China
e-mail: zjdxlinbin@zju.edu.cn; zhangminming@zju.edu.cn

H. Mao
Department of Radiology and Imaging Sciences, Emory University School of Medicine, Atlanta, GA, USA
e-mail: hmao@emory.edu

M. Zhang, B. Lin (eds.), *Diagnostic Imaging of Novel Coronavirus Pneumonia*, https://doi.org/10.1007/978-981-15-5992-1_1

has the characteristics of a global pandemic. At present, the origin of SARS-CoV-2 is still under investigation.

1.2 Etiological Characteristics

The coronavirus is named after its coronal-like spinous spike glycoproteins protruding from the viral envelope, which can be seen under the electron microscope as shown in Fig. 1.1. The first coronavirus was isolated from poultry in 1937. Until 1965, the coronavirus was first found in human. It is now known that the parasitic hosts of coronaviruses include bats, camels, birds, mice, hedgehogs, dogs, cats, and other mammals, as well as humans [1].

Based on the genetic characteristics, different coronaviruses can be divided into four genera: α, β, γ, and δ. SARS-CoV-2 belongs to the β coronavirus. The enveloped viral particles are round or oval in shape. It is often pleomorphic with a diameter of 60–140 nm. The genetic characteristics of SARS-CoV-2 infecting humans are significantly different from severe acute respiratory syndrome coronavirus (SARS-CoV) and Middle East respiratory syndrome coronavirus (MERS-CoV), previously discovered in humans and unlike any known coronaviruses [1, 2]. Current studies have shown that SARS-CoV-2 has more than 85% homology with bat-SL-CoVZC45. When isolated and cultured in vitro, SARS-CoV-2 can be found in human respiratory epithelial cells in about 96 h. Based on the prior knowledge on SARS-CoV and MERS-CoV, SARS-CoV-2 is considered to be sensitive to ultraviolet and heat. It is reported that exposure to 56 °C for 30 min or chemicals such as ether, 75% ethanol, peracetic acid, chloroform, and chlorine-containing disinfectant can effectively disinfect the SARS-CoV-2 [3].

1.3 Epidemiological Characteristics

1.3.1 Sources of Infection

The source of infection is mainly the symptomatic patients carrying SARS-CoV-2. Asymptomatic patients can be the source of infection; however, whether and how transmission of the virus from asymptomatic patients to the general population is still under investigation. Worth noting, there is still no confirmed report whether the virus can be transmitted from the animals to human or vice versa.

SARS-CoV-2 is highly contagious with a strong infectious power measured by the transmission efficiency. Epidemiology commonly uses the basic reproduction number (R0) to describe the infectious ability and transmission efficiency of a pathogen. R0 is the average number of cases that an infected person

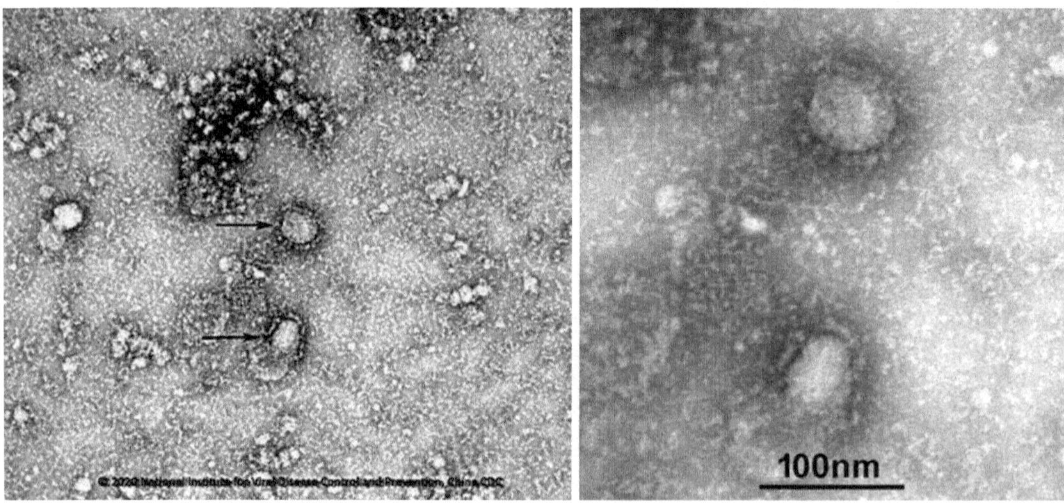

Fig. 1.1 Electron microscope images of 2019-nCoV. *Photo source*: National Resource Bank of Pathogenic Microorganisms (Institute for Virus Disease Prevention and Control, Chinese Center for Disease Control and Prevention)

or the host of virus can cause during his/her infectious period without the external intervention and immunity for all. The pathogen with a higher R0 is more contagious. According to the report from WHO [4], SARS-CoV-2 has an R0 between 2.0 and 3.5 in the early stage of disease prevalence. Several other studies estimated the R0 of SARS-CoV-2 between 3.8 and 4.7, or possibly even higher, reaching 5.7. By comparison, the R0 of SARS is 2.0–3.5 and MERS is less than 1.0 [5, 6].

1.3.2 Routes of Transmission

SARS-CoV-2 is primarily transmitted between people through respiratory droplets and contact routes. Individuals in close contact with infected person or virus carriers may inhale droplets containing the virus. Contact routes mean that the droplets emitted by patients with confirmed infection (including asymptomatic infection) are deposited on the surface, then touched by healthy individuals, and transferred to the mucous membrane of the mouth, nose, eyes, and so on. Therefore, the incidence of infection in persons with the household or the cluster in close contact is significantly higher. Wearing masks, washing hands frequently, and ventilating with constant fresh air are conducive to cutting off the transmission routes.

Aerosol transmission is considered to be a special type of droplet transmission, which means that the droplets containing viruses form aerosols under certain conditions, then suspend in the air for an extended period of time. Aerosol transmission may spread the virus to distant areas with the movement of the airflow. The possibility of aerosol transmission exists only when exposed to high concentrations of aerosols for a long time in a relatively closed environment.

As SARS-CoV-2 can be isolated in the feces, contact routes caused by fecal pollution may also contribute to the infection and disease spread [7].

1.3.3 Susceptible Population

It is reported that the probability of SARS-CoV-2 infection can be related to the amount of virus exposure [8]. The risk of getting infected increases as a person is exposed to a large number of viruses, even if their immune system is normal. However, immunocompromised and immunocompetent individuals are considered to be vulnerable to COVID-19.

Existing reports have shown that the age of COVID-19 patients is mainly 30–70 years old. Most of the critically ill patients are the elderly, obese, and those with underlying diseases [9]. The high-risk groups of severe illness and death are those over 60 years old and those with pre-existing diseases, such as hypertension, diabetes, chronic respiratory disease, and cancer. A small number of young and middle-aged patients were found to suffer from fulminant multiple system organ failure due to the strong inflammatory response (cytokine storm syndrome, CSS). Their prognosis is very poor. Cases of infection in children are relatively rare and mild.

1.4 Pathological Characteristics

The correlation between imaging findings and pathology is the base of radiological diagnosis. Every sign of imaging has its pathological basis. While there has been a significant amount of reports from COVID-19 research since the start of the pandemic, the report on pathological findings is still limited. Thus, the pathological characteristics of COVID-19 presented in this chapter are based on existing histopathological data collected from autopsy or biopsy.

1.4.1 The Specimen

Based on the chest X-ray computer tomography (CT) imaging descriptions and the autopsy report [10–12], COVID-19 is generally manifestation of interstitial pneumonia in the early stage, acute exudative pneumonia in the progressive stage, and focal pulmonary consolidation in the later stage. In the severe stage, interstitial pneumonia causes the lung lesions mixed with extravasated blood congestion, hemorrhage, and inflammatory exudation. The lung tissue loses its inherent spongy function and texture, appearing as a wet lung with bronze color. The severely infected lung becomes rigid, containing with white plaque or large consolidation found in the tissue section. A large amount of thick secretion and dark red liquid overflowing, and fiber streak-like changes can be seen in the tissue sections [12].

1.4.2 Histopathology and Stage

In the progress stage of COVID-19, the main involvement is pulmonary alveoli, which becomes inflamed and infiltrated with serous fluid, red blood cells, and macrophage. They are condensed and coagulated into a layer of red stained fibrin like membrane, i.e., the hyaline membrane attached to the inner surface of alveoli. In the severe stage, the epithelial cells in reactive hyperplasia alveolus become swelled or degenerated, necrotic, and eventually falling off. The pathological changes from acute exudative pneumonia to desquamation pneumonia involve proliferation of local fibroblasts. The reticular fibers are found proliferated and broke like glomerular hyperplasia. The fibrin deposition resulted from alveolar exudation exhibits the pattern as in the organizing pneumonia. Simultaneously, hypersecretion of mucus in goblet cells of the respiratory tract, mucoprotein dilution, disintegration of degradation system, and massive phlegm thrombus take places.

In early stage, the COVID-19 exhibited the general characteristics, which are similar with highly pathogenic viral pneumonia, such as exudation and consolidation. The details included proteinaceous exudate with globules, focal hyperplasia of pneumocytes with only patchy inflammatory cellular infiltration, and multinucleated giant cells. The exudate cells found were mainly monocytes and macrophages, some moderate multinucleated giant cells, a few lymphocytes, eosinophils, and neutrophils. The lymphocytes were mainly CD4 positive T cells. Type II alveolar epithelial cells were found proliferated significantly, which is not as obvious as in SARS [13]. Hyaline membranes were not prominent (Fig. 1.2).

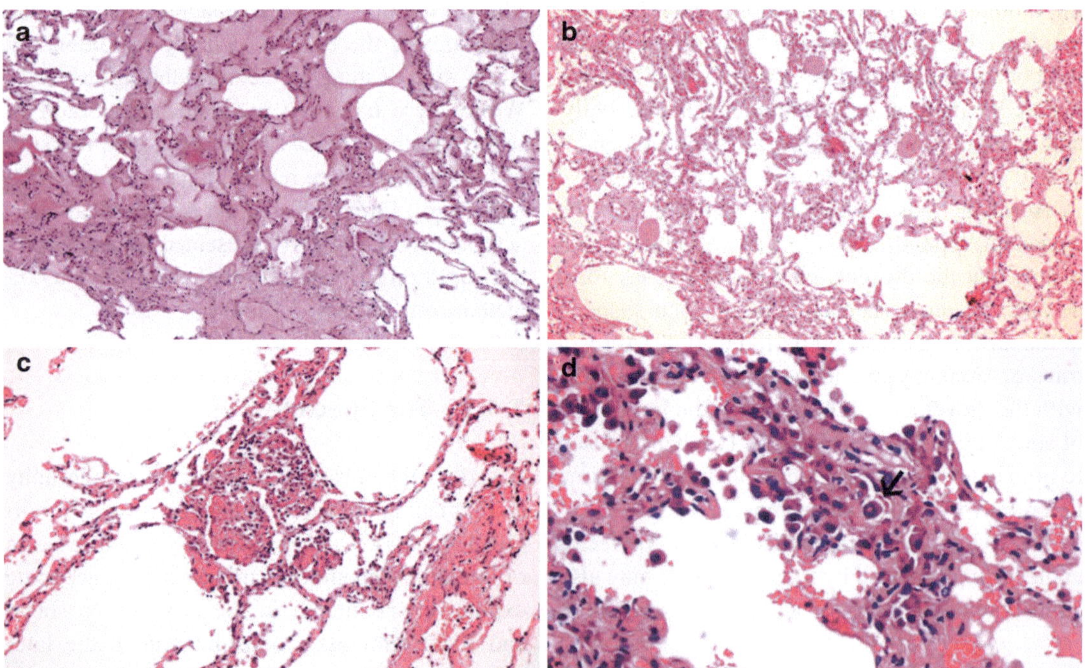

Fig. 1.2 The appearance of histological changes revealed in the early stage of COVID-19 involving focal proteinaceous exudates in alveolar spaces (**a**), scattered protein globules (**b**), granuloma-like nodules consisted of fibrin (**c**), inflammatory cells, and multinucleated giant cells inside the airspaces (**d**) [11]

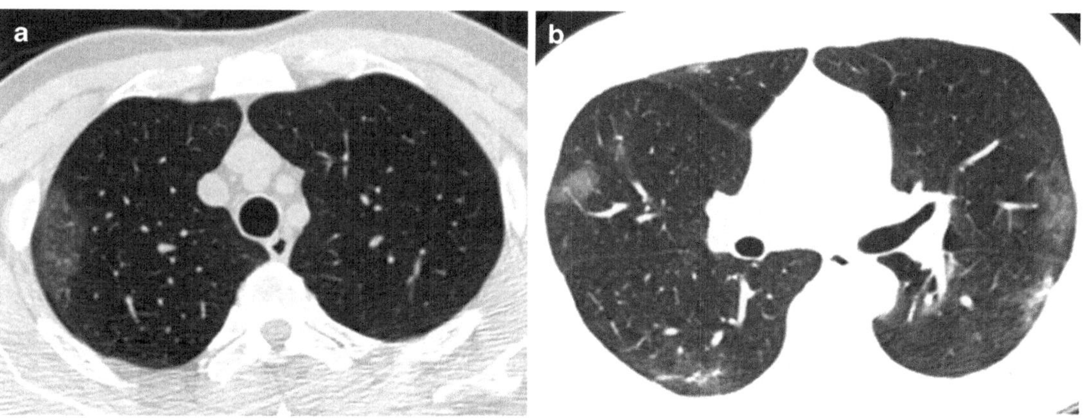

Fig. 1.3 The CT images from different patients with COVID-19 showed single GGO lesion (**a**) and multiple GGO lesions (**b**) separately

These pathological changes may present as single or multiple ground glass opacity (GGO) lesions in CT images as shown in Fig. 1.3.

In the later stage, substances in alveoli may disappear by liquefaction, absorption, and can be discharged from coughing. Pulmonary fibrosis can also be observed. If there is a secondary bacterial infection following COVID-19, neutrophil infiltration in alveoli and interstitium can be found. Reactive hyperplasia can be seen in the bronchial and alveolar epithelium with cytoplasmic bisexuality, nuclear enlargement, prominent nucleoli, and even formation of multinuclear giant cells. The post-mortem examination presented scattered oval protein globules in the local alveolar cavity, which may indicate disintegrating hemoglobin. Myozyme and myoglobin were found increased in some patients. The increased troponin was also reported in a case. In severe COVID-19 patients, D-dimer is typically increased likely due to the destruction of red blood cell membrane caused by hemolysis, and gradually reduced peripheral blood lymphocytes as the results of virus inhibition or even destruction of cellular immunity in the early stage [10].

With the COVID-19 progresses, the surrounding lung parenchyma showed patchy but evident proteinaceous and fibrin exudate (Fig. 1.4a). There was diffuse thickening of alveolar walls (Fig. 1.4b), focal small organization (not shown), and interstitial fibroblastic hyperplasia (Fig. 1.4c, arrow), indicating varying degrees of proliferative phase. Focally, abundant polymorphonuclear cells and macrophages infiltrating the airspaces can also be observed (Fig. 1.4d). Corresponding CT findings can be described as signs of thickened vascular passage (n = 32, 78.0%), GGO with interlobular septal thickening (n = 19, 46.3%) shown in Fig. 1.5a, b, and prickly pear sign (n = 3, 7.3%) in Fig. 1.5c, d in patients confirmed with COVID-19.

CT images on day 3 post symptoms revealing heterogeneous lesions bilaterally with interlobular septal thickening within GGO (Fig. 1.5a, b) and prickly pear sign (Fig. 1.5c, d) in COVID-19 patients (white arrows).

Severe disease onset might result in death due to massive alveolar damage and progressive respiratory failure. Different from acquired immune deficiency syndrome (AIDS), some severe COVID-19 patients may have acute respiratory deficiency syndrome (ARDS). ARDS can be caused by alveolar epithelial exfoliation and hyaline membrane formation in lung tissue. Once bilateral diffuse alveolar injury with mucinous exudation occurred, pulmonary edema and hyaline membrane formation can be observed in the pulmonary tissue, suggesting early ARDS. Inflammatory infiltration of mononuclear cells, mainly lymphocytes, can be seen in the lung. In the alveolus cavity, viral cytopathic like changes can be found as multinucleated giant cells and atypical enlarged alveoli cells. The atypical enlarged alveoli cells have large nuclei,

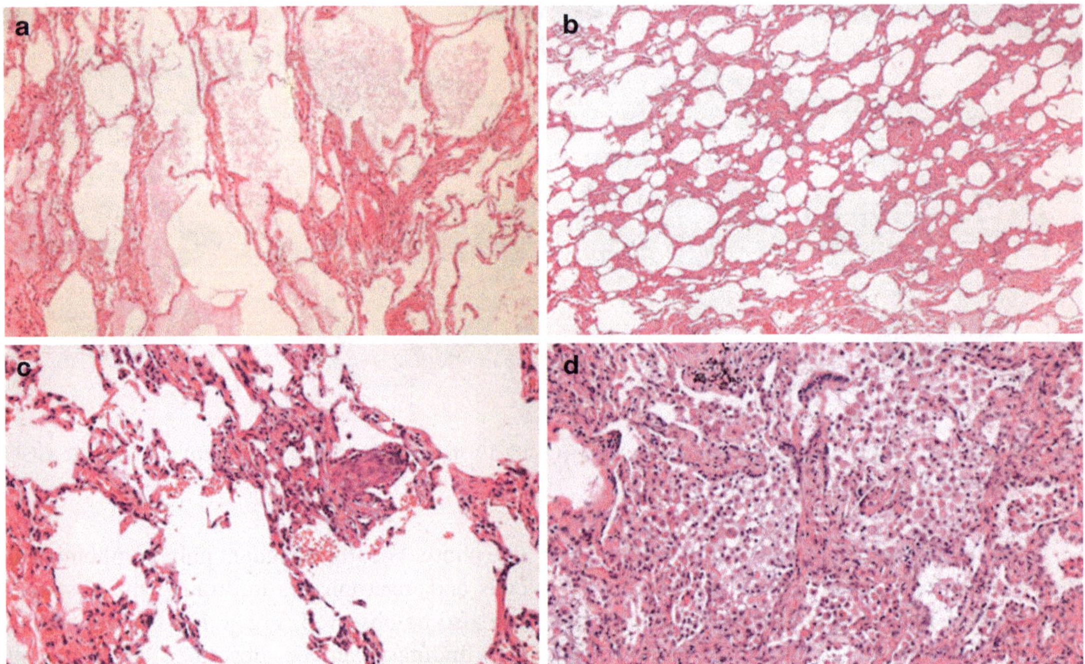

Fig. 1.4 Histologic changes from COVID-19 case. (**a**) Evident proteinaceous and fibrin exudate; (**b**) diffuse expansion of alveolar walls and septa owing to fibroblastic proliferations and type II pneumocyte hyperplasia; (**c**) plugs of proliferating fibroblasts or "fibroblast balls" in the interstitium; (**d**) abundant macrophages infiltrating airspaces and type II pneumocyte hyperplasia

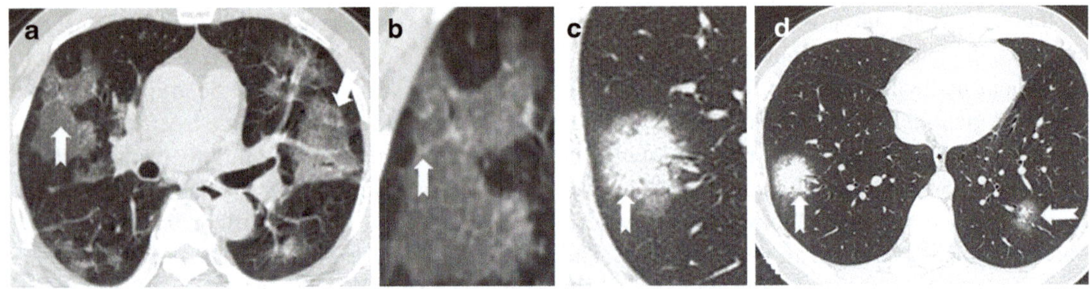

Fig. 1.5 Representative images of COVID-19 cases in chest high resolution CT scan

double cytoplasmic granules, and obvious nucleoli. No obvious intranuclear or cytoplasmic virus inclusions in the lung are reported.

In conclusion, the pathological characteristics of COVID-19 are similar to those caused by SARS. The main pathological changes occur in the lungs, immune system (spleen, lymph nodes), and blood vessels of various organs, but the severity and universality of the pathological changes in the lungs, spleen, and organs are less than that of SARS.

References

1. Zhu N, Zhang D, Wang W, et al. A novel coronavirus from patients with pneumonia in China, 2019. N Engl J Med. 2020;382(8):727–33.
2. Zhou P, Yang X, Wang X, et al. A pneumonia outbreak associated with a new coronavirus of probable bat origin. Nature. 2020;579(7798):270–3.
3. National Health Commission of the People's Republic of China. Diagnosis and treatment protocols of pneumonia caused by a novel coronavirus (trial version 7) [EB/OL]. [2020-03-03]. Retrieved

from: http://www.nhc.gov.cn/yzygj/s7653p/202003/46c9294a7dfe4cef80dc7f5912eb1989/files/ce3e6945832a438eaae415350a8ce964.pdf
4. World Health Organization. Modes of transmission of virus causing COVID-19: implications for IPC precaution recommendations [EB/OL] (2020-03-29). Retrieved from: https://www.who.int/news-room/commentaries/detail/modes-of-transmission-of-virus-causing-COVID-19-implications-for-ipc-precaution-recommendations
5. Li Q, Guan X, Wu P, et al. Early transmission dynamics in Wuhan, China, of novel coronavirus-infected pneumonia. N Engl J Med. 2020;382(13):1199–207.
6. Park SE. Epidemiology, virology, and clinical features of severe acute respiratory syndrome -coronavirus-2 (SARS-CoV-2; Coronavirus Disease-19). Clin Exp Pediatr. 2020;63(4):119–24.
7. Tian Y, Rong L, Nian W, et al. Review article: Gastrointestinal features in COVID-19 and the possibility of faecal transmission. Aliment Pharmacol Ther. 2020;51(9):843–51.
8. Koo HJ, Lim S, Choe J, et al. Radiographic and CT features of viral pneumonia. Radiographics. 2018;38(3):719–39.
9. Tu YF, Chien CS, Yarmishyn AA, et al. A review of SARS-CoV-2 and the ongoing clinical trials. Int J Mol Sci. 2020;21(7) pii: E2657.
10. Xu Z, Shi L, Wang Y, et al. Pathological findings of COVID-19 associated with acute respiratory distress syndrome. Lancet Respir Med. 2020;8(4):420–2.
11. Tian S, Hu W, Niu L, et al. Pulmonary pathology of early-phase 2019 novel coronavirus (COVID-19) pneumonia in two patients with lung cancer. J Thorac Oncol. 2020;15(5):700–4.
12. Liu Q, Wang RS, Qu GQ, et al. Gross examination report of a COVID-19 death autopsy. J Forensic Med. 2020;36(1):21–3.
13. Yao XH, Li TY, He ZC, et al. A pathological report of three COVID-19 cases by minimal invasive autopsies. Zhonghua bing li xue za zhi = Chinese Journal of Pathology. 2020;49(5):411–7.

2 Clinical Classification and Diagnosis of COVID-19

Nan Lu, Bin Lin, Hui Mao, and Minming Zhang

2.1 Clinical Manifestations [1]

The latency of coronavirus disease 2019 (COVID-19) is usually 1–14 days. Most patients show symptoms within 3–7 days based on the report from the current epidemiological survey. In the early stage of the disease, fever, dry cough, and fatigue are the main manifestations. Some patients may also experience additional symptoms such as nasal congestion, runny nose, pharyngeal pain, myalgia, and diarrhea. However, there are a significant number of individuals carrying SARS-CoV-2 who may not exhibit these symptoms. It is particularly important to identify these asymptomatic patients (asymptomatic infections) due to their potential close contact with healthy populations and possible transmission of SARS-CoV-2. COVID-19 patients in the severe condition often have dyspnea and/or hypoxemia one week after the disease onset. Severe patients can rapidly develop acute respiratory distress syndrome (ARDS), septic shock, metabolic acidosis, coagulation dysfunction, and multiple organ failure (MOF). It is worth noting that severe and critical patients may only present moderate and low fever, or even no obvious fever. The symptoms of children are relatively mild. Some children and newborns may have atypical symptoms, such as vomiting, diarrhea, and other abnormal digestive tract conditions, or only show poor energy and shortness of breath. Mild cases may only show low fever, mild fatigue, and other symptoms, such as mild weakness, without pneumonia. Overall, most patients have a good prognosis, while a few patients were in the critical condition. The prognosis of the elderly and those with chronic basic diseases is poor. The clinical progress of COVID-19 in maternal women is similar to that of the same age group.

2.2 Laboratory Examinations

2.2.1 General Examinations [1]

Patients with COVID-19 have normal or decreased number of peripheral blood lymphocytes, and a low total number of lymphocytes at the beginning of the disease. Most patients have a normal level of procalcitonin with increased levels of C-reactive protein (CRP) and erythrocyte sedimentation rate (ESR). In some cases, myoglobin and liver enzymes, including lactate dehydrogenase (LDH)

N. Lu · B. Lin · M. Zhang (✉)
Department of Radiology, the Second Affiliated Hospital, Zhejiang University School of Medicine, Hangzhou, China
e-mail: zjdxlinbin@zju.edu.cn; zhangminming@zju.edu.cn

H. Mao
Department of Radiology and Imaging Sciences, Emory University School of Medicine, Atlanta, GA, USA
e-mail: hmao@emory.edu

M. Zhang, B. Lin (eds.), *Diagnostic Imaging of Novel Coronavirus Pneumonia*,
https://doi.org/10.1007/978-981-15-5992-1_2

and muscle enzyme may increase. In severe cases, D-dimer is elevated whereas the peripheral blood lymphocyte decreased progressively. Troponin can be found increased in some patients in the critical condition. The expression levels of inflammatory markers, including tumor necrosis factor (TNF)-α, interleukin (IL)-2R, and IL-6, are often increased in severe and critical patients.

2.2.2 Etiology and Serological Examinations

2.2.2.1 Etiology Examinations [1, 2]

Etiology examination is based on the sequence specific ribonucleic acid (RNA) from SARS-CoV-2. The viral RNAs can be detected in the specimens of nasopharyngeal swabs, sputum and other lower respiratory tract secretions, blood, and feces by the reverse transcription-polymerase chain reaction (RT-PCR) assay with the assistance of next generation sequencing (NGS).

The target genes of SARS-CoV-2 by RT-PCR include open reading frame 1a/b (ORF1a/b), nucleocapsid protein (N), and (or) envelope protein (E) genes. The results of nucleic acid testing (NAT) or RT-PCR test are determined according to the following criteria: For a negative case, ORF1a/b gene should be negative, and N gene/E gene are also negative; for a positive case, both ORF1a/b gene and N gene/E gene are positive. For a highly suspicious case, ORF1a/b gene is positive, but N gene/E gene are negative. When the case is uncertain, ORF1a/b gene is negative, N gene/E gene are found to be either negative or positive. If NGS is applied, the sequencing results should be compared with the known SARS-CoV-2 sequence for homology analysis.

In particular, viral nucleic acid testing is greatly affected by a number of factors, such as the time after infection, the method and experience of specimen collection, the origin of the specimen, the quality and preservation of the samples, possible contamination, and sensitivity of the methods. Specimen samples collected from lower respiratory tract (sputum or airway extracts) usually contain a high load of viral nucleic acids, thus are most likely yield the accurate test results. Regardless, the specimen samples shall be sent for examination as soon as they are collected. It should be noted that negative results from RT-PCR tests cannot be the only basis for exclusion of infection.

2.2.2.2 Serological Test for Detection of the Antibody to SARS-CoV-2 [1, 3–5]

As any viral infection, the antibody against the specific infection is depended subsequently. In COVID-19 patients, specific IgM is typically detectable 3–5 days after symptom onset. Specific IgG antibody titer in the recovery phase is found to increase to ≥4 times higher than that in the acute phase. Compared to RT-PCR assays, the detection of antibody assays has several advantages, including faster, less expensive, easy-to-use, and accessible to staff without laboratory training. Considering that confirming suspected COVID-19 cases faster with the help of serological test could reduce exposure risk during repeated sampling and save valuable RT-PCR tests, virus-specific antibody detection for COVID-19 is important as a complement to NAT for the diagnosis of suspected cases, and also in examining asymptomatic infection in close contacts.

2.3 Thoracic Imaging Findings

Multiple patchy shadows and interstitial changes occur early, particularly at the lung periphery. The conditions further develop into multiple ground-glass opacities and infiltrates in both lungs. In severe cases, the patient may have lung consolidation and rare pleural effusion.

2.4 Diagnosis [1]

2.4.1 Suspected Case Diagnosis

The patient meets 1 epidemiological history and 2 clinical manifestations can be diagnosed as suspected case. The patient who has no epidemiological history but meets 3 clinical manifestations can also be diagnosed as suspected case. Epidemiological history and clinical manifestations are shown in Table 2.1.

2.4.2 Confirmed Case Diagnosis

Suspected cases with one of the following etiological or serological evidences can be diagnosed as confirmed cases:

- Detection of SARS-CoV-2 nucleic acid is positive by real-time fluorescence RT-PCR.
- The virus gene sequences are highly homologous to SARS-CoV-2.
- Serum specific IgM antibody and IgG antibody are positive; serum specific IgG antibody is positive from negative, or in the recovery phase ≥4 times higher than that in the acute phase.

Table 2.1 Epidemiological history and clinical manifestations of suspected case

Epidemiological history	Clinical manifestations
1. Within 14 days before the onset of the disease, the patient has a travel or residence history in the high-risk regions or countries	1. The patient has fever and/or respiratory symptoms
2. Within 14 days before the onset of the disease, the patient has a history of contact with those infected with SARS-CoV-2 (those with a positive NAT result)	2. The patient has the CT imaging features of COVID-19 mentioned above
3. Within 14 days before the onset of the disease, the patient had direct contact with patients with fever or respiratory symptoms in high-risk regions or countries	3. The white blood cells count in the early stage of the disease is normal or decreased, with the lymphocyte count normal or decreased
4. Disease clustering (2 or more cases with fever and/or respiratory symptoms occur at such places as homes, offices, and school classrooms within 2 weeks)	

2.4.3 Clinical Classifications

2.4.3.1 Cases with Mild Condition

The clinical symptoms are mild with no image manifestations of pneumonia in chest X-ray or CT examinations. Low-grade fever and mild weakness can be seen as the only symptoms. The first CT examination usually shows no abnormality, which may be due to the fact that the early virus is mainly located in the upper respiratory tract and does not cause exudative lesions in the lung. These patients can be contagious and must be treated with medical isolation once diagnosed. It should be noted that some patients with the mild disease had no abnormal imaging findings during the entire course of the disease, while some had no abnormal imaging in the early stage of the disease, but presented moderate imaging manifestations as the disease progressed.

Case 1

Medical History and Clinical Manifestations

A 25-year-old male was admitted in the hospital with diarrhea, fever, and chills for 1 day (highest body temperature: 38.9 °C). Results from the laboratory tests indicated a normal white blood cell count of 9.7×10^9/L, 81% neutrophils, and 11.4% lymphocytes. C-reactive protein was elevated to 17.61 mg/L. This patient is the resident in the city of Jingzhou in Hubai, but stayed in Wuhan for a half-day before traveling to the city where he was admitted after the symptom onset. The RT-PCR test for novel coronavirus was positive.

Imaging Features

Initial chest CT and follow-up chest CT scans showed no obvious abnormality in both lungs for 3 times (Fig. 2.1).

Case 2

Medical History and Clinical Manifestations

A 41-year-old female was admitted in the hospital reporting occasional dry cough, but no fever or chills. Results from the laboratory tests showed a normal white blood cell count of

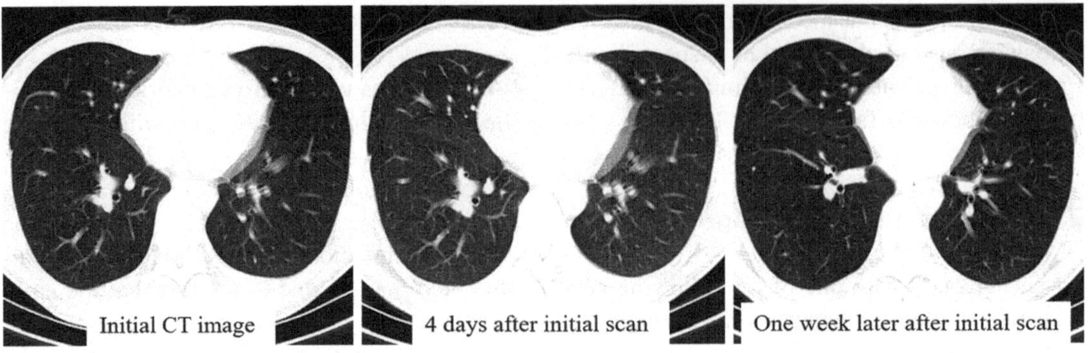

Fig. 2.1 Initial and follow-up chest CT images of a patient with mild COVID-19

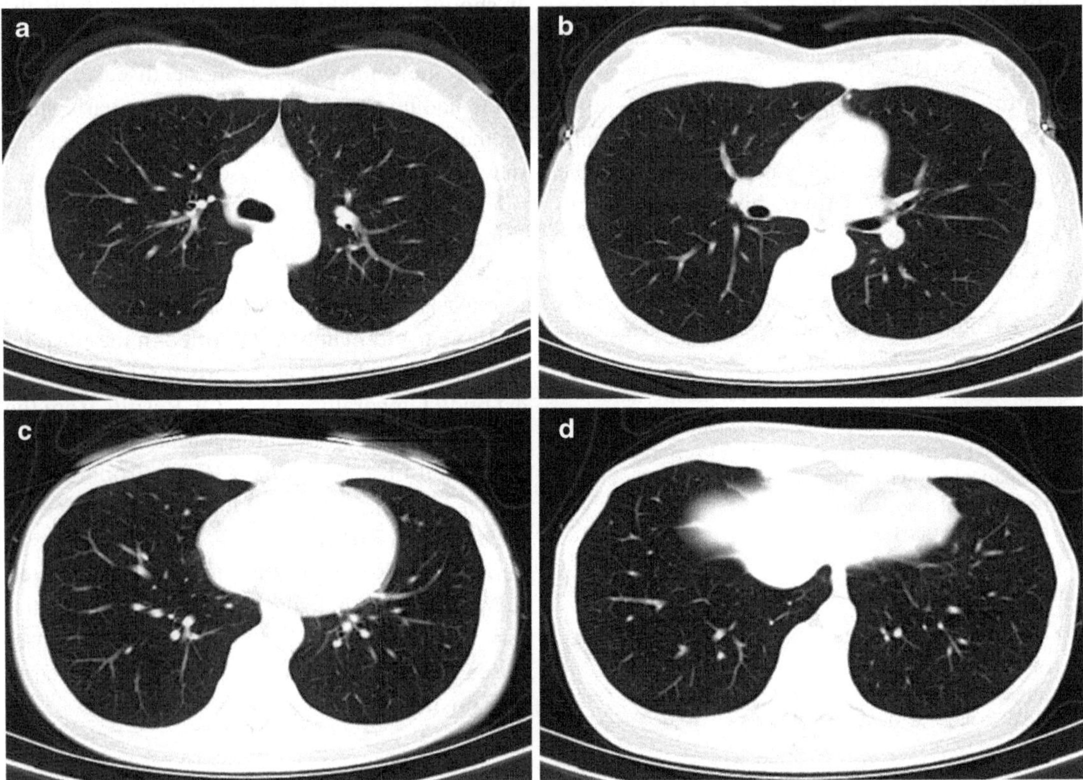

Fig. 2.2 Initial CT images of a patient with mild COVID-19 showed no obvious abnormality

4.2×10^9/L, 65.1% neutrophils, and 19% lymphocytes. The C-reactive protein level was less than 0.499 mg/L. The RT-PCR nucleic acid test for novel coronavirus was positive. The husband of this patient was diagnosed with COVID-19 after he had contacted a COVID-19 patient who came from the city of Wuhan.

Imaging Features

Initial chest CT showed no obvious abnormality (Fig. 2.2). Follow-up chest CT 5 days later showed subpleural nodular and patchy ground-glass shadows with fuzzy edge in the left upper lobe and both lower lobes (white arrows) (Fig. 2.3). Compared with the previous images,

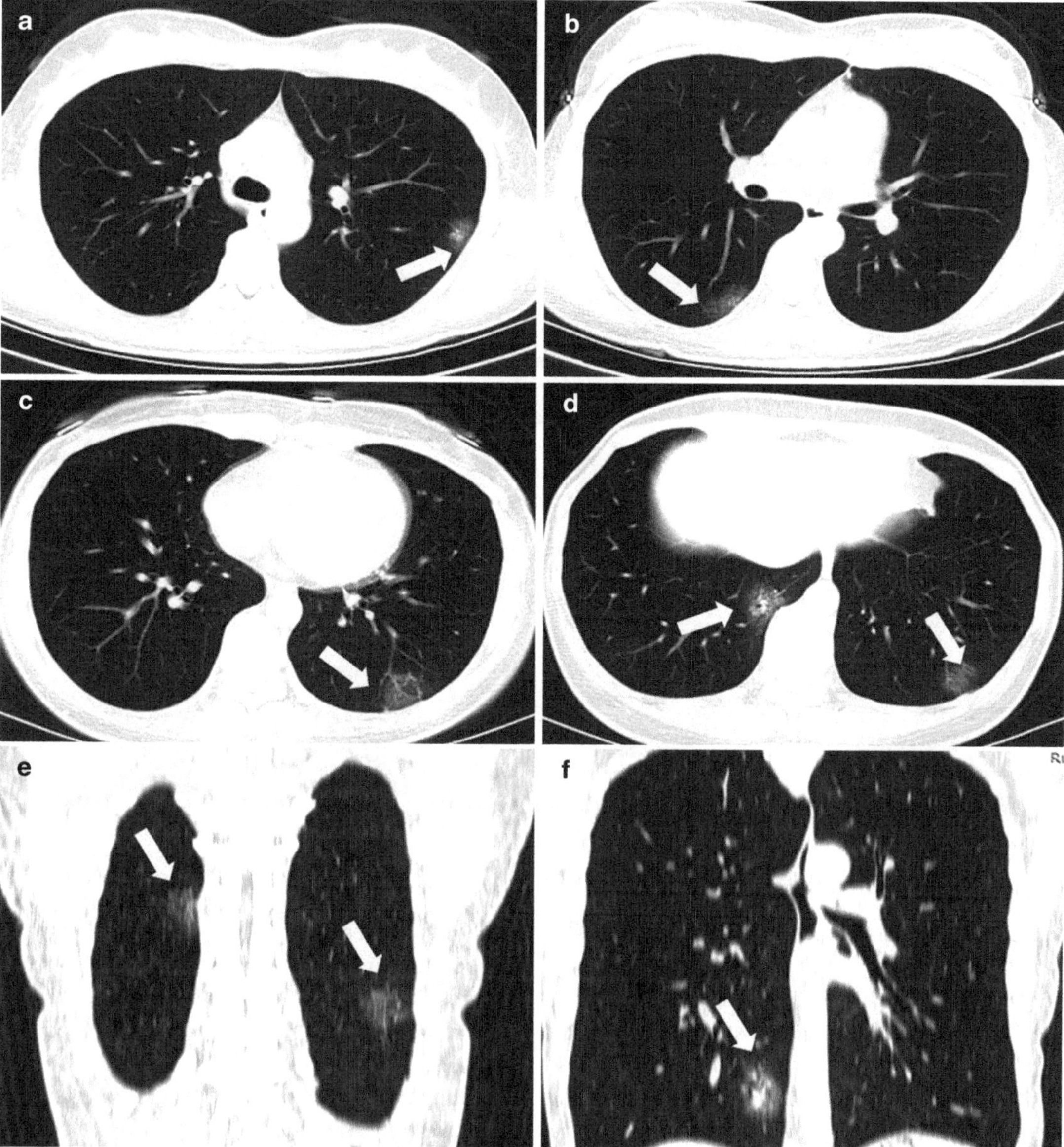

Fig. 2.3 Follow-up CT images of the same patient with mild COVID-19 collected 5 days after the initial scan

small reticular shadows or thickened vascular emerged in some lesions.

Twelve days after initial CT examination, the second follow-up chest CT showed multiple subpleural strip shadows in the left upper lobe and both lower lobes of the lung, which were smaller comparing to those seen in initial CT images (white arrows) (Fig. 2.4).

2.4.3.2 Cases with Moderate Conditions

The moderate cases are developed from the mild cases. Patients with the moderate conditions usually have symptoms such as fever and abnormal respiratory tract conditions. Pneumonia manifestations can be seen in chest X-ray or CT imaging, presenting as multiple foci located in the

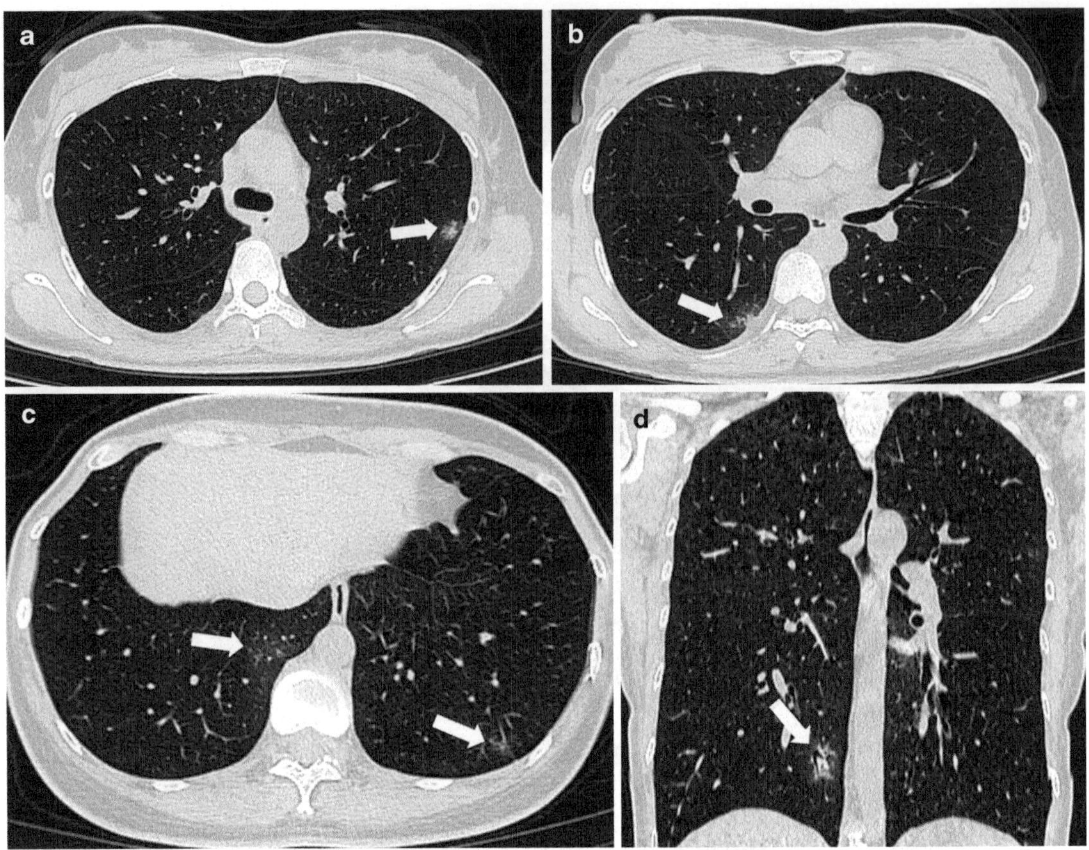

Fig. 2.4 Follow-up CT images 12 days after initial scan of the same patients with mild COVID-19

lung periphery, subpleural area, and both lower lobes. Lung abnormalities are rarely seen as a single lesion on chest CT scans. The density of the foci is not uniform, and most of them are seen as ground-glass shadows, in which blood vessel thickening or air bronchogram can be found. Ground-glass nodule may be accompanied by the halo sign, along with ground-glass patchy shadows or reversed halo sign, with or without interlobular septal thickening, which typically present as a "crazy paving" pattern. A small number of cases may show consolidation or fibrosis. Pleural effusion is rare.

Case 3

Medical History and Clinical Manifestations

A 60-year-old female was admitted in the hospital with cough and low fever for 5 days (highest body temperature: 37.5 °C). The patient had no contact or residential history with Wuhan. The results from RT-PCR test of the throat swab sample were negative. A normal white blood cell count of 3.8×10^9/L, 69.1% neutrophils, and 21.4% lymphocytes were reported in the laboratory tests. The second RT-PCR test after admission was positive.

Imaging Features

Initial chest CT showed the subpleural patchy ground-glass shadow in the right lower lobe (white arrow) (Fig. 2.5).

Follow-up chest CT (5 days after initial CT examination) showed multiple patchy ground-glass shadows with fuzzy boundary, mostly in the subpleural area of the right upper lobe and both lower lobes, with line grid shadows and consolidation (white arrows) (Fig. 2.6). The progressive

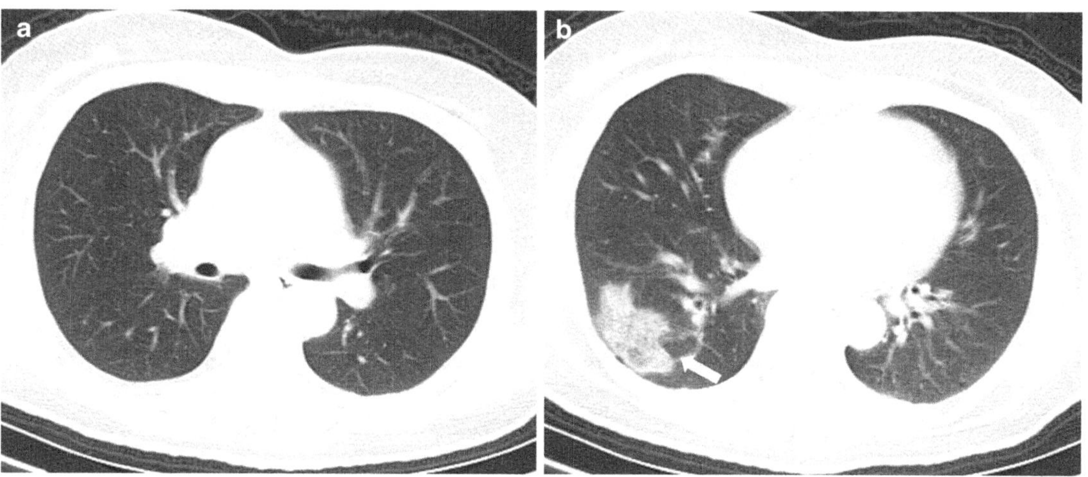

Fig. 2.5 Initial CT images of a female patient with moderate COVID-19

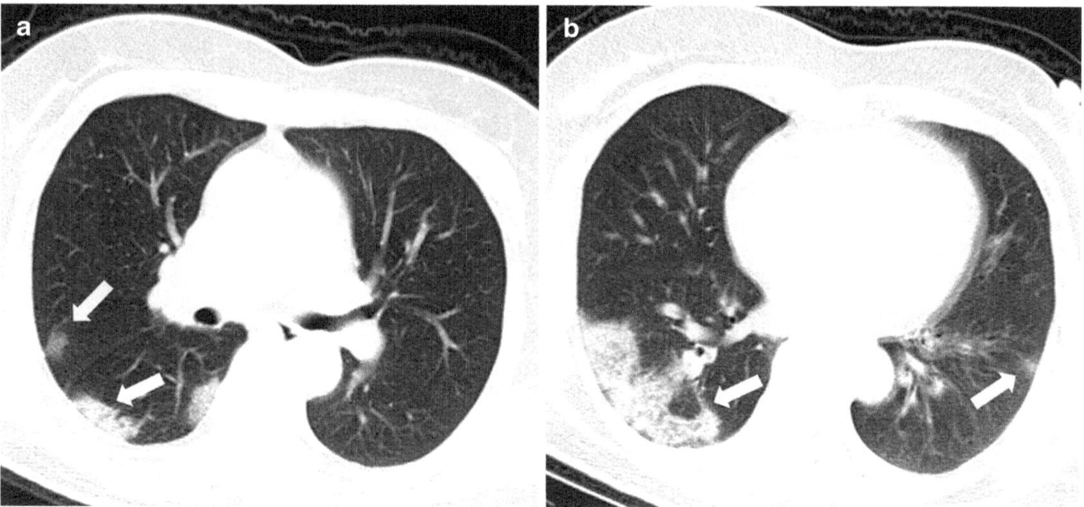

Fig. 2.6 Follow-up CT images of the patient with moderate COVID-19 5 days after initial scan

changes are seen from these lesions comparing to the first set of images.

Follow-up chest CT at 9 days after initial CT examination showed multiple patchy ground-glass shadows with fuzzy boundary, mostly in the subpleural area of the right upper lobe and both lower lobes, with local fine grid shadows, which have been absorbed compared to the images from prior CT scans (white arrows) (Fig. 2.7).

2.4.3.3 Severe Cases

Adult patients who meet any of the following criteria can be classified as severe cases: (1) respiratory rate ≥30 breaths/min; (2) oxygen saturation ≤93% at a rest state; and (3) arterial partial pressure of oxygen (PaO_2)/oxygen concentration (FiO_2) ≤ 300 mmHg (1 mmHg = 0.133 kPa). The PaO_2/FiO_2 shall be corrected for areas with the high altitude (over 1000 meters above the sea

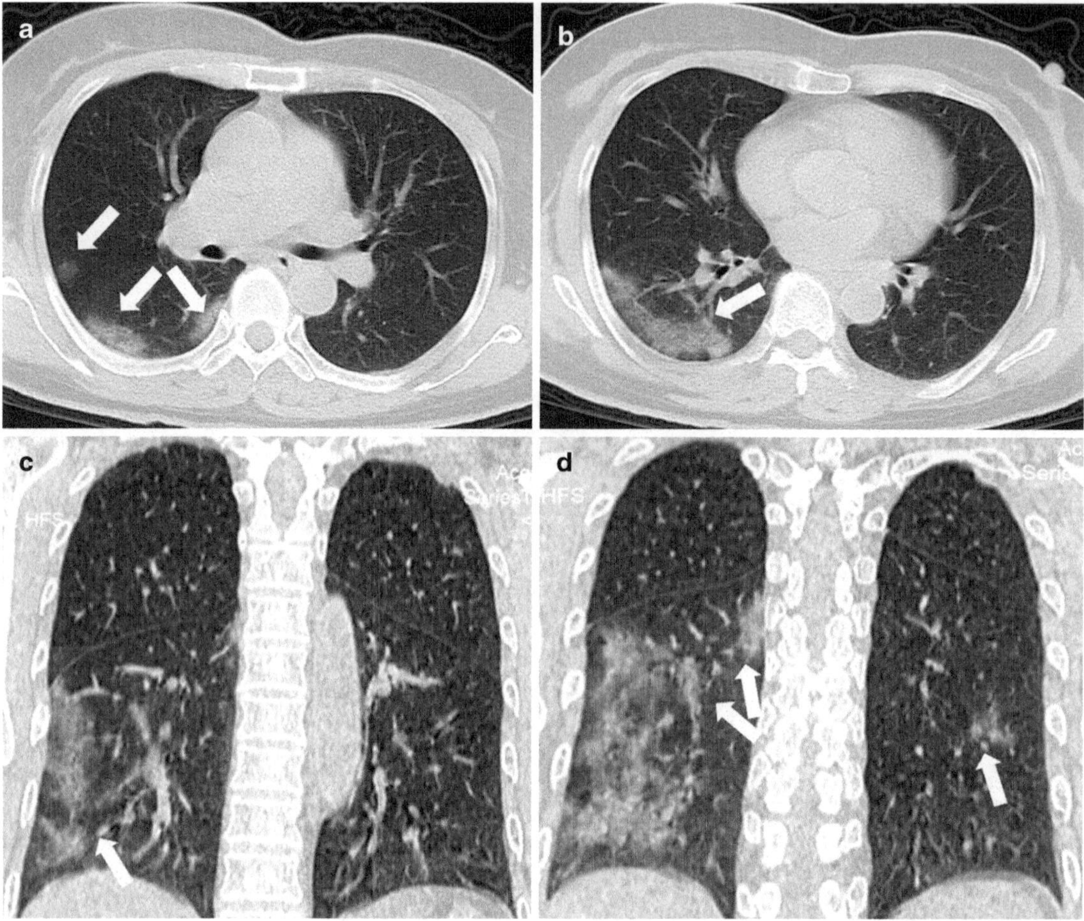

Fig. 2.7 Follow-up CT images of the patient with moderate COVID-19 9 days after initial scan

level) according to the following formula: PaO_2/FiO_2 × [atmospheric pressure (mmHg)/760].

Patients with >50% increase of lesions in lung CT within 24–48 h should be treated as severe cases.

Children with any conditions meeting the following criteria can be classified as severe cases: (1) respiratory rate ≥60 breaths/min (<2 months old), ≥50 breaths/min (2–12 months old), ≥40 breaths/min (1–5 years old), or ≥30 breaths/min (>5 years old), exclude the effect of fever or crying; (2) oxygen saturation ≤92% at the rest state; (3) assisted breathing (moaning, fluttering of the alar, and tri-retraction sign), cyanosis, intermittent apnea; (4) lethargy and convulsions; and (5) antifeedant or feeding difficulties, with sign of dehydration.

Case 4

Medical History and Clinical Manifestations

A 48-year-old male came to the hospital with fever (highest body temperature: 39 °C) and chills for 6 days, and cough and expectoration for 3 days. Initial laboratory tests indicated a normal white blood cell count of 5.7×10^9/L, 73.5% neutrophils, and 18.8% lymphocytes. Elevated

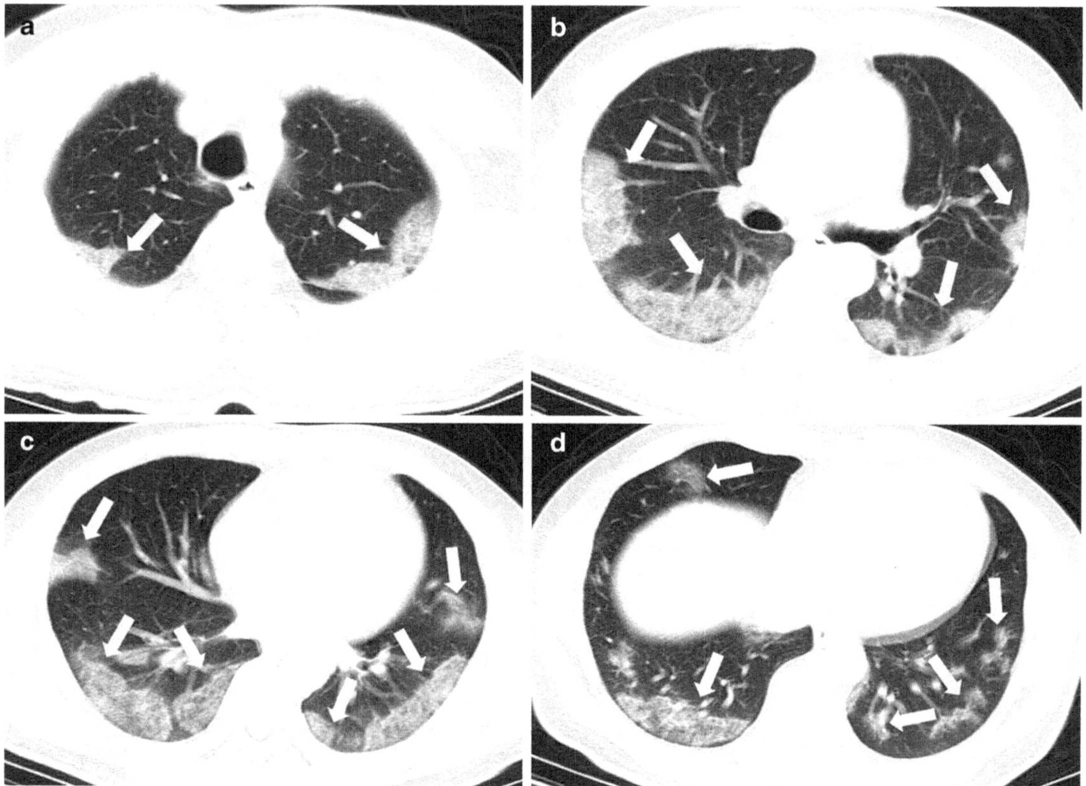

Fig. 2.8 Initial CT images of a male patient with severe COVID-19

C-reactive protein level (14.85 mg/L) was also reported. The patient had close contact with his son who traveled from Wuhan. The RT-PCR test for novel coronavirus was positive.

Three days later, the results from his follow-up laboratory tests on the day of his admission indicated a normal white blood cell count of 5.4×10^9/L, 75.4% neutrophils, and 20.3% lymphocytes. The C-reactive protein level was elevated further to 114.9 mg/L. On the third day of admission, the patient had high fever, severe cough, feeling of fatigue, and poor appetite. Initial chest CT and follow-up scans showed the gradually increased multi-foci in the lung, exceeding 50% area of the lung. His oxygenation index decreased about 300 mmHg. Subsequently, he was classified as a severe patient.

Imaging Features

The initial chest CT scan showed multiple dense subpleural patchy ground-glass shadows with fuzzy edges in both lungs, with the fine grid shadow and "crazy paving" pattern (white arrows) (Fig. 2.8).

Diffuse subpleural patchy ground-glass density shadows with fuzzy edges in both lungs remained in the follow-up chest CT scan 3 days after initial CT examination. The "crazy paving" pattern, thickening of vessels, and air bronchogram became more obvious than those seen in the previous scan (white arrows) (Fig. 2.9).

Follow-up chest CT on the 13 days after initial CT examination showed multiple subpleural strips and patchy shadows with high density,

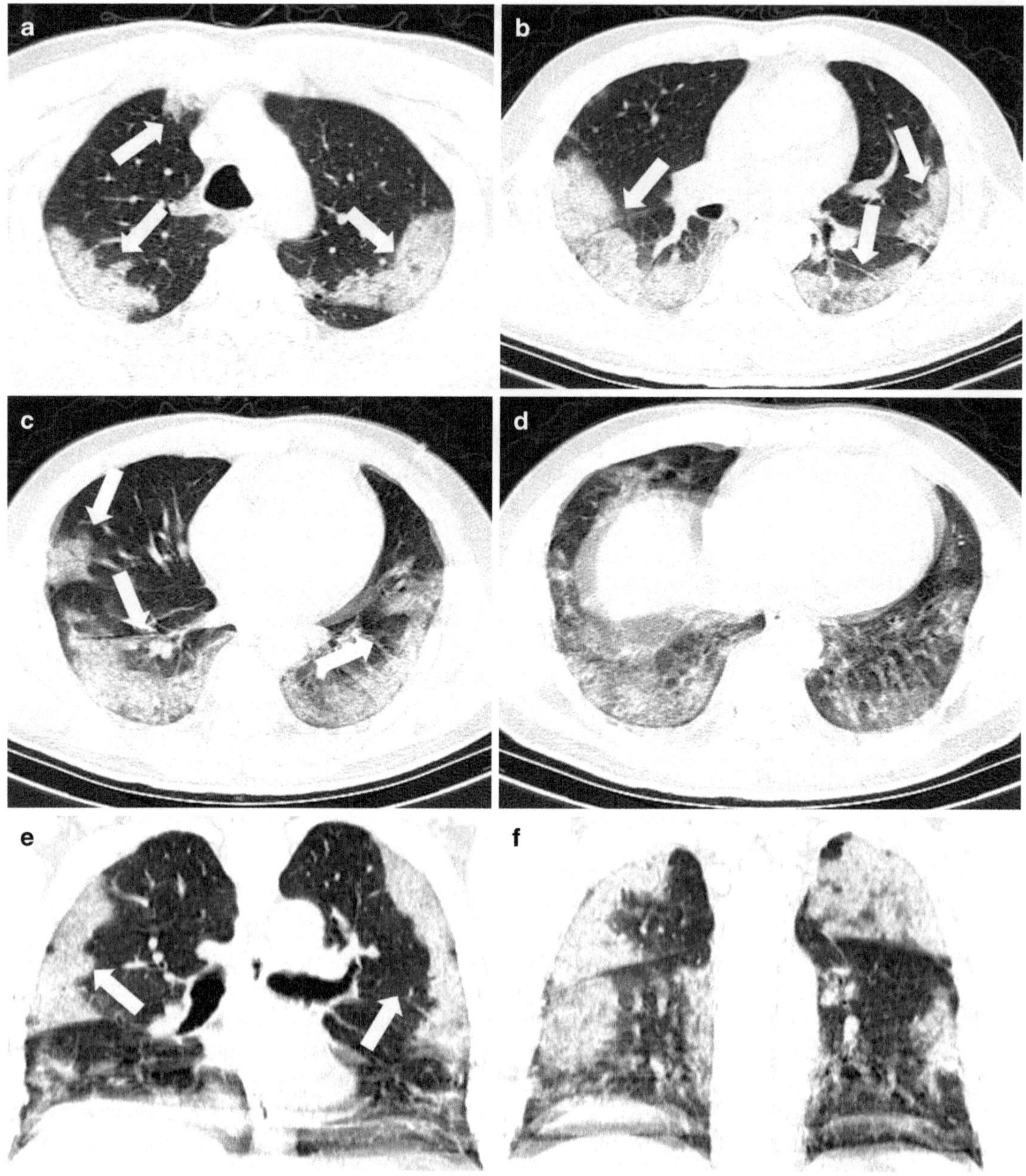

Fig. 2.9 Follow-up CT images of a male patient with severe COVID-19 5 days after initial scan

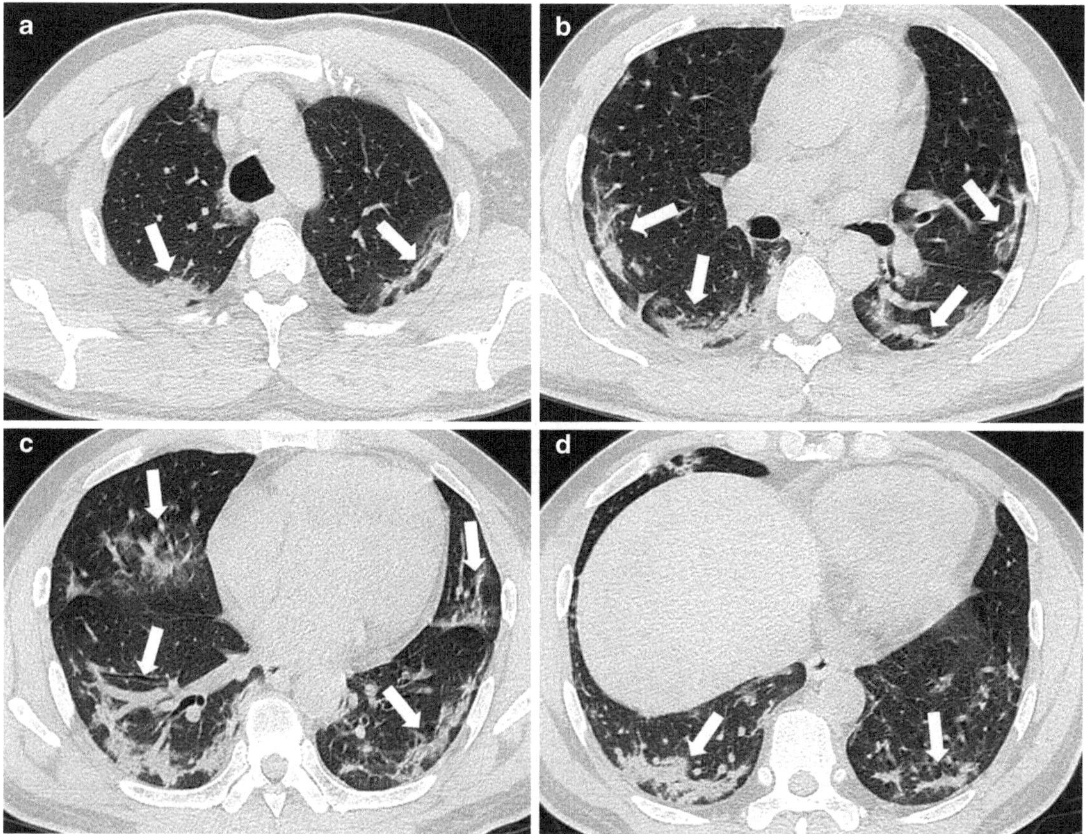

Fig. 2.10 Follow-up CT images of a male patient with severe COVID-19 on 13 days after the initial scan

some of which were absorbed and some transitioned to fibrosis comparing to those seen in prior images (white arrows) (Fig. 2.10).

Follow-up chest CT at 29 days after initial CT examination) showed multiple subpleural high density strips with relatively clear edge, which were absorbed further with more fibrosis developed (white arrows) (Fig. 2.11).

2.4.3.4 Critical Cases

Critical cases should meet any of the following criteria: (1) occurrence of respiratory failure requiring mechanical ventilation; (2) presence of shock; and (3) other organ failure that requires monitoring and treatment in the ICU.

Critical cases may show expanded consolidation, with the whole lung density showing increased opacity, sometimes known as a "white lung."

Case 5

Medical History and Clinical Manifestations

A 79-year-old female was admitted in the hospital for low fever (highest body temperature: 37.5 °C) for 6 h. The results from the laboratory tests indicated a normal white blood cell count of 4.43×10^9/L, 62.4% neutrophils, 26.9% lymphocytes. Elevated levels of erythrocyte sedimentation rate (41 mm/h) and C-reactive protein (10.54 mg/L) were reported. The patient is a resident of Wuhan for a long time. She had been in a hospital in Wuhan and traveled to the city where she was admitted in the hospital a few days prior to the symptom onset. The RT-PCR test for the novel coronavirus was positive. The patient developed respiratory failure during the hospitalization and was on the ventilation.

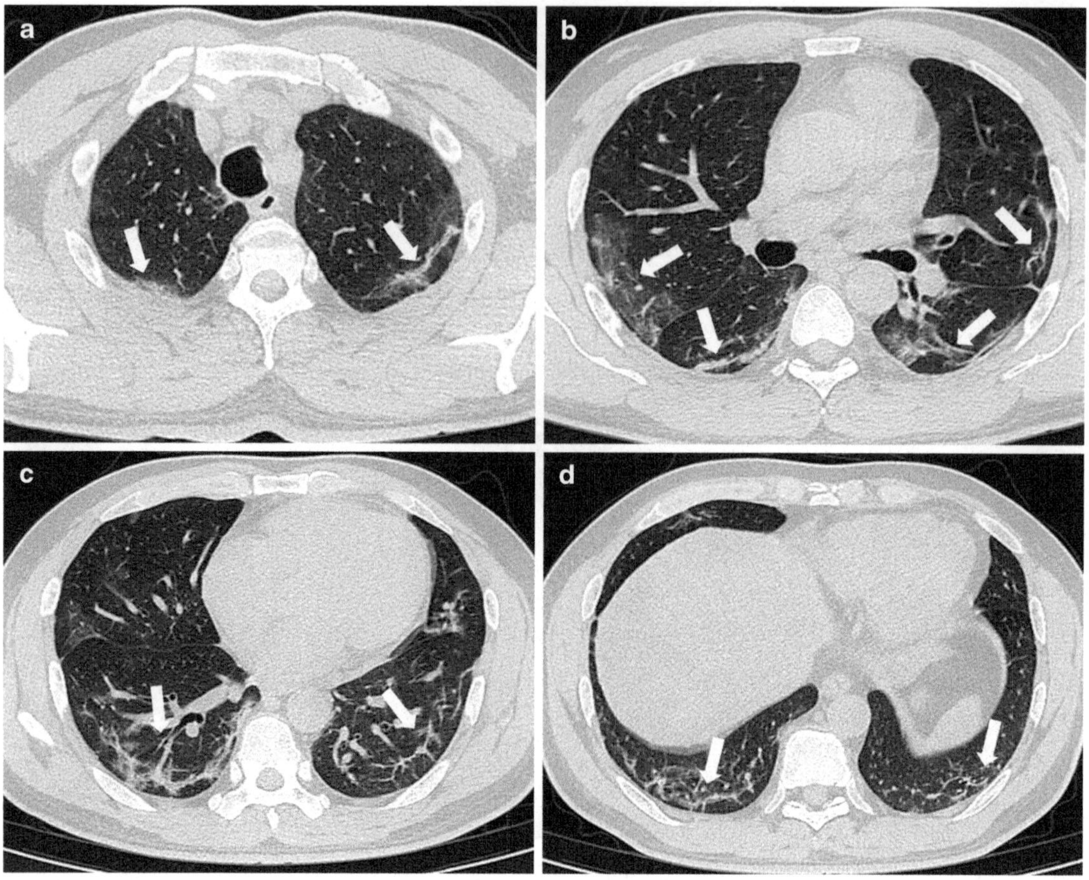

Fig. 2.11 Follow-up CT images of a male patient with severe COVID-19 at 29 days after initial scan

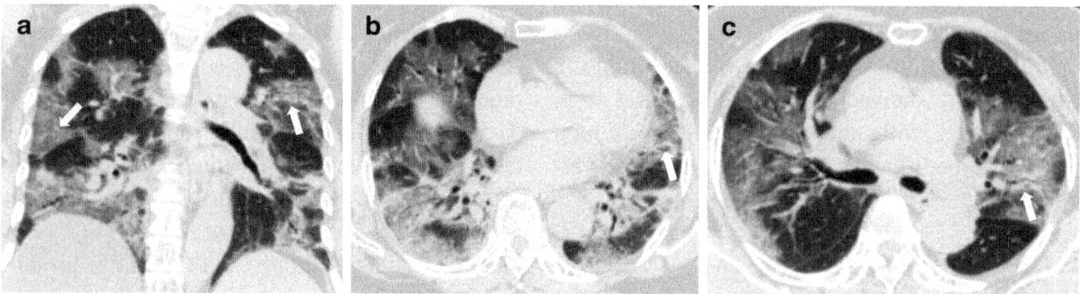

Fig. 2.12 Chest CT of a patient with critical COVID-19

Imaging Features

Chest CT of this patient showed multiple ground-glass patchy shadows and consolidation in bilateral lungs. The lesions had grid like changes and thickening of small vessels, with all lung lobes involved (white arrows) (Fig. 2.12).

References

1. National Health Commission of the People's Republic of China. Diagnosis and treatment protocols of pneumonia caused by a novel coronavirus (trial version 7). [EB/OL]. [2020-03-03]. http://www.nhc.gov.cn/yzygj/s7653p/202003/46c9294a7dfe4cef80dc7f5912eb1989/files/ce3e6945832a438eaae415350a8ce964.pdf
2. He C, Jiang H, Xie Y, et al. Discussion on laboratory test pathways for diagnosis and treatment of COVID-19. Chin J Respir Crit Care Med. 2020;19(02):125–7.
3. Qin C, Zhou L, Hu Z, et al. Dysregulation of immune response in patients with COVID-19 in Wuhan, China. Clin Infect Dis. 2020;71(15):762–8. ciaa248.
4. Long Q, Liu B, Deng H, et al. Antibody responses to SARS-CoV-2 in patients with COVID-19. Nat Med. 2020;26(6):845–8.
5. Xiang F, Wang X, He X, et al. Antibody detection and dynamic characteristics in patients with COVID-19. Clin Infect Dis. 2020:ciaa461.

3 Imaging Manifestations of COVID-19

Lihua Wang, Chao Wang, Bin Lin, Hui Mao, and Minming Zhang

3.1 Chest X-Ray Findings

Without sufficient in vitro diagnostic tests available in the initial period of the pandemic, CT was the commonly used first-line examination for COVID-19 in China [1, 2]. However, the practice led to an unusual challenge to control infection in the CT suite. The American College of Radiology indicates that decontamination of the CT facility required after scanning COVID-19 patients may disrupt radiological services, thus recommending to use portable chest X-ray to minimize the risk of cross-infection [3]. However, chest X-ray (also called chest radiography) has lower sensitivity than CT for diagnosis of COVID-19 due to its lower density resolution; therefore, it can be used for screening possible COVID-19 but cannot replace CT for evaluation of the disease [4]. It is important for clinicians, especially radiologists, to recognize chest X-ray features of COVID-19.

In the early stage, COVID-19 lesions with little pulmonary exudation are often difficult to be detected by chest X-ray [4, 5]. The chest X-ray findings of COVID-19 patients with clinically moderate condition, as shown in Figs. 3.1 and 3.2, include localized patchy fuzzy opacity or multiple segmental patchy opacity in the medium, periphery, and subpleural areas of both lungs. Patients with clinically severe condition present much pronounced X-ray findings, including multiple large flaky opacity shadows in both lungs, sometimes accompanied by a small amount of pleural effusion [6–8]. Finally, clinically critical patients often exhibit diffuse consolidation, presenting as "white lung" on chest X-ray images (Fig. 3.3). COVID-19 patients in the critical condition may develop significant dyspnea and decrease of the oxygen saturation [8, 9].

L. Wang · C. Wang · B. Lin · M. Zhang (✉)
Department of Radiology, the Second Affiliated Hospital, Zhejiang University School of Medicine, Hangzhou, China
e-mail: lihuawang@zju.edu.cn; wangchaosmart@zju.edu.cn; zjdxlinbin@zju.edu.cn; zhangminming@zju.edu.cn

H. Mao
Department of Radiology and Imaging Sciences, Emory University School of Medicine, Atlanta, GA, USA
e-mail: hmao@emory.edu

M. Zhang, B. Lin (eds.), *Diagnostic Imaging of Novel Coronavirus Pneumonia*,
https://doi.org/10.1007/978-981-15-5992-1_3

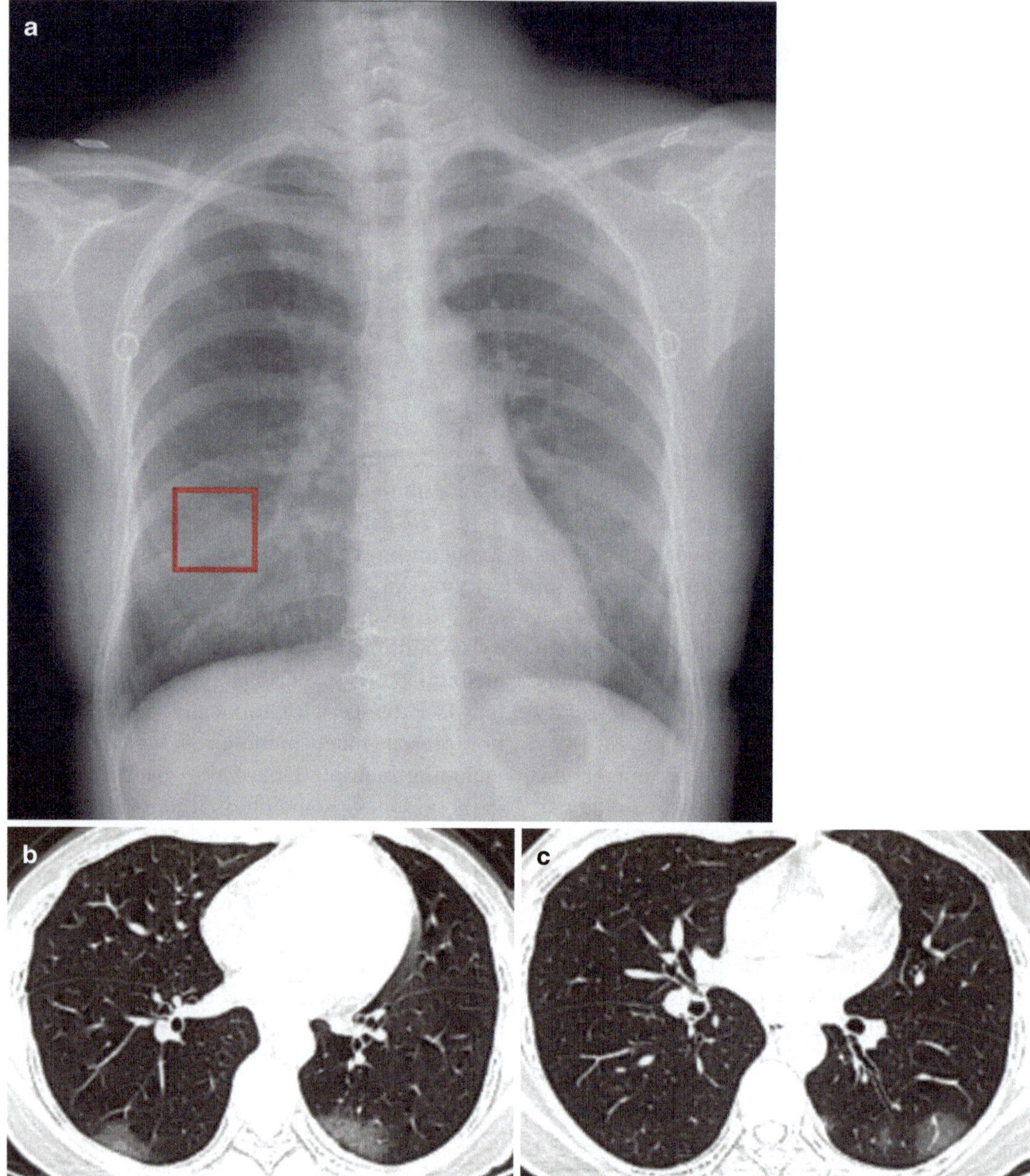

Fig. 3.1 Chest X-ray (**a**) and CT images (**b**, **c**) of a COVID-19 patient (43-year-old female)

Chest X-ray (**a**) showed patchy opacity shadows in the right lower lung fields, partly overlapped with the breast shadow, which made it difficult to determine the boundary of the lesion (**a**, red frame). The boundary was blurred. In comparison, chest CT (**b**, **c**) showed multiple ground-glass opacities (GGOs) in both lower lobes with a subpleural distribution. The microvasculature was seen thickened within GGO (**c**).

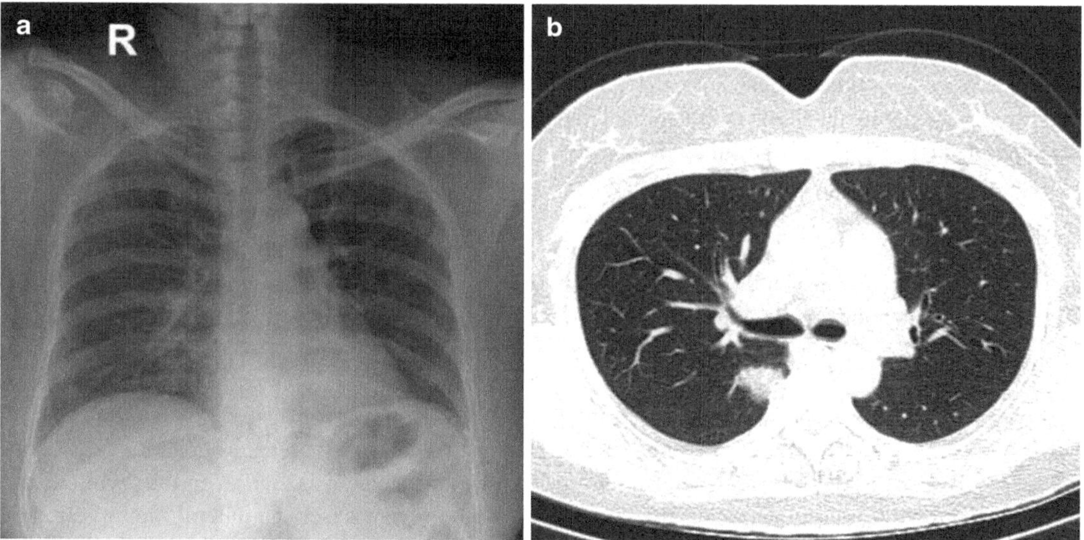

Fig. 3.2 Chest X-ray (**a**) and CT images (**b**) of a COVID-19 patient (36-year-old female)

At admission of this patient, no obvious abnormality on the chest radiograph (**a**) was observed. Five days later, chest CT (**b**) showed small patchy of consolidation in the subpleural area of the posterior segment of the right upper lobe adjacent to the oblique fissure, with blurred margin.

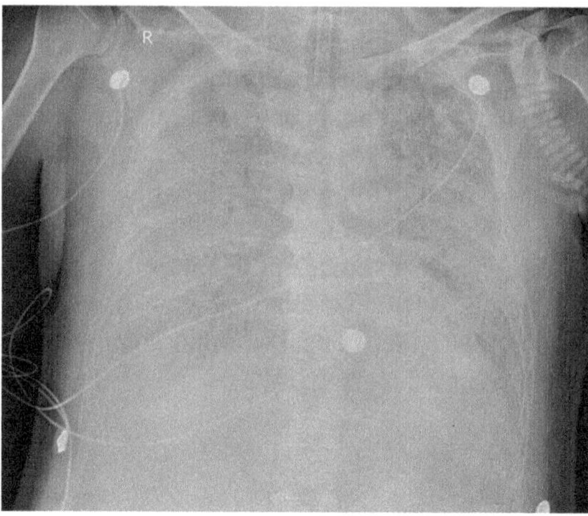

Fig. 3.3 Chest X-ray of a COVID-19 patient with clinically critical condition (69-year-old male)

The X-ray image of this patient in critical conditions shows the diffuse consolidation of both lungs, referred to as "white lung," invisible heart shadow, and costa-phrenic angle, noticing the air bronchogram sign in the central airways (red arrow).

3.2 Chest CT Findings

In the early stage of the epidemic, chest CT findings were once deployed as the major indications for clinical diagnosis in the hard-hit epidemic area with large numbers of severe and critical patients, such as Hubei, China [3]. The volumetric CT scan with 5 mm slice thickness (16 slices CT and above) followed by reconstruction to 1.0–1.5 mm slice is recommended. Multi-plane reconstruction (axial, sagittal, and coronal) then can be performed based on thin-slice CT images [1, 3, 4]. This process is essential to the early detection of the lesions, especially subtle lesion that cannot be seen in chest radiograph, and determination of the extent of the lesion. However, the current guidelines by different organizations and agencies have not reached an agreement on the timing of using low-dose CT (LDCT) and the follow-up interval for COVID-19 patients [1].

Some COVID-19 patients presented negative findings in pulmonary CT in the early stage, while abnormalities in the lung gradually emerged as the disease progressed [4]. Other early stage patients' can present image features of single or multiple nodular, patchy, or flake GGO which may have a peripheral/subpleural distribution, mainly in the lower lobes of the lung. Localized lesions can be seen distributed mostly in subsegments or segments, with or without reticular shadow and interlobular septum thickening, in which expanding microvascular shadow appears as a "grid-like change." Mosaic-like perfusion with interlobular septa thickening can be seen as a "crazy-paving sign" [4]. GGO lesions may become more pronounced in 3–7 days with an increased number and enlarged area. GGO lesions may gradually change into consolidation, or co-exist with consolidation or strip shadows. The air bronchogram sign can be found within the lesion. Furthermore, bronchiectasis is found within consolidation, with or without subsegmental or lobular atelectasis. The latter may present as a fusiform, flat, or stripy dense shadow connected to bronchovascular bundle. After treatment, GGO or consolidation lesions become fused or partially absorbed. The size of the lesion is often reduced while the density is focally increased due to fibroid change inside. In some patients progressed to the critical stage, CT showed diffuse consolidation of both lungs, sometimes with heterogeneous GGO, subsegmental atelectasis, and even the "white lung" in some severe cases. Unilateral pleural effusion is rarely present [4–6].

3.2.1 Common CT Manifestations

3.2.1.1 GGO

Pulmonary CT findings of COVID-19 patients include single or multiple patchy GGO of different sizes, clear or unclear edges, and peripheral/subpleural distribution (Fig. 3.4). GGO lesions often show a slight increase in density and a hazy, cloudy appearance, without covering the pulmonary vascular shadow (Fig. 3.5). The corresponding pathological changes of the lesion are alveolar effusion with partially filled air cavity [1]. The effusion is mainly serous and fibrin, as the type II alveolar epithelial cells proliferate significantly and some cells shed, causing the microvascular congestion and edema in the alveolar septa [1].

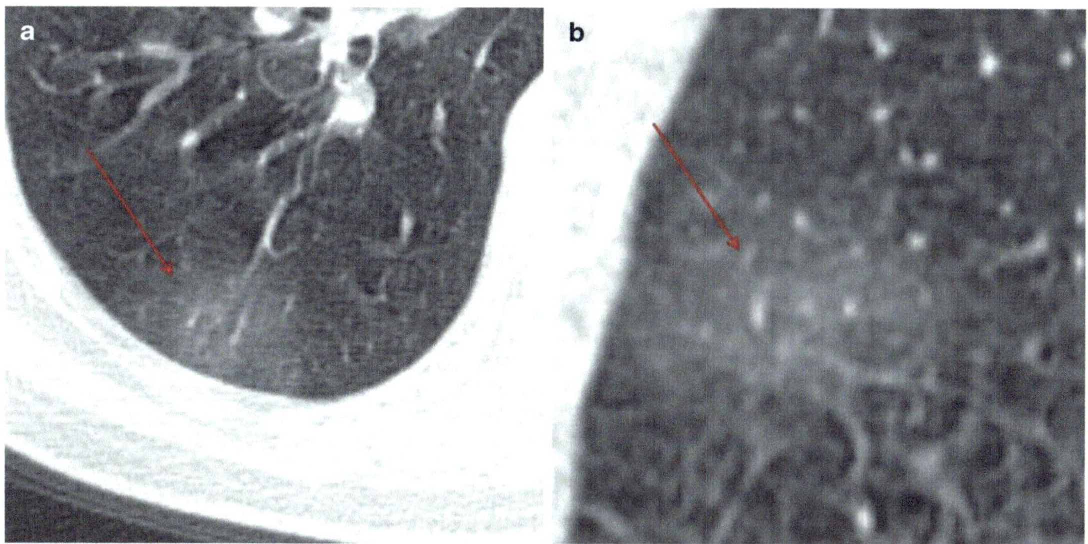

Fig. 3.4 Axial chest CT (**a**) and a reconstructed coronal image (**b**) of a COVID-19 patient (37-year-old male)

A selected chest CT image shows blurred patchy subpleural GGO in the posterior basal segment of the right lower lobe (red arrows).

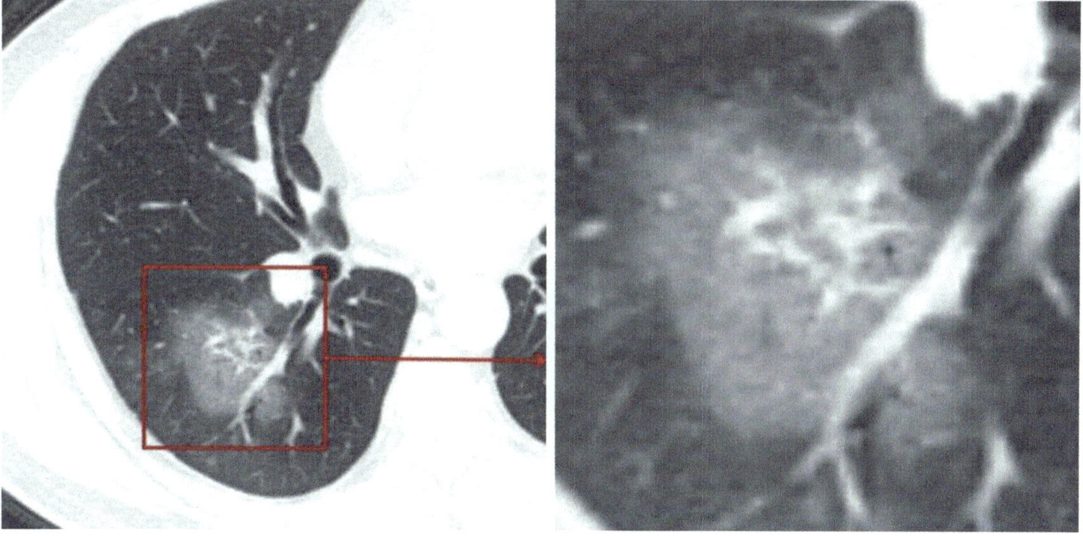

Fig. 3.5 Chest CT images of a COVID-19 patient (50-year-old male)

The chest CT image demonstrates a patchy GGO in the right lower lobe with thickened microvascular inside (red frame).

3.2.1.2 Consolidation

Consolidation on pulmonary CT indicates increased pulmonary parenchymal density. Pulmonary vessels and airway wall are obscured due to the lack of contrast from the alveolar gas. Acinar, lobular, pulmonary segment, or lobe involvement can be found in the COVID-19, but the volume reduction of involved lung is not obvious. Pathologically, the air in the alveolar is replaced by exudate or other substance from the infected tissue [1]. Lung consolidation lesion often develops from GGO, sometimes with the air bronchogram sign observed inside (Figs. 3.6, 3.7, and 3.8).

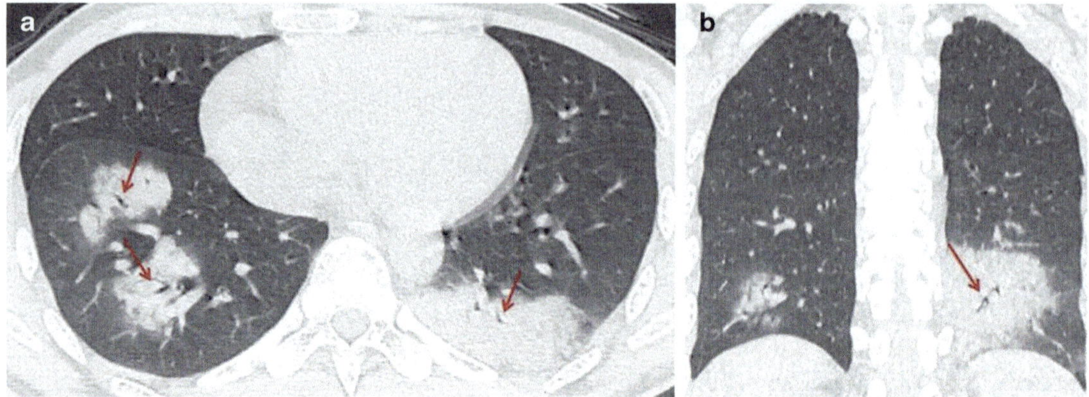

Fig. 3.6 Axial chest CT (**a**) and a reconstructed coronal image (**b**) of a COVID-19 patient (29-year-old male)

A chest CT image shows patchy consolidation in both lower lobes along the subpleural area, noticing the air bronchogram sign (red arrow).

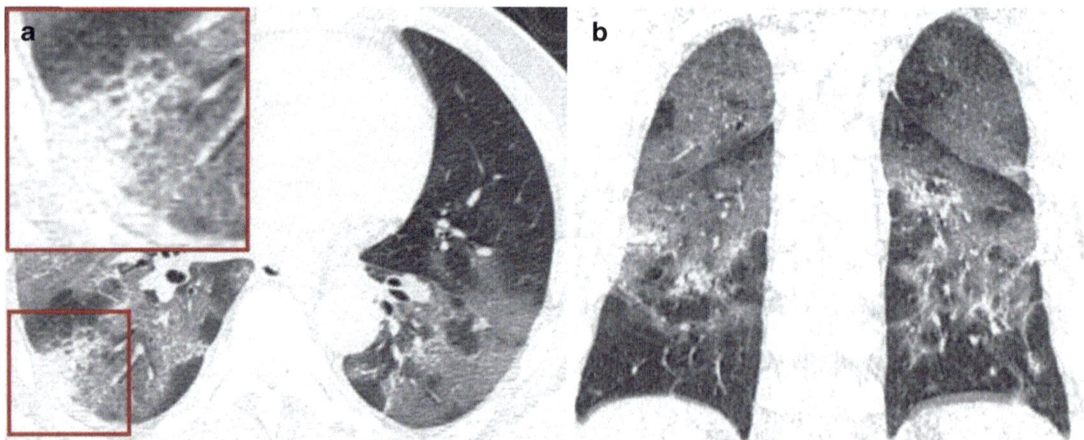

Fig. 3.7 Axial chest CT (**a**) and a reconstructed coronal image (**b**) of a COVID-19 patient (57-year-old male)

A chest CT image shows multiple GGOs in both lungs, thickened interlobular septa, local consolidation with mosaic-like perfusion (red frame), and the line shadow in both lower lung fields which indicates fibrosis.

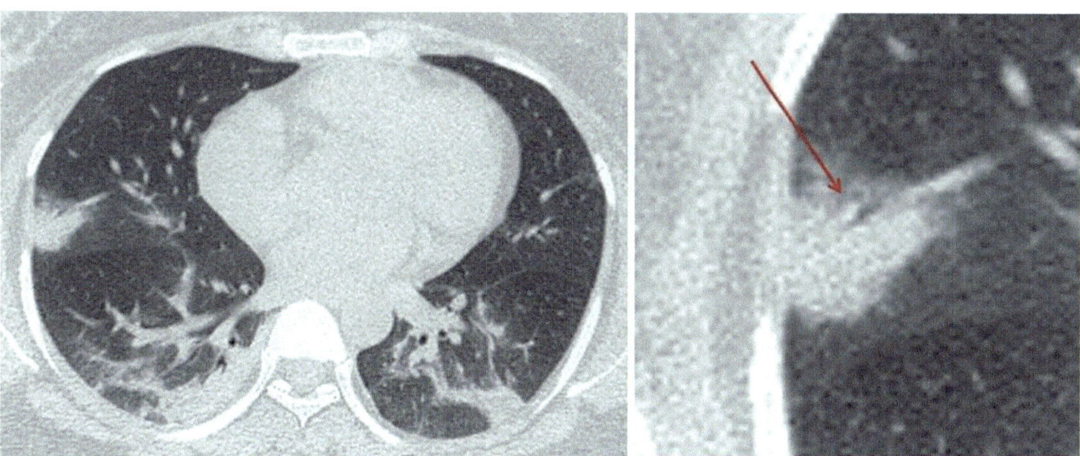

Fig. 3.8 Chest CT of a COVID-19 patient (32-year-old female)

A chest CT image shows multiple patchy consolidation. Air bronchogram (red arrow) can be seen within the lesion in the middle lobe of right lung. Lobular atelectasis can be observed in the lower lobes of both lungs.

3.2.1.3 Reticular and Crazy-Paving Pattern

Multiple linear shadows of pulmonary lobules within GGO lesions may present a "reticular pattern," while the combination with interlobular septal thickening may present a "crazy-paving pattern" (Figs. 3.9 and 3.10). Early pathological changes in the lungs of COVID-19 patients include pulmonary edema, protein exudation, pulmonary interstitial thickening, and infiltration with multinucleated giant cells and macrophages in the alveolar cavity [1].

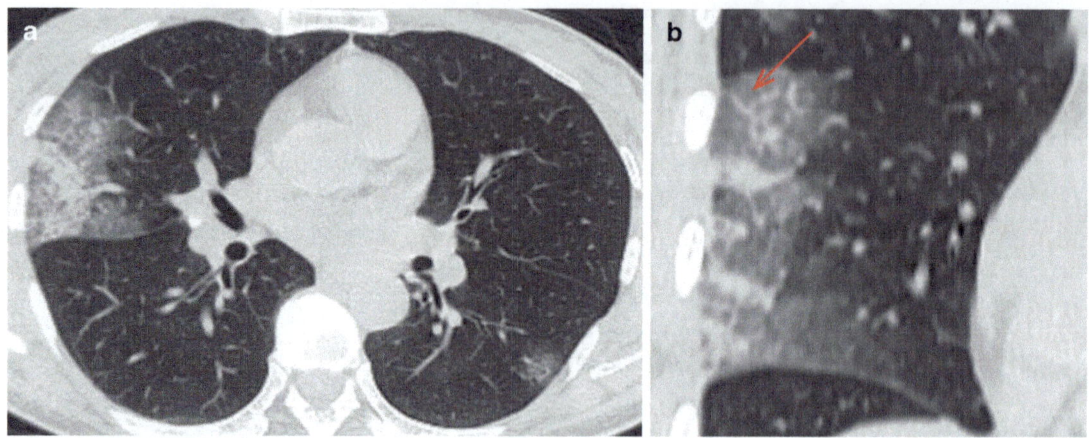

Fig. 3.9 Axial chest CT (**a**) and a reconstructed coronal image (**b**) of a COVID-19 patient (51-year-old female)

CT images of lung show scattered GGO in both lungs, mosaic-like shadow with thickened interlobular septa, and interlobular linear shadow (red arrow), presenting a "crazy-paving pattern."

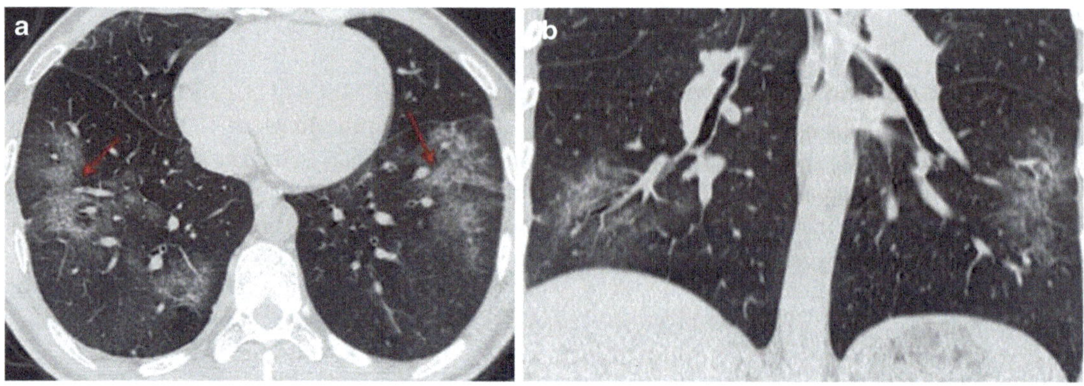

Fig. 3.10 Axial chest CT (**a**) and a reconstructed coronal image (**b**) of a COVID-19 patient (51-year-old female)

Scattered GGO in bilateral lower lobes, appearing as a "reticular pattern" (red arrow), can be seen in this chest CT image.

3.2.2 Other CT Findings of COVID-19

3.2.2.1 Fibrous Lesions

Fibrous lesions may develop as line shadow in patients with COVID-19 in a short time (Figs. 3.11 and 3.12). However, most fibrous lesions can be completely absorbed. Gross observations from the autopsy of COVID-19 patients showed that, in addition to a large amount of viscous secretions spilling from the alveoli, fibrous cords were also seen on the general section.

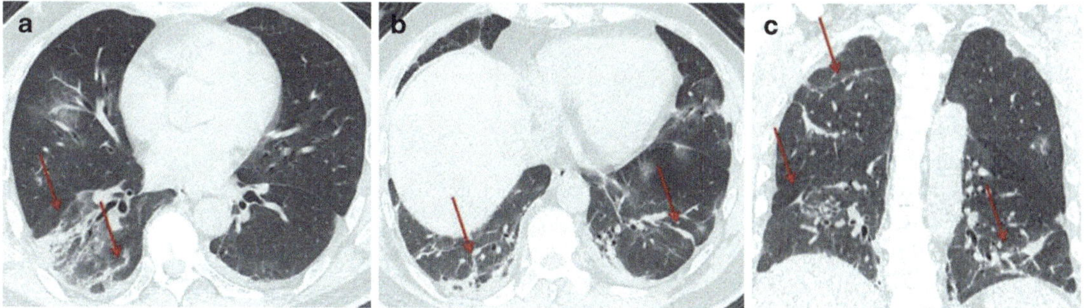

Fig. 3.11 Axial chest CT (**a**, **b**) and a reconstructed coronal image (**c**) of a COVID-19 patient (51-year-old male)

Chest CT showed multiple patchy GGO and partial consolidation. Fibrous cords were visible around the lesions (red arrow).

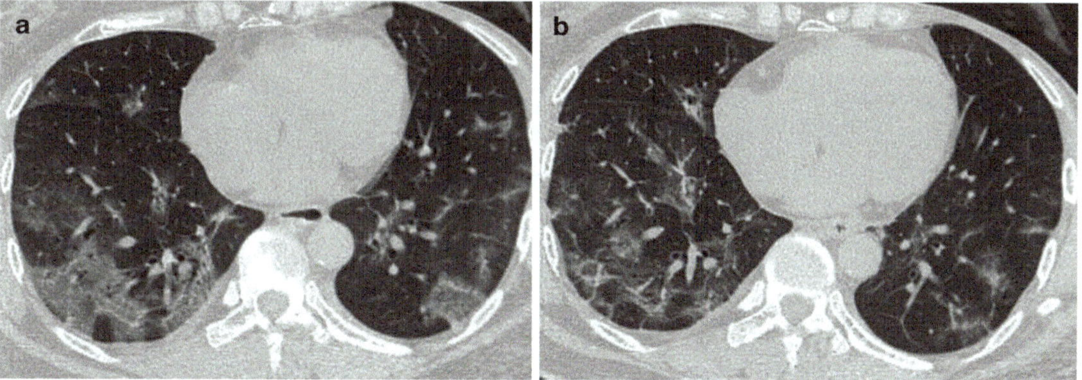

Fig. 3.12 Chest CT (**a**) of a COVID-19 patient (60-year-old female) and her follow-up CT (**b**)

Chest CT showed scattered GGO in both lobes with a subpleural distribution (**a**) at admission. The follow-up CT 5 days later showed obvious absorption of lung lesions and increased fibrosis shadow within the lesions (**b**).

3.2.2.2 Air Bronchogram Sign

Air bronchogram sign refers to the air-filled shadow of the bronchoalveolar cavity protruding from the lining of opaque (high-density) and gas-free lung tissues (Fig. 3.13).

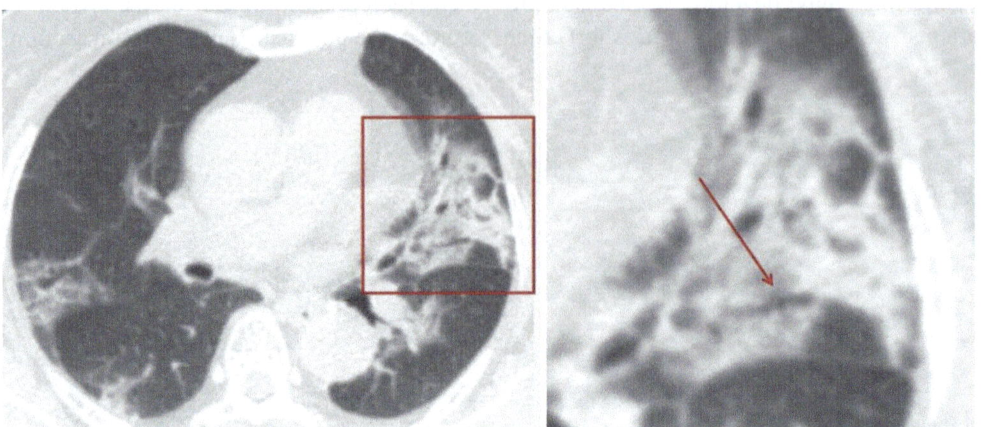

Fig. 3.13 Chest CT of a COVID-19 patient (79-year-old female)

Chest CT showed multiple patchy GGOs and subsegmental or segmental consolidation in both lungs (red frame), note the air bronchogram sign within the consolidation (red arrow).

3.2.2.3 Microvascular Thickening

In patients with COVID-19, there are dilated microvasculature shadows within or near the lesions appearing on CT (Fig. 3.14), which are typically visible at all stages of the disease.

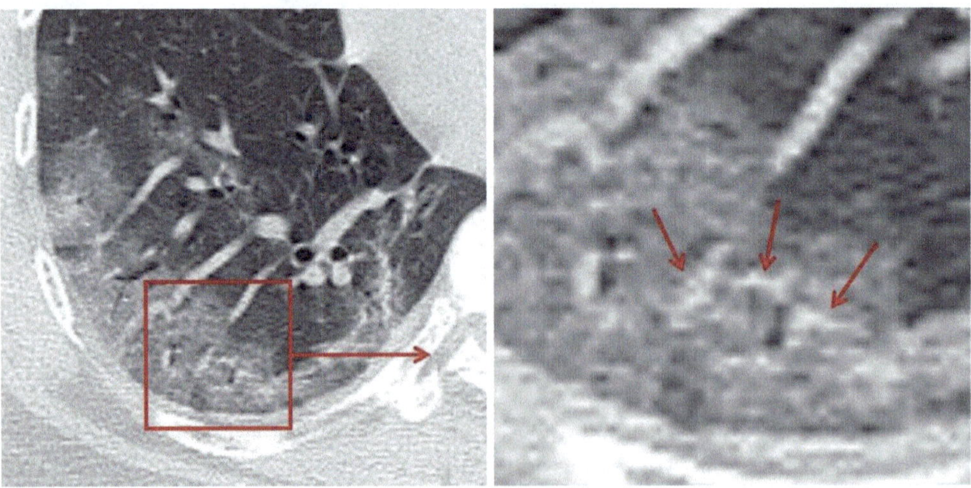

Fig. 3.14 Chest CT of a COVID-19 patient (60-year-old female)

Chest CT showed subpleural flaky GGO in the right lower lobe of the lung, note the dilated microvascular shadows (red arrow).

3.2.2.4 Halo Sign

Halo sign on CT of COVID-19 refers to the appearance of a circle of GGO around the lesion, presenting a halo-like change (Fig. 3.15). Halo was first used to describe the GGO around focal invasive aspergillus nodule caused by perifocal hemorrhage, which is a nonspecific sign. The perifocal halo sign of COVID-19 is different from the traditional one, mainly manifested as the change of mist-like inflammatory exudate around the lesion. Currently, we defined it as a halo sign. However, the pathological interpretations remain to be clarified.

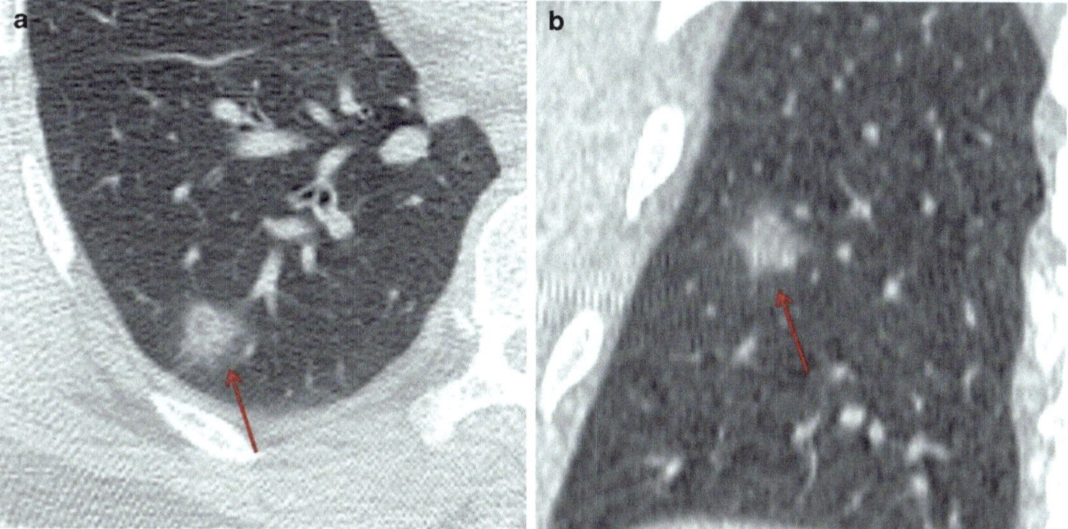

Fig. 3.15 Axial chest CT (**a**) and a reconstructed coronal image (**b**) of a COVID-19 patient (50-year-old male)

Chest CT showed a nodule in the right lower lobe with halo sign around it (red arrow).

3.2.2.5 Reversed Halo Sign

Reversed halo sign refers to the appearance of GGO at the center of the lesion. The surrounding appearance is a ring or crescent shape of high-density strip shadow (Fig. 3.16). Reversed halo sign was initially recognized as a specific sign of cryptogenic organizing pneumonia (COP). Reversed halo sign has been found to be associated with a variety of diseases, including infectious, non-infectious, and neoplastic diseases. It rarely appears in the viral pneumonia but not uncommon in the COVID-19. Its pathological interpretations are not established. A more faint GGO-like rim seen on CT images may be present in COP, and sometimes it may appear as a target-like center.

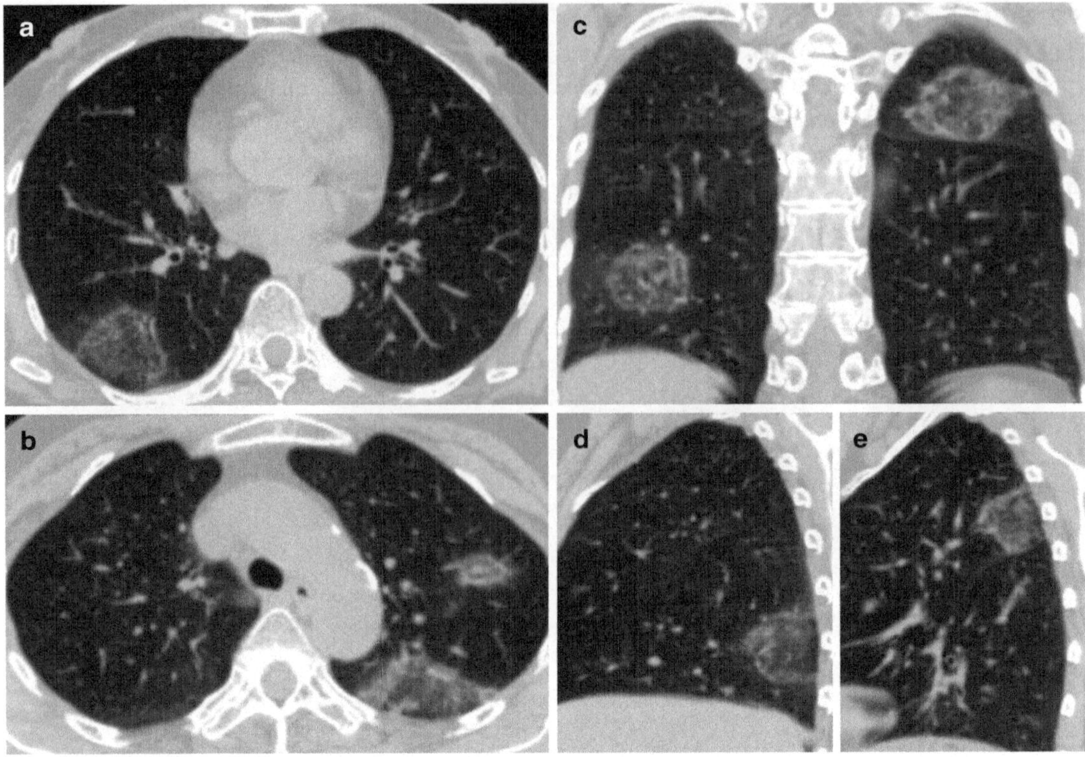

Fig. 3.16 Axial chest CT (**a**, **b**), reconstructed coronal (**c**), and sagittal (**d**, **e**) images of a COVID-19 patient

A chest CT image shows patchy opacity in the right lower lobe and the left upper lobe. There was a GGO shadow with slightly dotted high density in the center of the lesion and ring-like high-density strip or line shadow rim, presenting a reversed halo sign (red arrow).

3.2.2.6 Tractive Bronchiectasis

Traction bronchiectasis may be seen in the consolidation or fiber cords shadow on CT images of COVID-19 patients. This nonspecific sign may be resulted from surrounding fibrosis (Fig. 3.17).

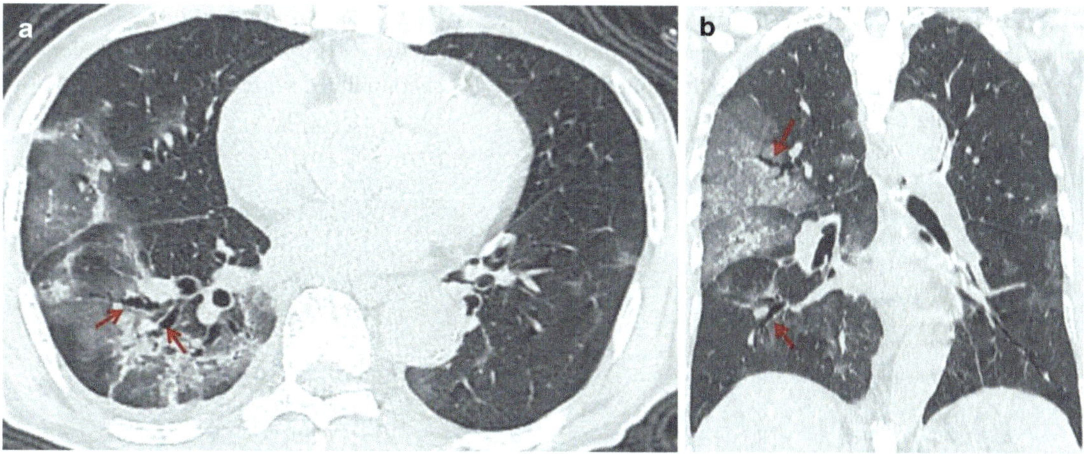

Fig. 3.17 Axial chest CT (**a**) and a reconstructed coronal image (**b**) of a COVID-19 patient

Chest CT showed multiple GGO in both lungs, local consolidation, irregular dilated bronchus with slightly thickened bronchial wall (red arrow), and fibrosis around the lesions. There is a small amount of pleural effusion at the right side.

3.2.2.7 Atelectasis

Atelectasis refers to complete collapse or incomplete expansion of lung tissues caused by bronchial obstruction or contraction of scar tissue. Most atelectasis observed in the COVID-19 patients was subsegmental or lobular atelectasis (Fig. 3.18).

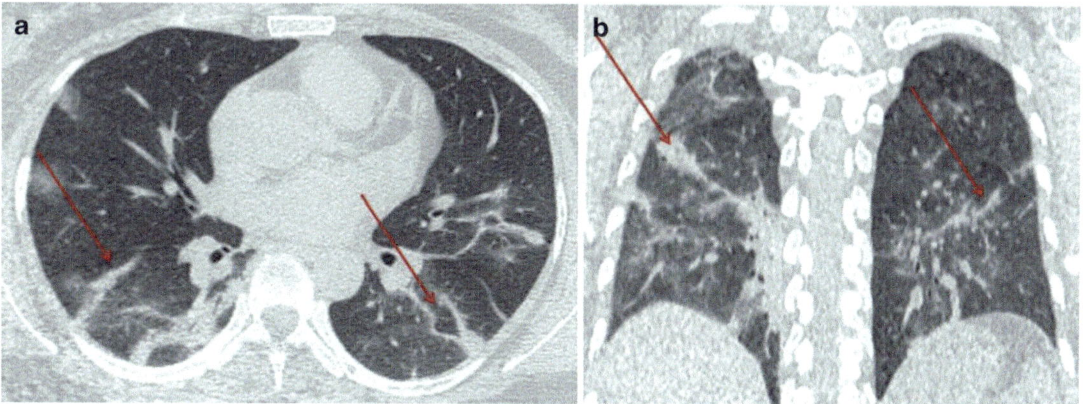

Fig. 3.18 Axial chest CT (**a**) and a reconstructed coronal image (**b**) of a COVID-19 patient (82-year-old male)

Chest CT showed multiple stripe-like shadows in both lungs, which were dominated by consolidation. There were striated shadows of reduced volume (red arrows) in the lower lobes, suggesting subsegmental atelectasis or lobular atelectasis.

3.2.2.8 Nodule

In the early stage of COVID-19 infection, pulmonary CT can detect lung nodules with diameter ≤ 3 cm, including solid nodules, partial solid nodules, or pure ground-glass nodules with clear or fuzzy boundaries (Figs. 3.19 and 3.20). Nodules may be accompanied with the halo sign.

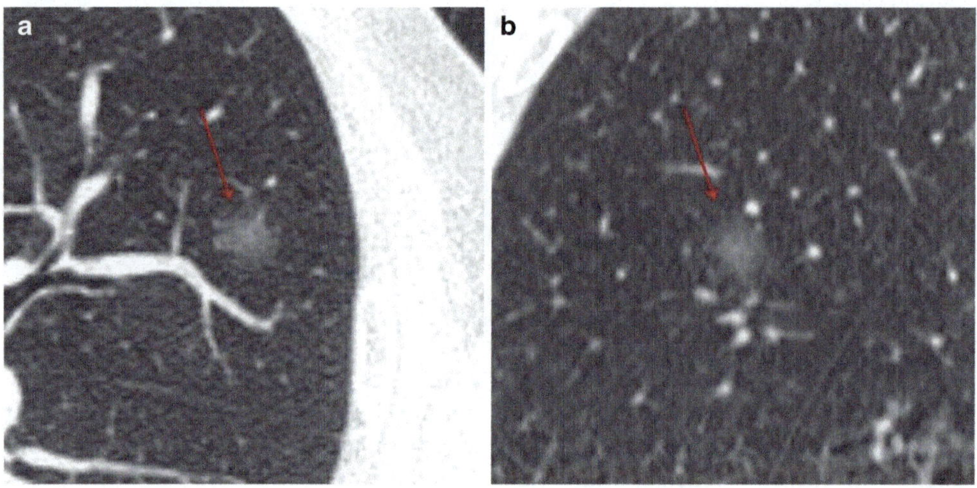

Fig. 3.19 Axial chest CT (**a**) and a reconstructed coronal image (**b**) of a COVID-19 patient (32-year-old female)

Chest CT showed a pure ground-glass nodule with blurred boundaries in the apicoposterior segment of left upper lobe (red arrow).

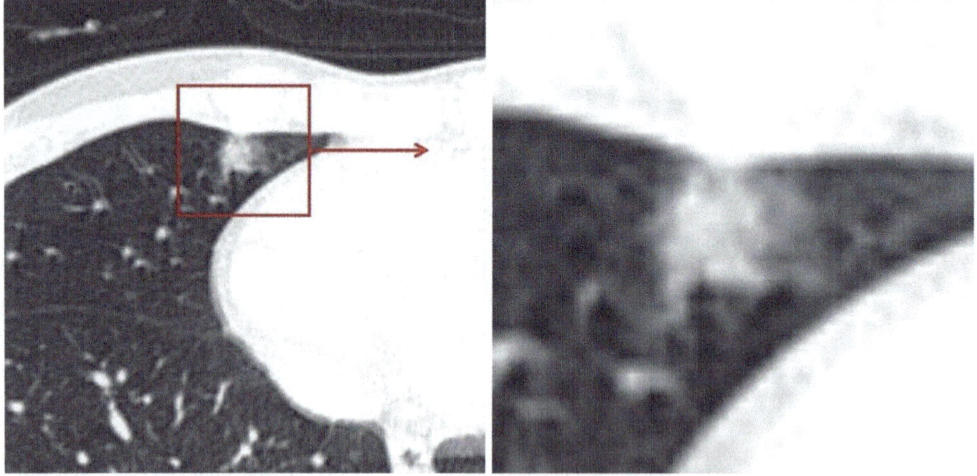

Fig. 3.20 Chest CT of a COVID-19 patient (50-year-old male)

Chest CT showed a subpleural solid nodule in the right middle lobe with blurred boundaries (red frame).

3.2.2.9 Tree-in-Bud Sign

The sign of tree-in-bud (TIB) on chest CT images appears as bud-like shadow formed when central lobular bronchioles are dilated and filled with mucus, pus, or fluid. TIB sign has been reported in a few COVID-19 cases (Fig. 3.21) and is considered to be mainly caused by the distal airway and alveolar injury due to inflammation with the involvement of bronchioles.

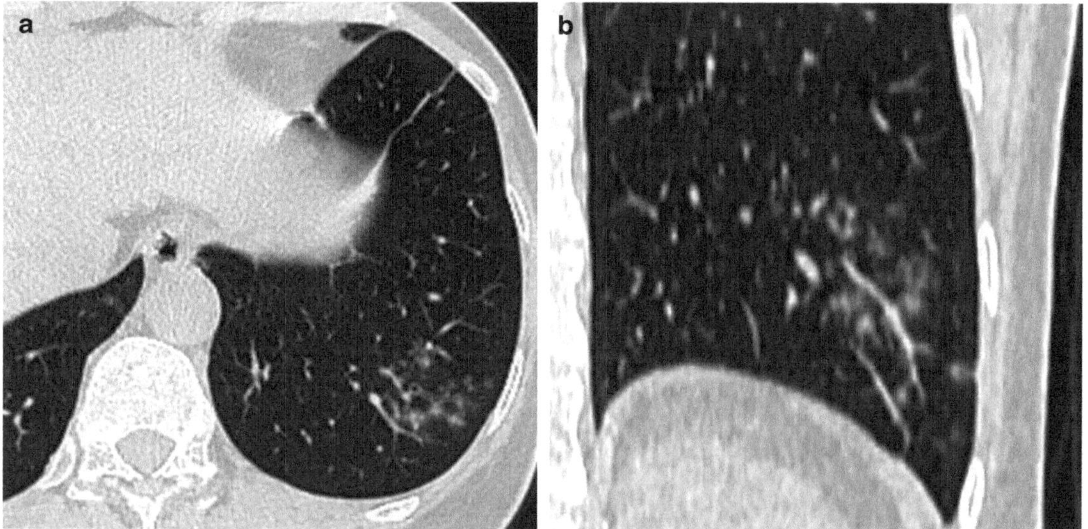

Fig. 3.21 Axial chest CT (**a**) and a reconstructed sagittal image (**b**) of a COVID-19 patient (23-year-old male)

Chest CT showed small nodules along bronchi with blurred boundaries in the left lower lobe, presenting a tree-in-bud sign.

3.2.2.10 Other Findings

Interlobar fissure and bilateral pleural thickening can also be observed on chest CT of some cases (Fig. 3.22). In addition, pleural effusion and enlarged mediastinal lymph nodes were also occasionally reported.

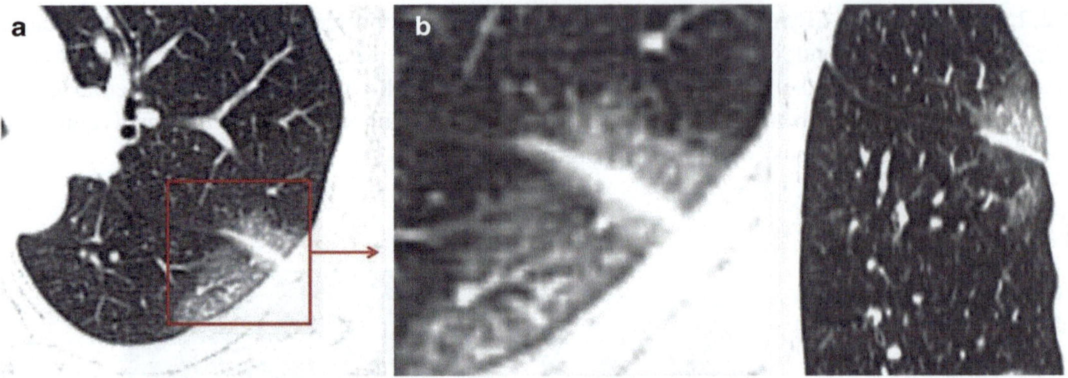

Fig. 3.22 Axial chest CT (**a**) and a reconstructed sagittal image (**b**) of a COVID-19 patient (53-year-old female)

Chest CT showed multiple GGO in the left lung with localized thickening of the left oblique fissure (red frame).

Due to limited biopsy and autopsy done during the pandemic, there is still lack of comparison and correlation between pathological characterization of the lesions and imaging findings in the current COVID-19 cases [1]. In addition, the evolution and natural history of COVID-19 is still under investigation with new data and findings continuing to be collected. Therefore, the pulmonary CT imaging features and interpretation in the patients with COVID-19 pneumonia may be reviewed and revised in the future. We may continue to supplement and revise the contents of this book in the future.

References

1. National Health Commission of the People's Republic of China. Diagnosis and treatment protocols of pneumonia caused by a novel coronavirus (trial version 7). [EB/OL]. [2020-03-03].http://www.nhc.gov.cn/yzygj/s7653p/202003/46c9294a7dfe4cef80dc7f5912eb1989/files/ce3e6945832a438eaae415350a8ce964.pdf
2. Huang C, Wang Y, Li X, et al. Clinical features of patients infected with 2019 novel coronavirus in Wuhan, China. Lancet. 2020;395(10223):497–506.
3. Zhu N, Zhang D, Wang W, et al. A novel coronavirus from patients with pneumonia in China, 2019. N Engl J Med. 2020;382(8):727–33.
4. Wong HYF, Lam HYS, Fong AH, et al. Frequency and distribution of chest radiographic findings in COVID-19 positive patients. Radiology. 2019 Mar;27:201160.
5. Li Q, Guan X, Wu P, et al. Early transmission dynamics in Wuhan, China, of novel coronavirus-infected pneumonia. N Engl J Med. 2020;382(13):1199–207.
6. Lili R, Yeming W, Zhiqiang W, et al. Identification of a novel coronavirus causing severe pneumonia in human: a descriptive study. Chin Med J. 2020;133(9):1015–24.
7. Chen N, Zhou M, Dong X, et al. Epidemiological and clinical characteristics of 99 cases of 2019 novel coronavirus pneumonia in Wuhan, China: a descriptive study. Lancet. 2020;395(10223):507–13.
8. Wang Z, Yang B, Li Q, et al. Clinical features of 69 cases with coronavirus disease 2019 in Wuhan, China. Clin Infect Dis. 2020;71(15):769–77. a272.
9. Zhou L, Liu HG. Early detection and disease assessment of patients with novel coronavirus pneumonia. Chin J Tuberculosis Respir Dis. 2020;43:E003.

Typical Cases of COVID-19 Pneumonia in Adult

4

Minming Zhang, Hui Mao, Lihua Wang, Pingding Kuang, Xiqi Zhu, Hanpeng Zheng, Qiyuan Wang, Fan Yang, Lulu Gao, Jian Lv, Yongchou Li, Bin Lin, Zhujing Shen, Nan Lu, and Haisheng Zhou

4.1 Mild Typical Case and Its Outcome

Case 1

Medical History and Clinical Manifestation

A 27-year-old man was admitted in the hospital with fever (highest body temperature: 38.7 °C) for 1 day. Laboratory test results indicated normal white blood cell and neutrophil count, decreased lymphocyte count, eosinophil count and lymphocyte percentage, and increased C-reactive protein and interleukin 6 (IL-6). Exposure history: The patient returned hometown from Wuhan, China. The SARS-CoV-2 nucleic acid test was positive 4 days after admission.

Imaging Features

Initial chest CT scan of the lungs showed no obvious abnormalities (Fig. 4.1).

Follow-up chest CT (3 days after initial CT examination) showed patchy ground-glass opacities (GGOs) in apical segment of the right upper lobe and left lower lobe of the lungs, with blurred boundary. In the lesion of the left lower lobe, there were dilated blood vessels (**b**: white arrow) and air bronchi signs (**b**: red arrow). Consolidation can be seen locally in the left inferior lobe of the mediastinal window (Fig. 4.2).

After 5 days follow-up and reexamination, CT showed that the lesions in the right upper lobe and the left lower lobe were slightly more absorbed than before, while the reversed halo sign (**c**: red arrow) became obvious (Fig. 4.3).

Follow-up chest CT (8 days after initial CT examination) showed obvious absorption of lesions in the lower lobe of the left lung and complete absorption of lesions in the right upper lobe (Fig. 4.4).

Follow-up chest CT (13 days after initial CT examination) showed complete absorption of two lung lesions (Fig. 4.5).

M. Zhang (✉) · L. Wang · P. Kuang · Q. Wang
F. Yang · B. Lin · Z. Shen · N. Lu
Department of Radiology, the Second Affiliated Hospital, Zhejiang University School of Medicine, Hangzhou, China
e-mail: zhangminming@zju.edu.cn; lihuawang@zju.edu.cn; zjdxlinbin@zju.edu.cn; shenzhujing@zju.edu.cn

H. Mao
Department of Radiology and Imaging Sciences, Emory University School of Medicine, Atlanta, GA, USA
e-mail: hmao@emory.edu

X. Zhu · J. Lv
Department of Radiology, Nanxishan Hospital of Guangxi Zhuang Autonomous Region, Guilin, China

H. Zheng · H. Zhou
Department of Radiology, YueQing People's Hospital, WenZhou, China

L. Gao
Department of Radiology, Zhejiang Hospital, Hangzhou, China

Y. Li
Department of Radiology, the Third Affiliated Hospital of Wenzhou Medical University, Ruian, China

M. Zhang, B. Lin (eds.), *Diagnostic Imaging of Novel Coronavirus Pneumonia*,
https://doi.org/10.1007/978-981-15-5992-1_4

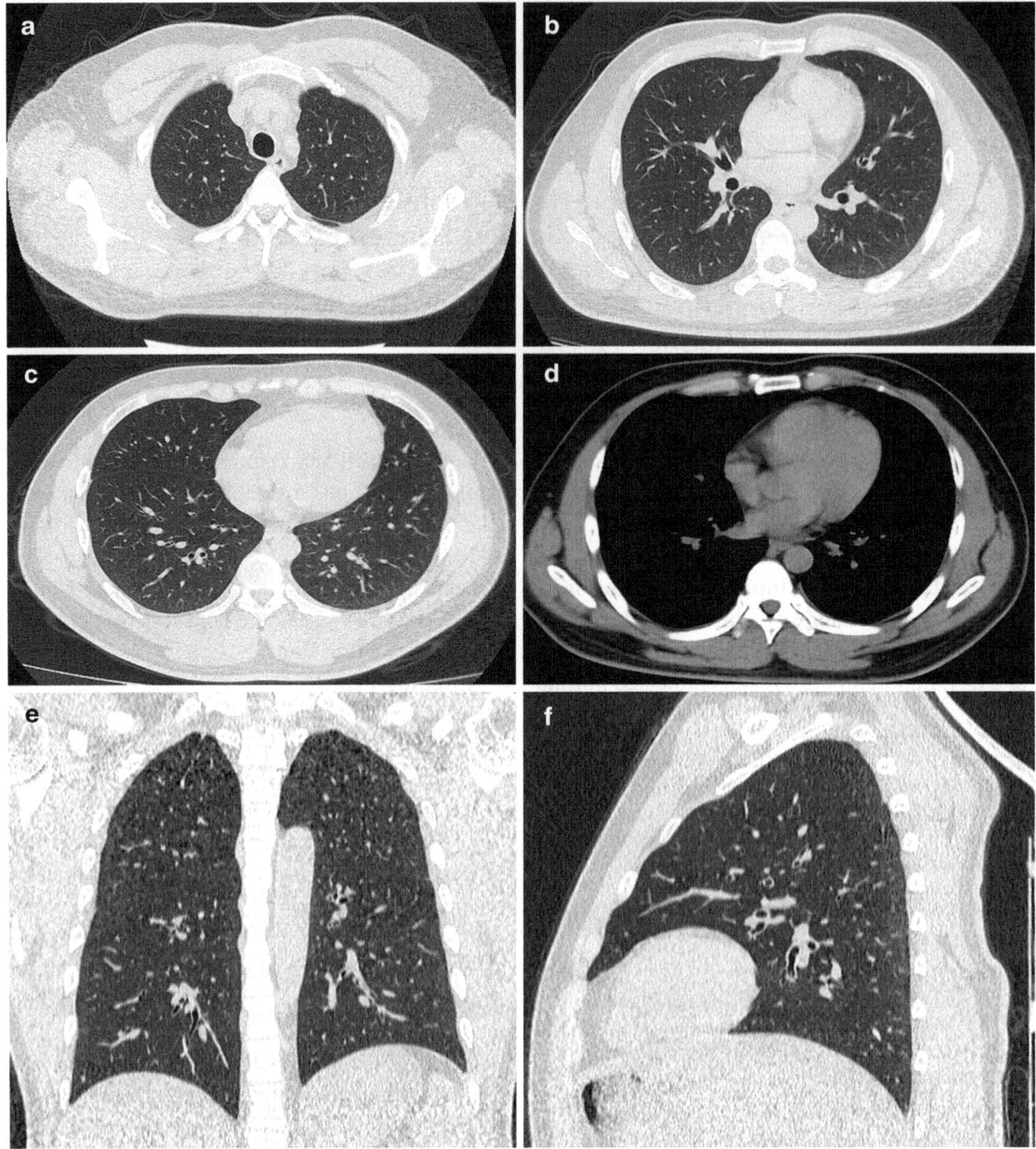

Fig. 4.1 Initial chest CT (**a–d**), reconstructed coronal (**e**) and sagittal (**f**) images of the patient

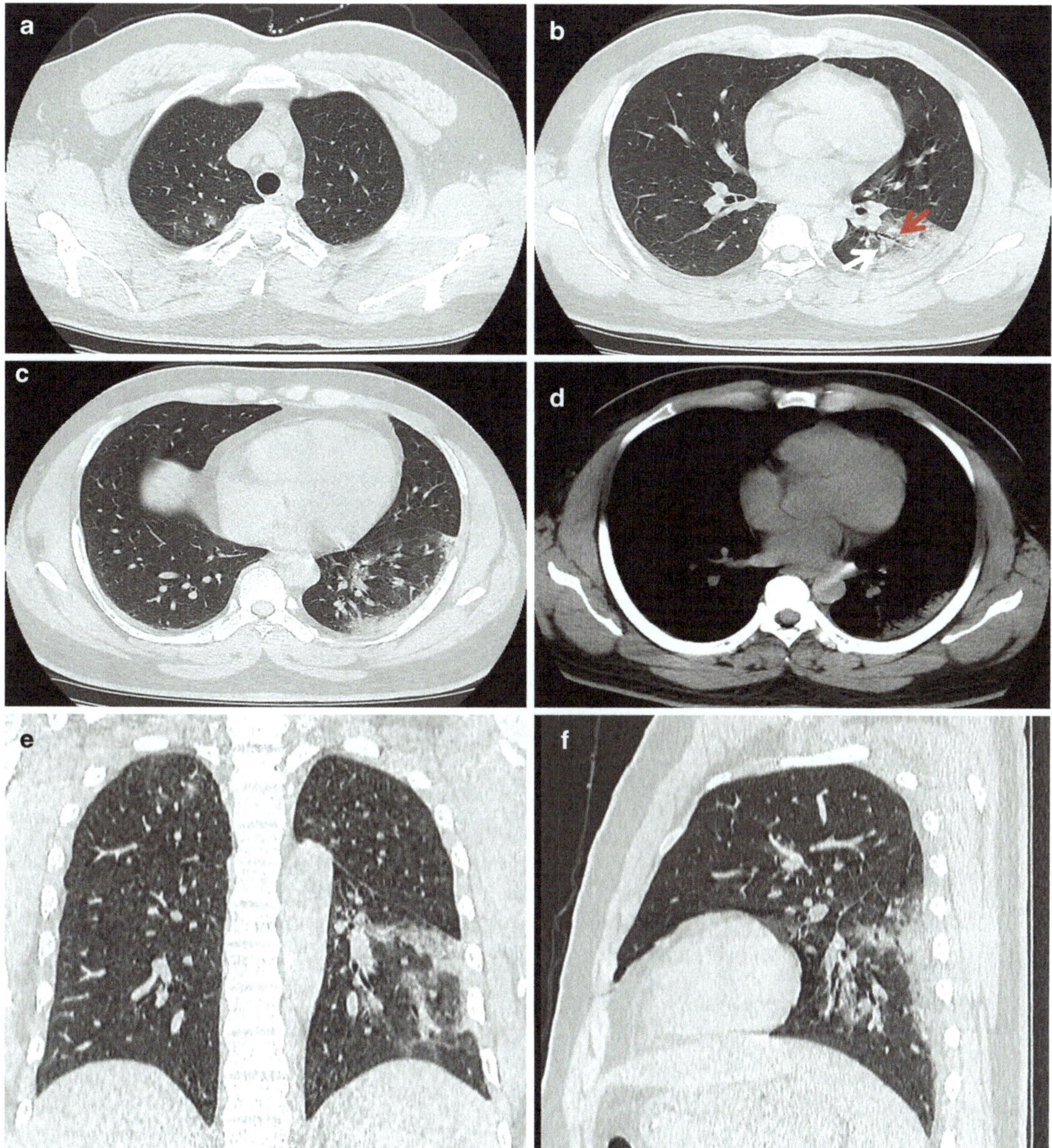

Fig. 4.2 Follow-up axial chest CT (**a–d**), reconstructed coronal (**e**) and sagittal (**f**) images 3 days after initial scan

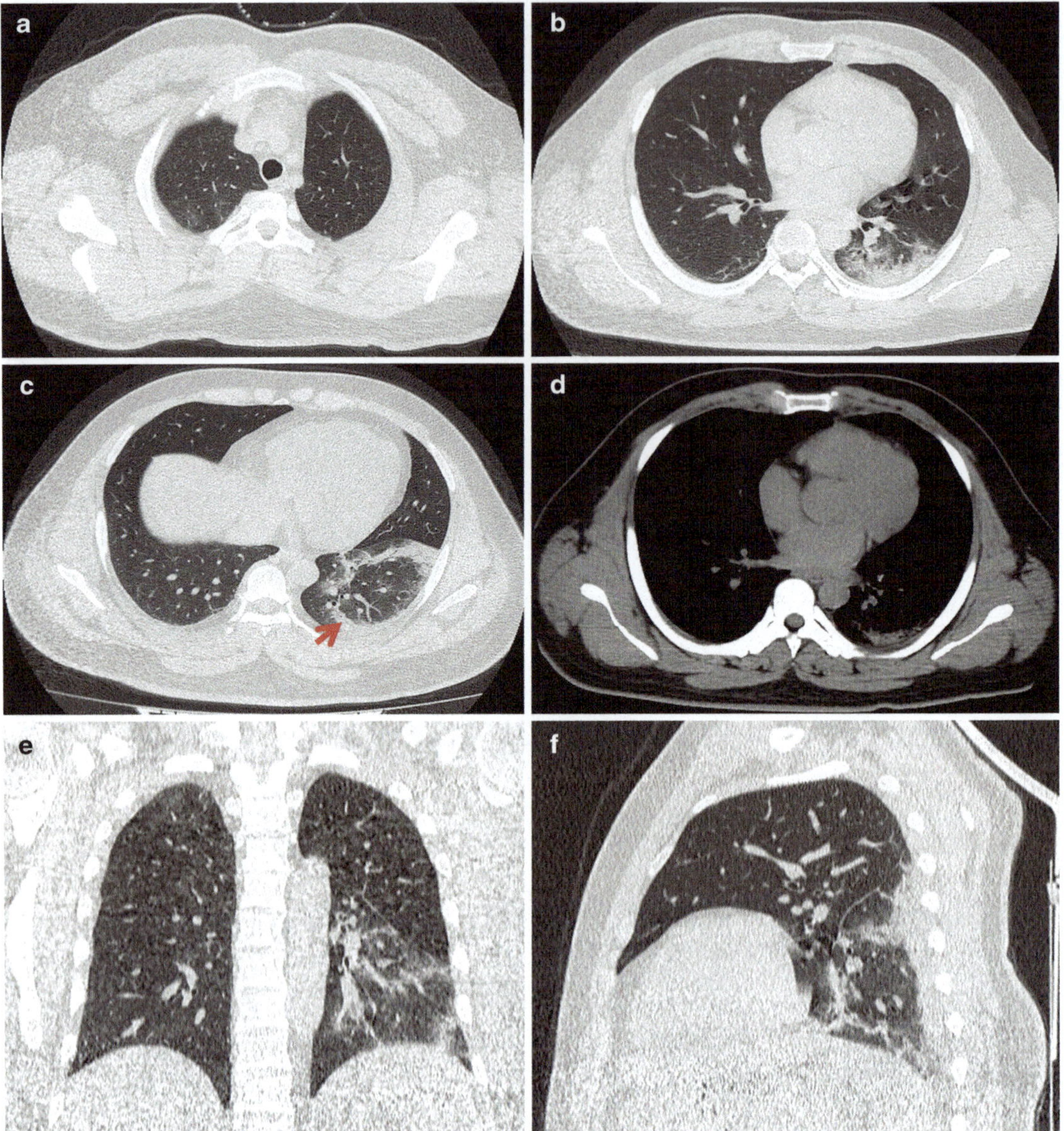

Fig. 4.3 Follow-up axial chest CT (**a–d**), reconstructed coronal (**e**) and sagittal (**f**) images 5 days after initial scan

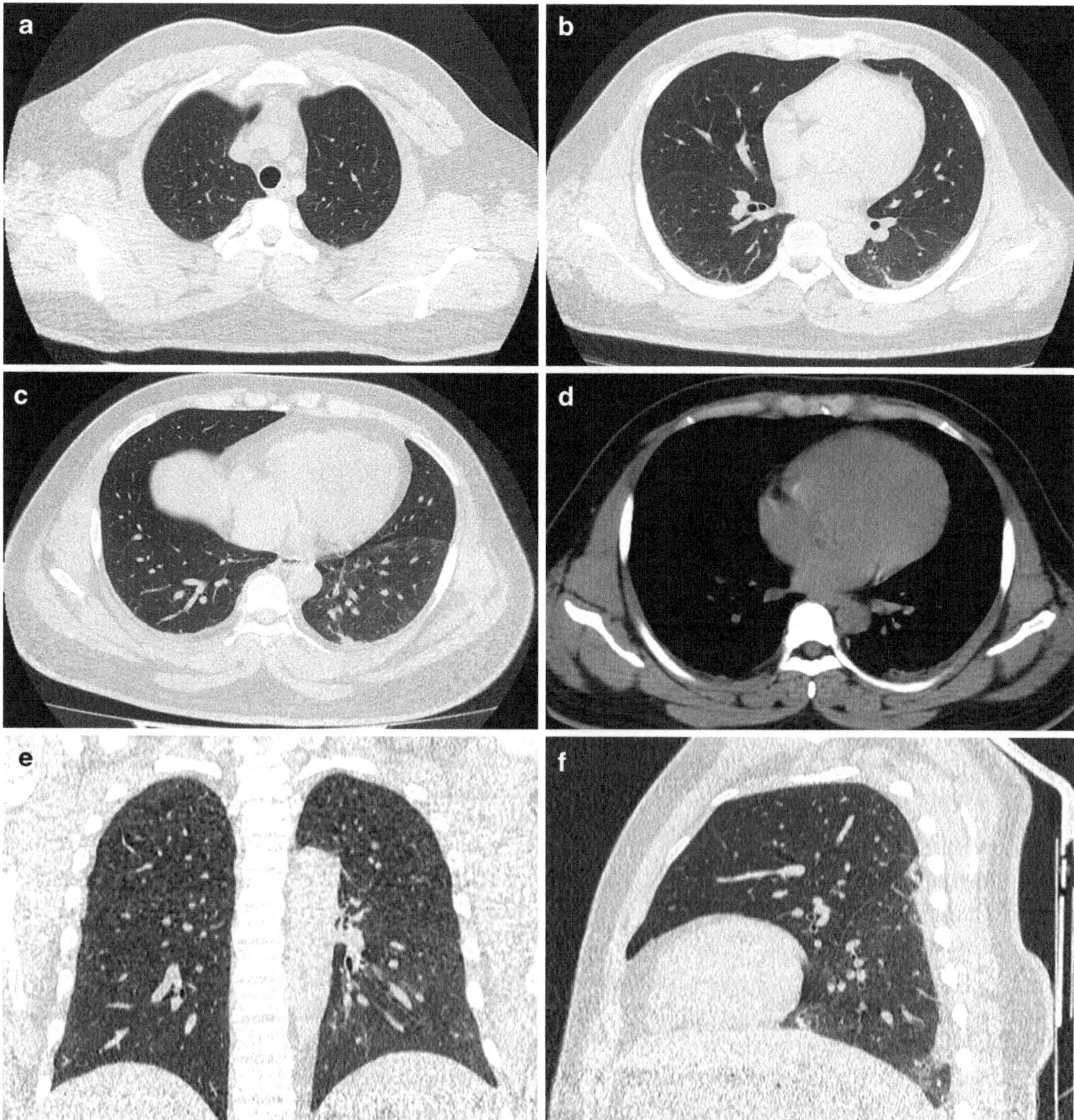

Fig. 4.4 Follow-up axial chest CT (**a–d**), reconstructed coronal (**e**) and sagittal (**f**) images 8 days after initial scan

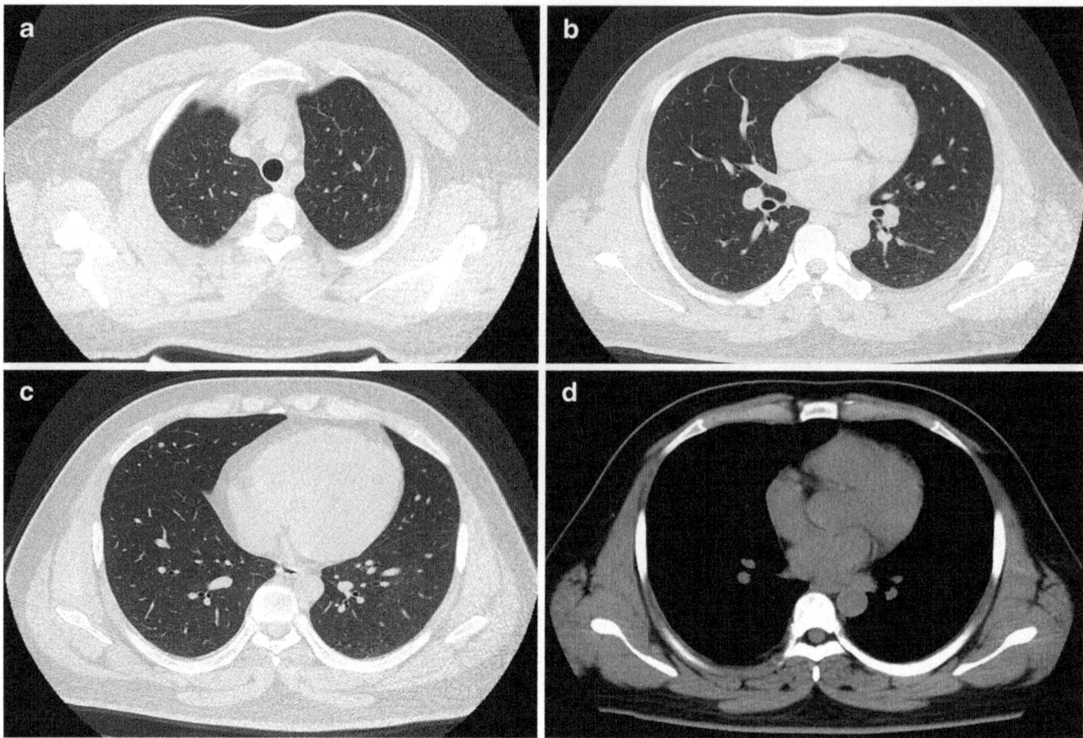

Fig. 4.5 Follow-up CT images 13 days after initial scan

Comments: In the early stage of the disease, the imaging performance of the patient was negative, and the SARS-CoV-2 nucleic acid test was also negative. Then, there were typical imaging manifestations, subpleural plaques, and reversed halo signs in the process of absorption and improvement. The lesions were absorbed 10 days after treatment. This dynamic development process is a common type of COVID-19.

4.2 Progressive Typical Case and Its Outcome

Case 2

Medical History and Clinical Manifestation

A 50-year-old man, with a history of AIDS, was admitted in the hospital with fever (highest body temperature: 38 °C) for 3 days, accompanied by cough and mild diarrhea. Laboratory test results indicated an increased neutrophil percentage, decreased lymphocyte count and percentage, increased blood sedimentation, increased C-reactive protein and IL-6. Exposure history: The patient has lived in Wuhan, China for a long time. He returned to his hometown by train from Wuhan to visit his relatives 9 days prior to symptom onset. The patient tested positive for SARS-CoV-2 nucleic acid test 5 days after admission.

Imaging Features

Initial chest CT showed multiple patchy ground-glass opacities in both lungs, dilated of small blood vessels (**b**: white arrow) and crazy-paving pattern (**b**: red arrow) were observed in the lesion, and some lesions were accompanied (Fig. 4.6).

Follow-up chest CT (2 days after initial CT examination) showed that the lesions were progressed. The lesions were slightly enlarged, and the density of the lesions was slightly increased (Fig. 4.7).

Follow-up chest CT (7 days after initial CT examination) showed the lesion was partially absorbed and the lesion was decreased compared with the previous CT (Fig. 4.8).

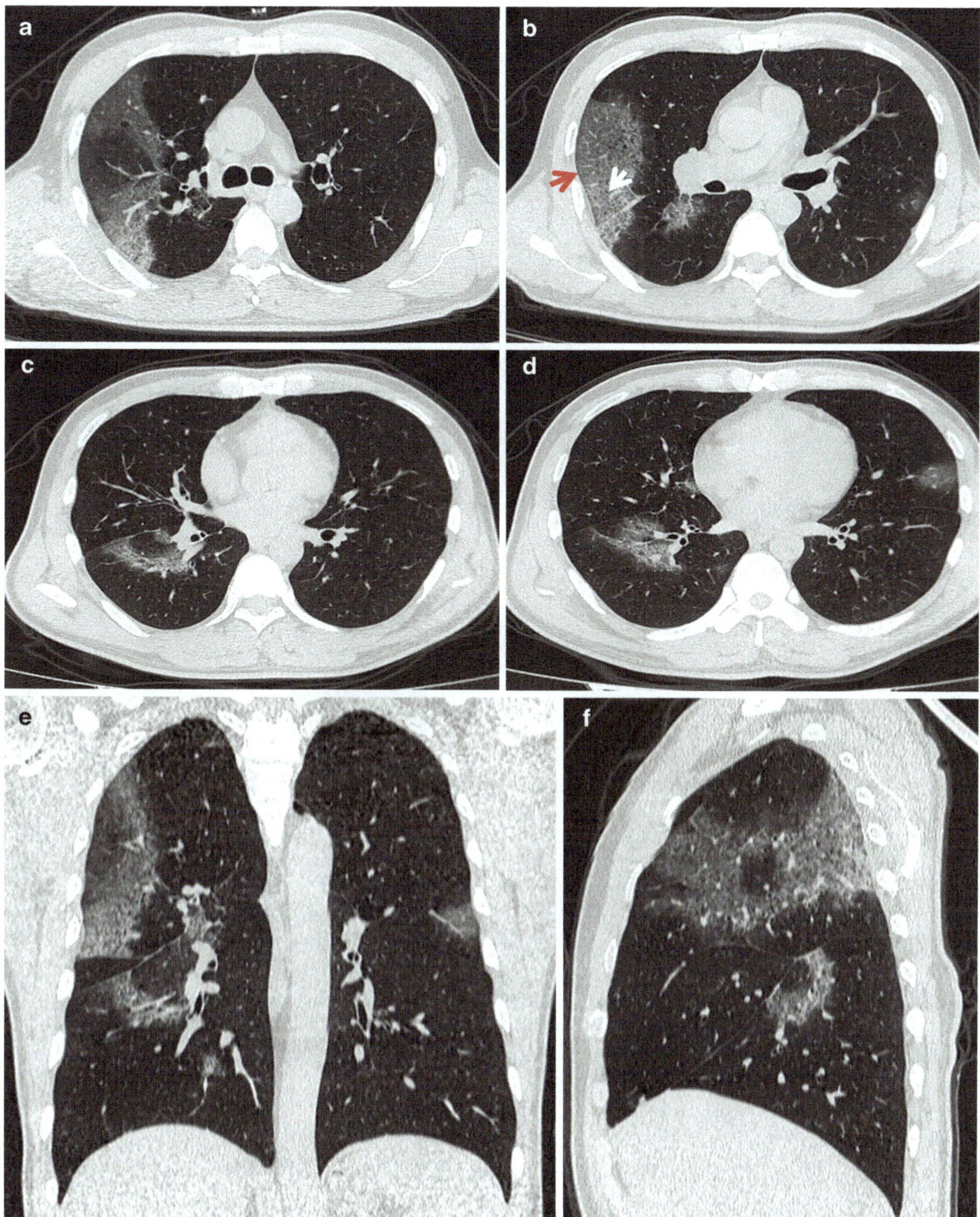

Fig. 4.6 Initial chest CT (**a–d**), reconstructed coronal (**e**) and sagittal (**f**) images of the patient

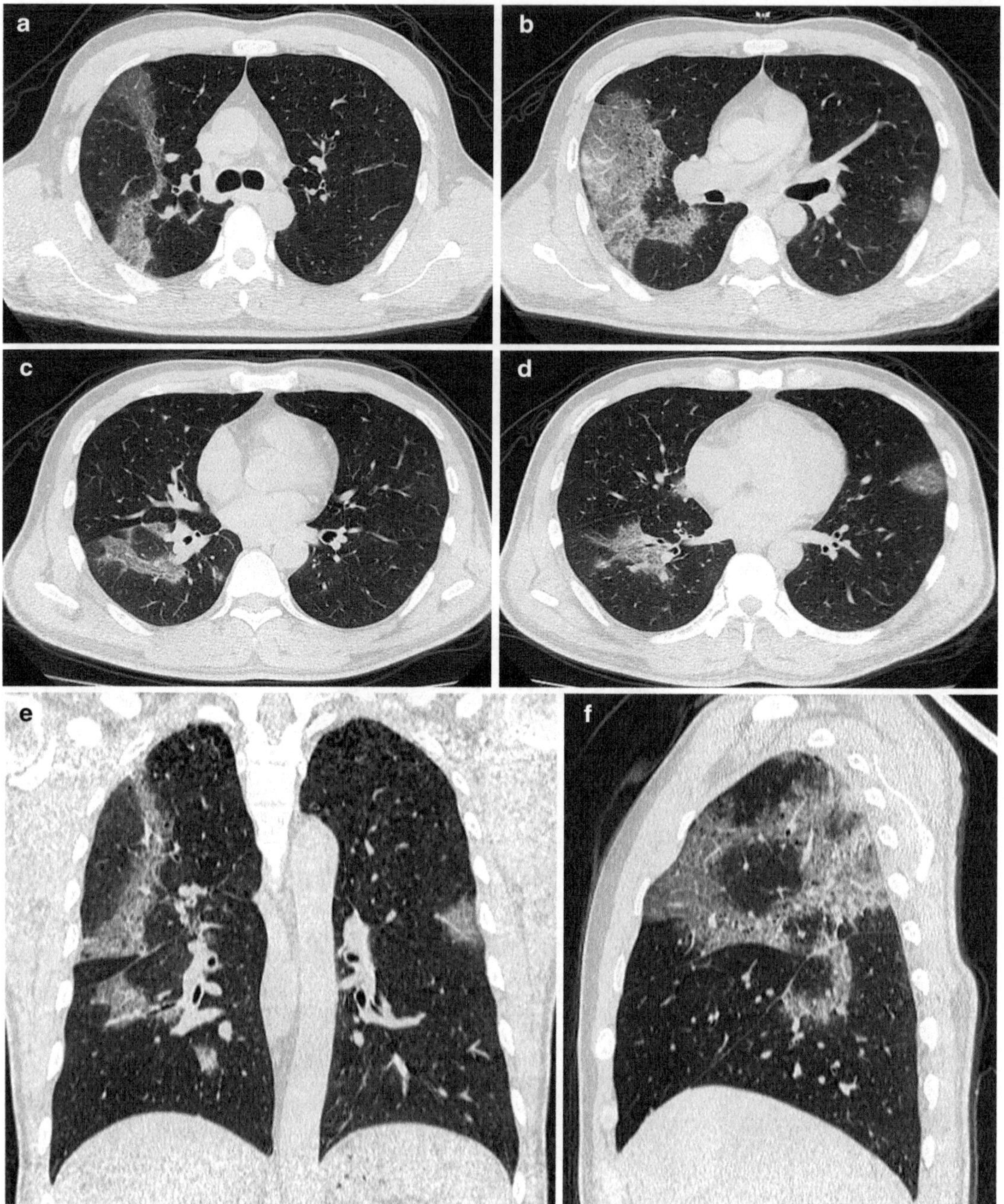

Fig. 4.7 Follow-up axial chest CT (**a–d**), reconstructed coronal (**e**) and sagittal (**f**) images 2 days after initial scan

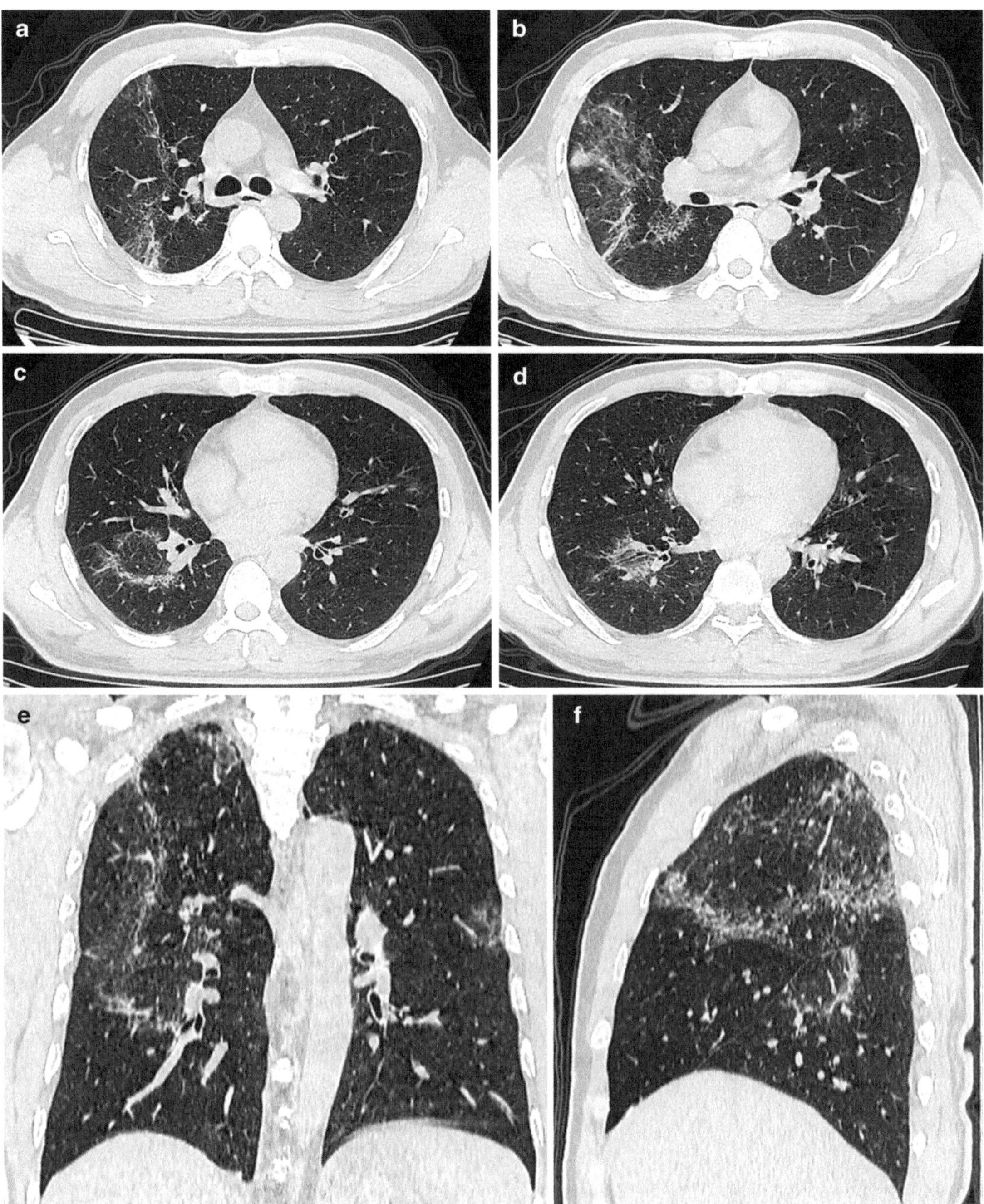

Fig. 4.8 Follow-up axial chest CT (**a–d**), reconstructed coronal (**e**) and sagittal (**f**) images 7 days after initial scan

After 14 days follow-up and reexamination, CT showed that the lesion was further absorbed, but not completely (Fig. 4.9).

Comments: The patient is a middle-aged male with a history of AIDS. The clinical manifestations and chest CT manifestations of the patient were typical. In the process of disease progress and improvement, the images showed patchy ground-glass shadow and reticular shadow accompanied with the expansion and reduction, without consolidation.

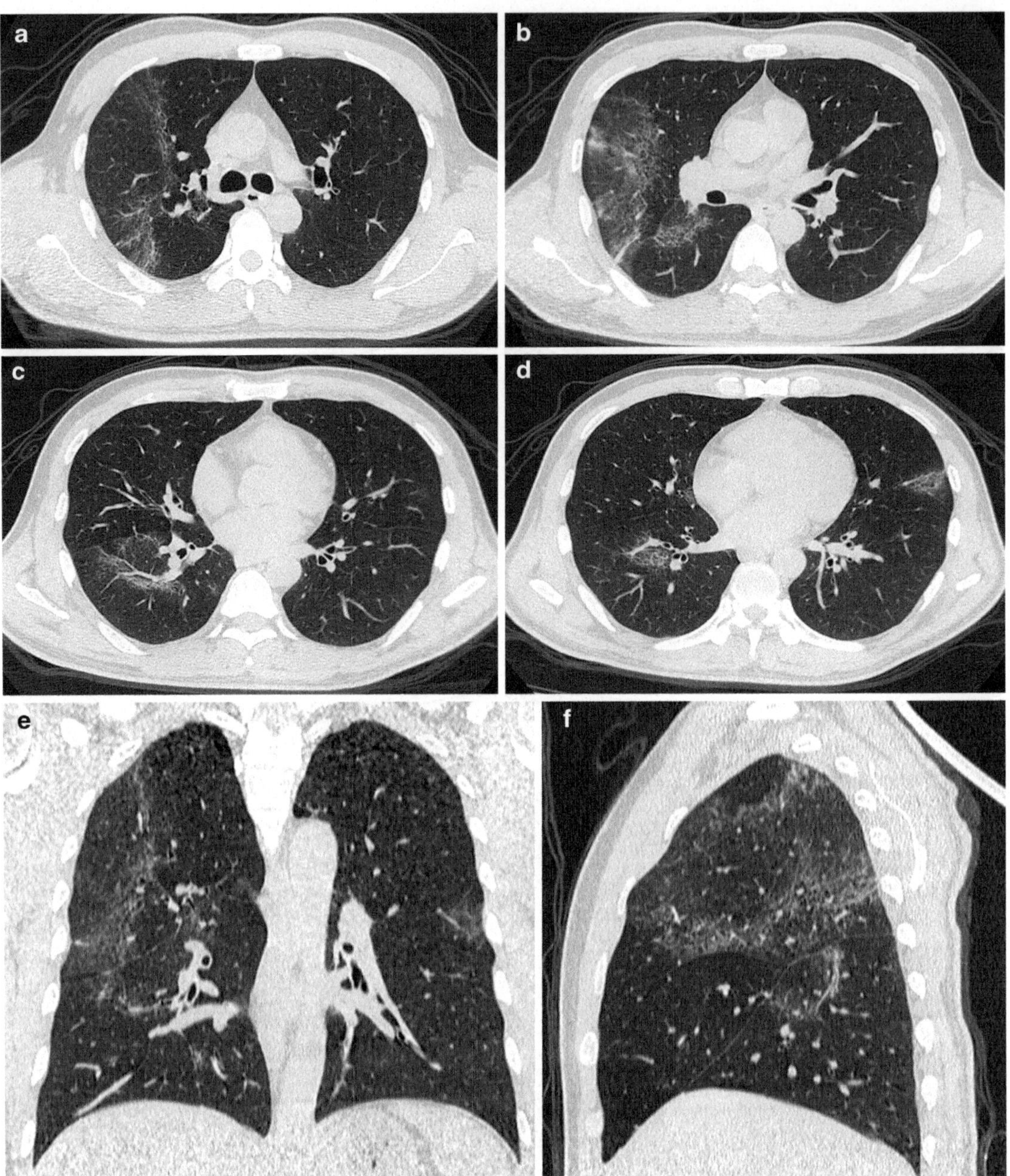

Fig. 4.9 Follow-up axial chest CT (**a–d**), reconstructed coronal (**e**) and sagittal (**f**) images 14 days after initial scan

Case 3

Medical History and Clinical Manifestation

A 43-year-old male was admitted in the hospital for cough for 3 days, mainly dry cough and fever once (highest body temperature: 38.3 °C). Laboratory test results indicated a normal blood routine, and elevated IL-6. Exposure history: The patient had lived in Wuhan, China for years and returned home from Wuhan prior to symptom onset. He was tested positive for SARS-CoV-2 nucleic acid test 2 days after admission. His SARS-CoV-2 nucleic acid test was negative for next five times during hospitalization. But SARS-CoV-2 nucleic acid test turned positive again 25 days after admission.

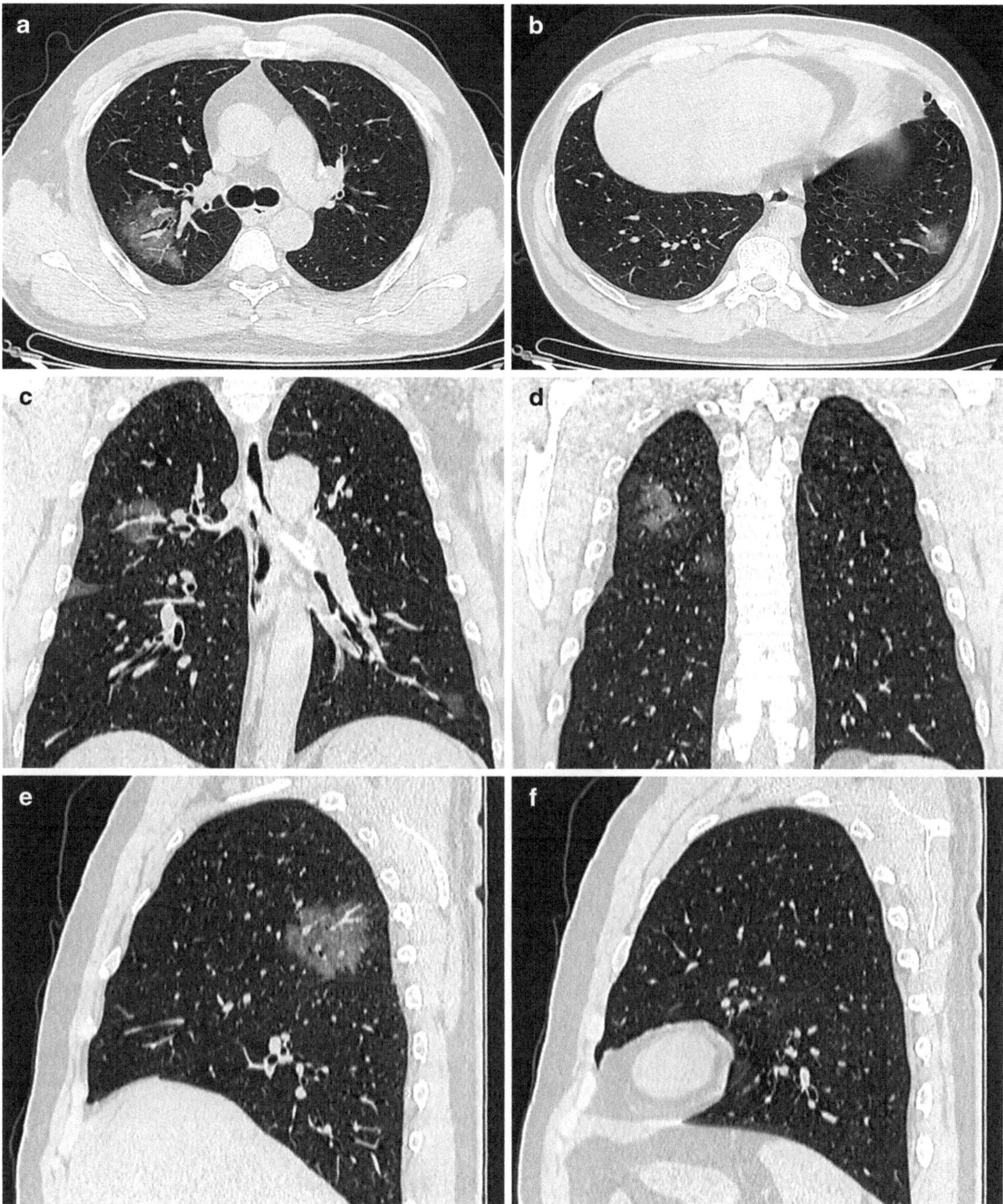

Fig. 4.10 Initial axial chest CT (**a**, **b**), reconstructed coronal (**c**, **d**) and sagittal (**e**, **f**) images of the patient

Imaging Features

Initial chest CT showed multiple nodules and patchy GGOs in both lungs. The lesion was distributed along the subpleural and surrounding bronchovascular tracts, with clear lesion boundaries. Dilated vascular and air bronchogram could be seen in the lesion (Fig. 4.10).

Follow-up chest CT (3 days after initial CT examination) showed that multiple patchy GGOs in bilateral lungs were slightly larger and denser than before, and new reticular changes appeared in the lesions (Fig. 4.11).

Follow-up chest CT (5 days after initial CT examination) showed that the density of most

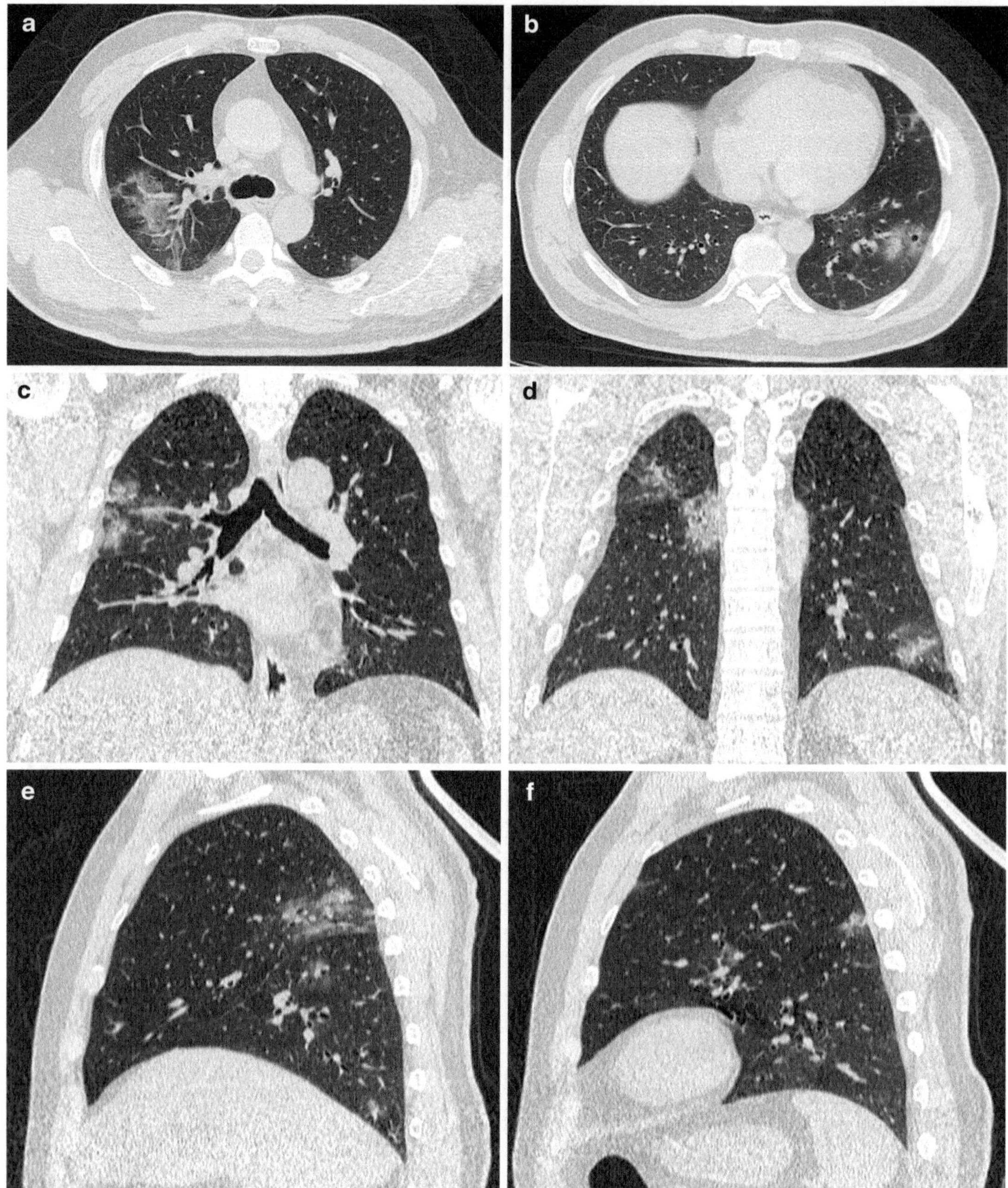

Fig. 4.11 Follow-up axial chest CT (**a**, **b**), reconstructed coronal (**c**, **d**) and sagittal (**e**, **f**) images 3 days after initial scan

lesions was reduced, while the lesion range of the left lower lobe was enlarged, and the left pleura was thickened (Fig. 4.12).

Follow-up chest CT (10 days after initial CT examination) showed that the multiple patchy GGOs were absorbed compared with the previous examination (Fig. 4.13).

Follow-up chest CT (26 days after initial CT examination) showed that the lesions were further absorbed (Fig. 4.14).

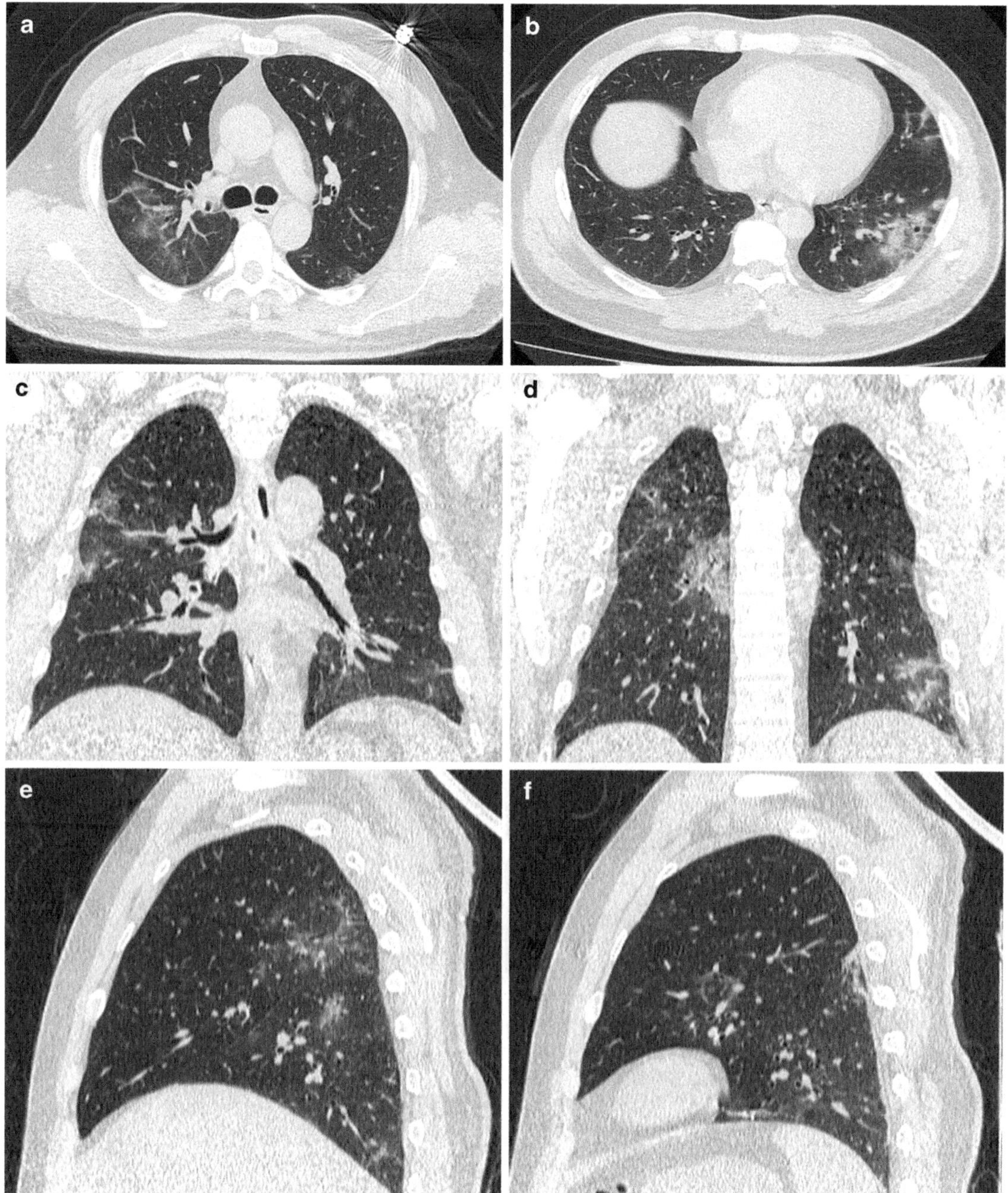

Fig. 4.12 Follow-up axial chest CT (**a**, **b**), reconstructed coronal (**c**, **d**) and sagittal (**e**, **f**) images 5 days after initial scan

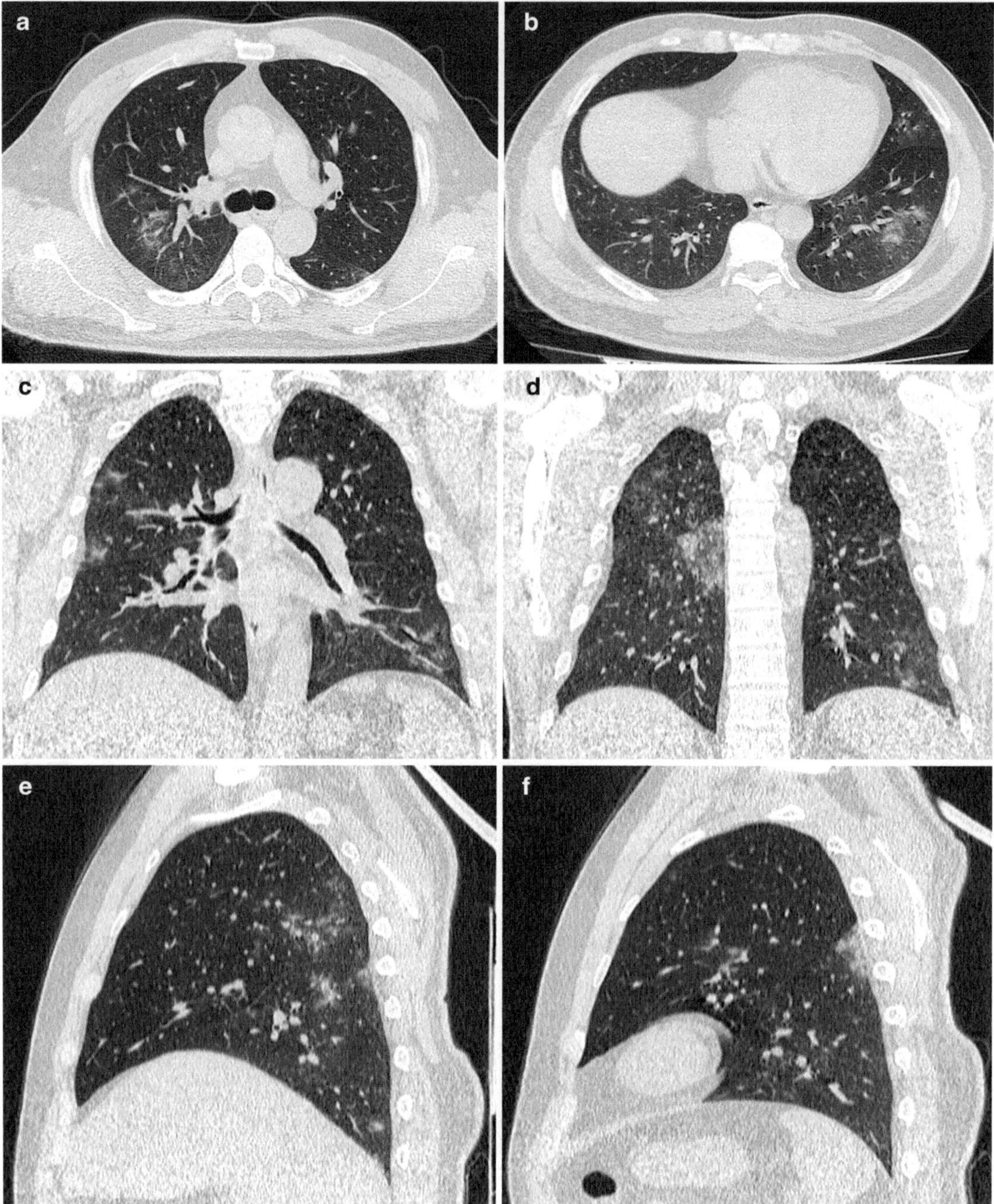

Fig. 4.13 Follow-up axial chest CT (**a**, **b**), reconstructed coronal (**c**, **d**) and sagittal (**e**, **f**) images 10 days after initial scan

Comments: This patient's SARS-CoV-2 nucleic acid test is very characteristic. The patient's SARS-CoV-2 nucleic acid test was positive 2 days after admission, but the next 5 times of nucleic acid test became negative, and turn into positive again 25 days after admission. However, the patient's CT examination was always positive, which posed a challenge to the clinical discharge standard, suggesting that it is necessary to determine whether to be discharged based on the absorption of CT lesions, even the patient's nucleic acid test was negative for 2 consecutive times.

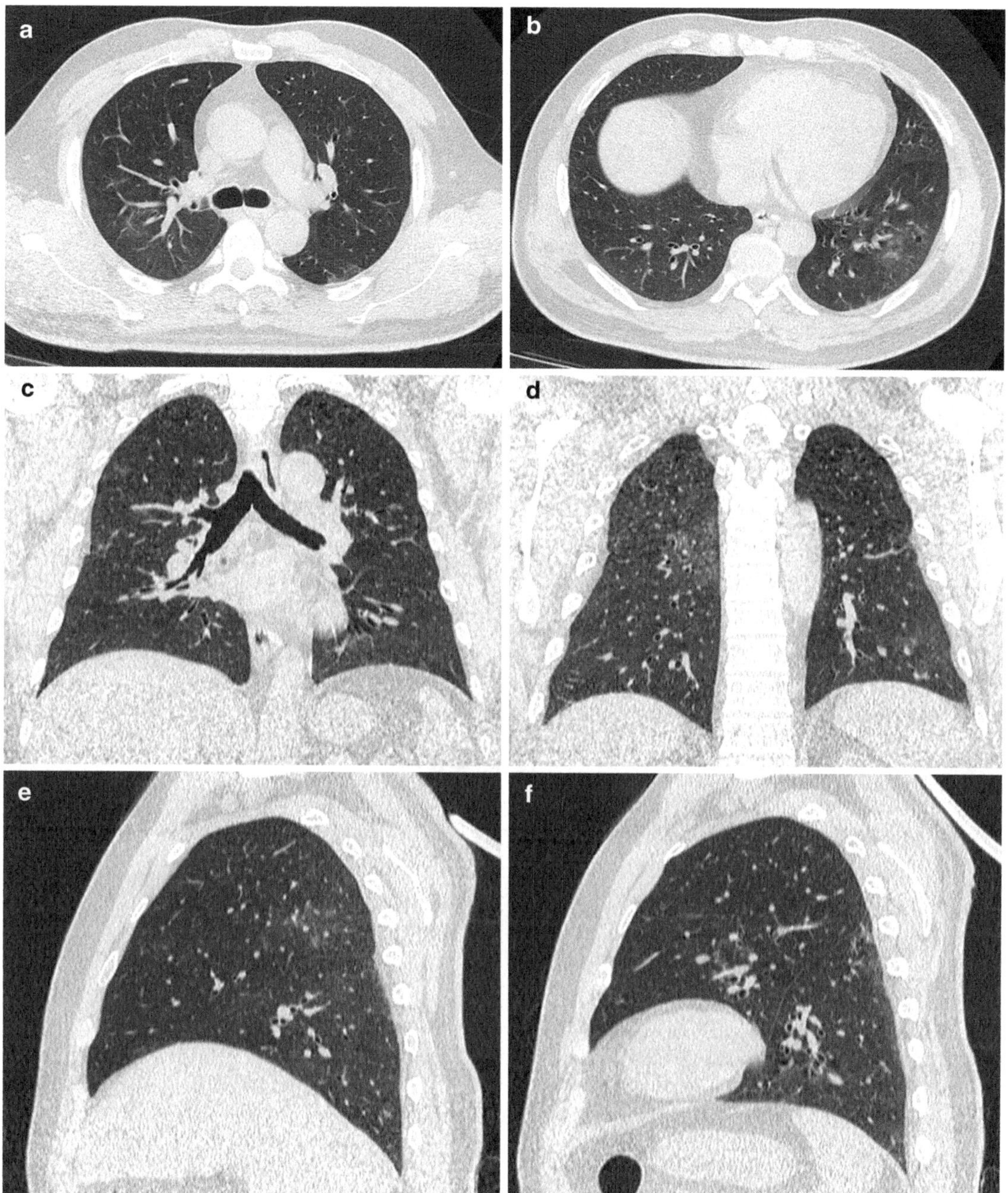

Fig. 4.14 Follow-up axial chest CT (**a**, **b**), reconstructed coronal (**c**, **d**) and sagittal (**e**, **f**) images 26 days after initial scan

Case 4

Medical History and Clinical Manifestation

A 43-year-old male was admitted in the hospital for 6 h for fatigue, soreness for 4 days, cough and fever (highest body temperature: 38 °C) for 1 day. Laboratory test results indicated a decreased white blood cell count. Exposure history: The patient denied close contact with COVID-19 patients within 2 weeks. Patient's SARS-CoV-2 nucleic acid test was positive. The patient had a history of hepatitis B for 10 years.

Imaging Features

Initial chest CT showed multiple patchy and nodular GGOs in both lungs accompanied by

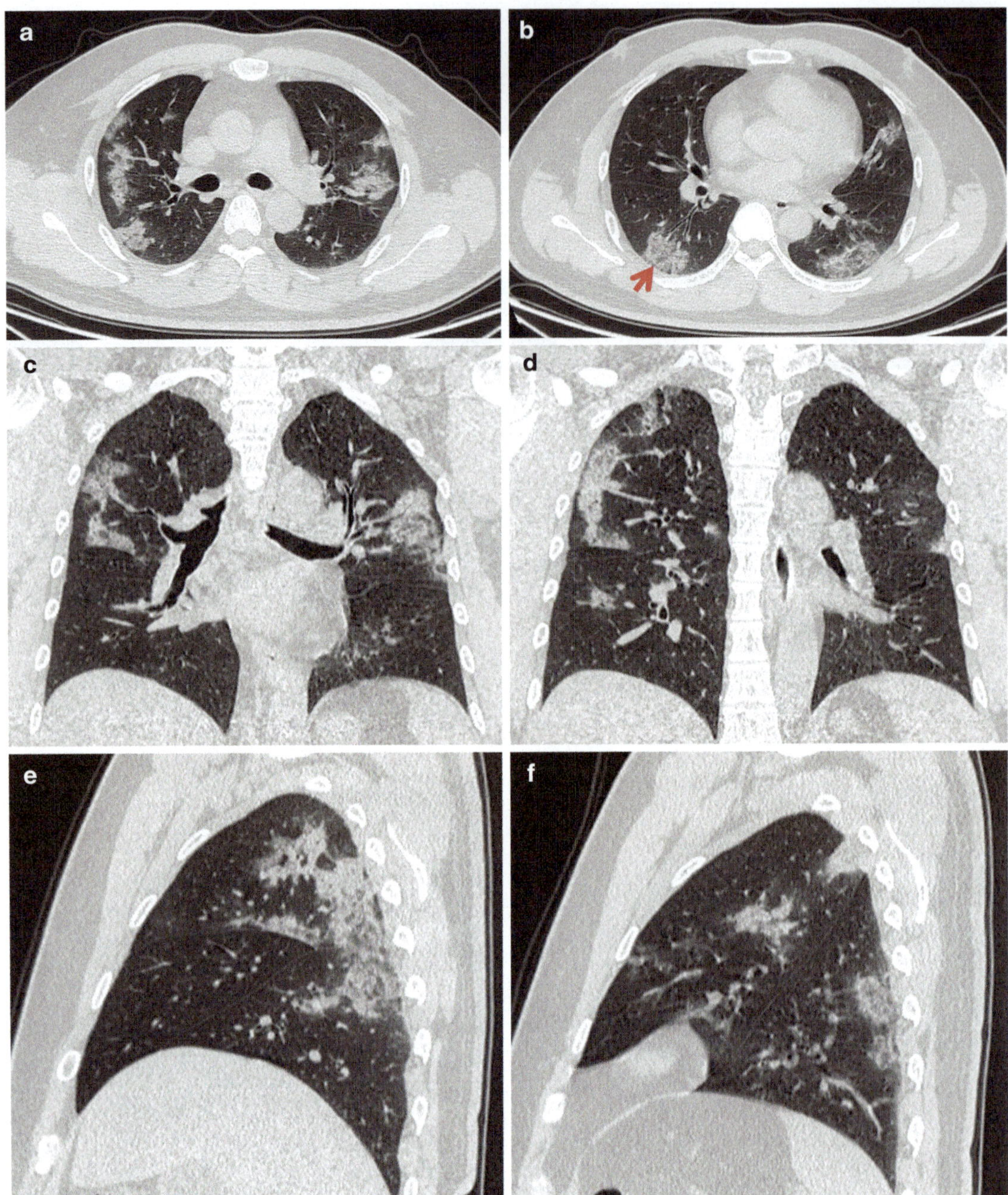

Fig. 4.15 Initial axial chest CT (**a**, **b**), reconstructed coronal (**c**, **d**) and sagittal (**e**, **f**) images of the patient

partial consolidation. The lesions were distributed along the subpleural and bronchovascular tracts, and the adjacent pleura was slightly thickened. Air bronchogenic signs, thickened blood vessel, and reticular changes could be seen in some lesions, while some GGOs showed reversed halo sign (red arrow) (Fig. 4.15).

Follow-up chest CT (24 days after initial CT examination) showed patchy GGOs in both lungs, with obvious absorption and dissipation (Fig. 4.16).

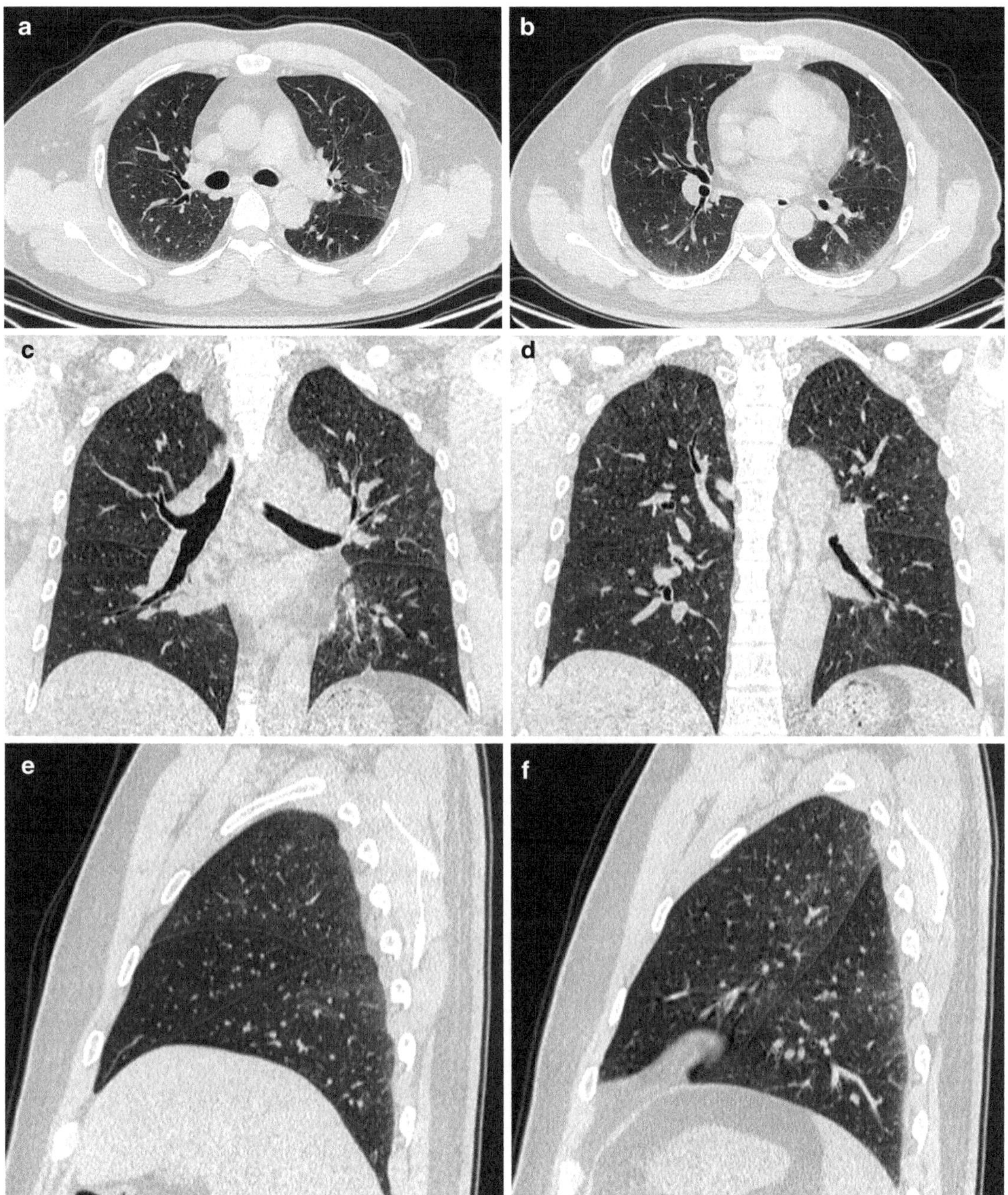

Fig. 4.16 Follow-up axial chest CT (**a**, **b**), reconstructed coronal (**c**, **d**) and sagittal (**e**, **f**) images 24 days after initial scan

Comments: The patient has no definite epidemiological history, but its clinical and imaging manifestations are typical. Positive SARS-CoV-2 nucleic acid test is the diagnostic standard.

Case 5

Medical History and Clinical Manifestation

A 37-year-old male was admitted in the hospital for fever with occasional cough and diarrhea for 1 day. Laboratory test results indicated a decreased lymphocyte count and increased mononuclear cell count and percentage. There was no exact contacting history with COVID-19 patient. He was tested positive for SARS-CoV-2 nucleic acid test 1 day after admission.

Imaging Features

Initial chest CT showed scattered solid nodules with halo sign (red arrow) in both lungs (Fig. 4.17).

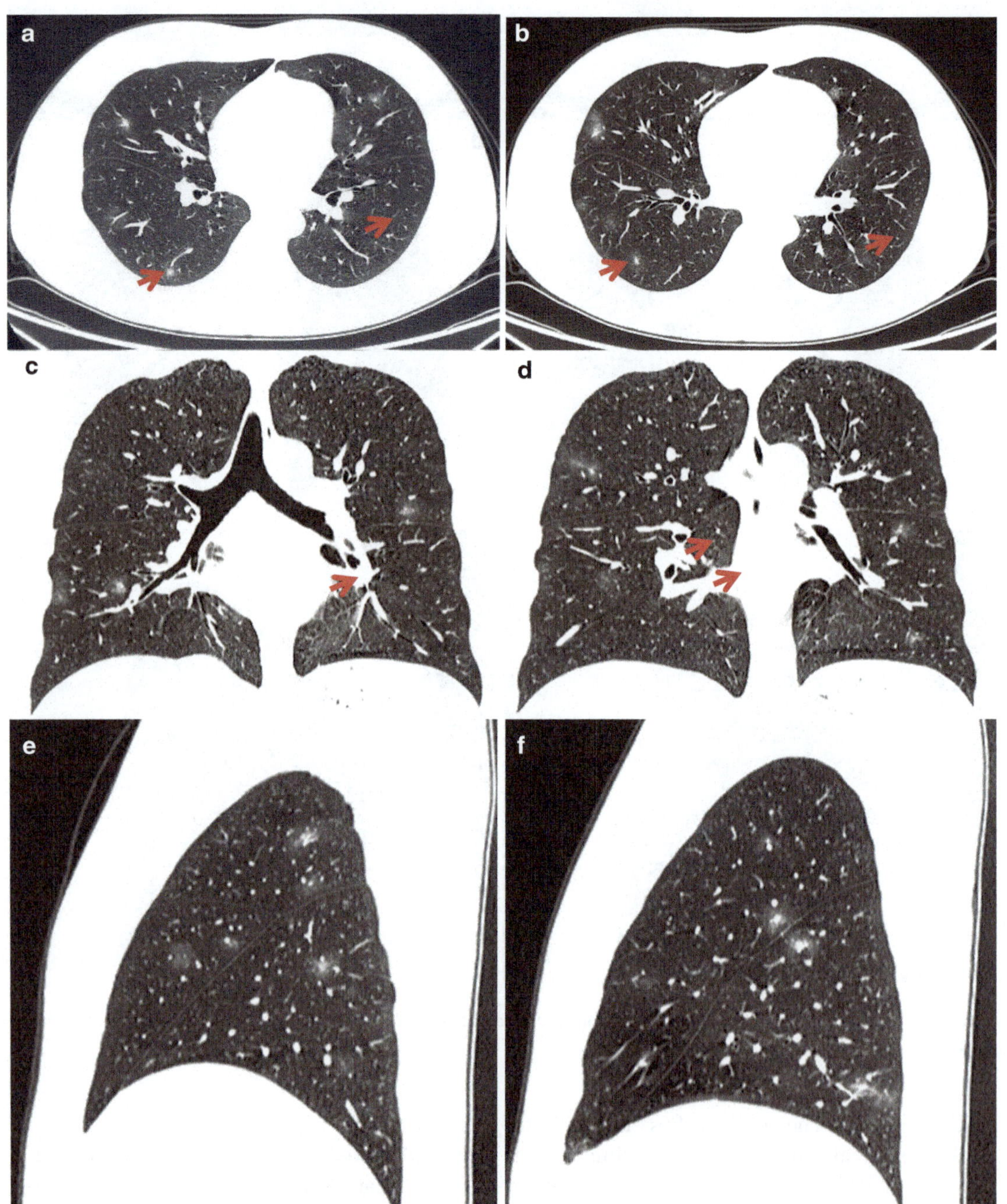

Fig. 4.17 Initial axial chest CT (**a**, **b**), reconstructed coronal (**c**, **d**) and sagittal (**e**, **f**) images of the patient

Follow-up chest CT (21 days after initial CT examination) showed that most of the scattered lesions turned to be pure GGOs, and some lesions with fiber cords (red arrow), which were significantly absorbed compared with the previous (Fig. 4.18).

Comments: The patient had no definite epidemiological history, and CT showed multiple solid nodules with halo sign. This is an uncommon image sign in COVID-19, which needs to be differentiated from fungal pneumonia.

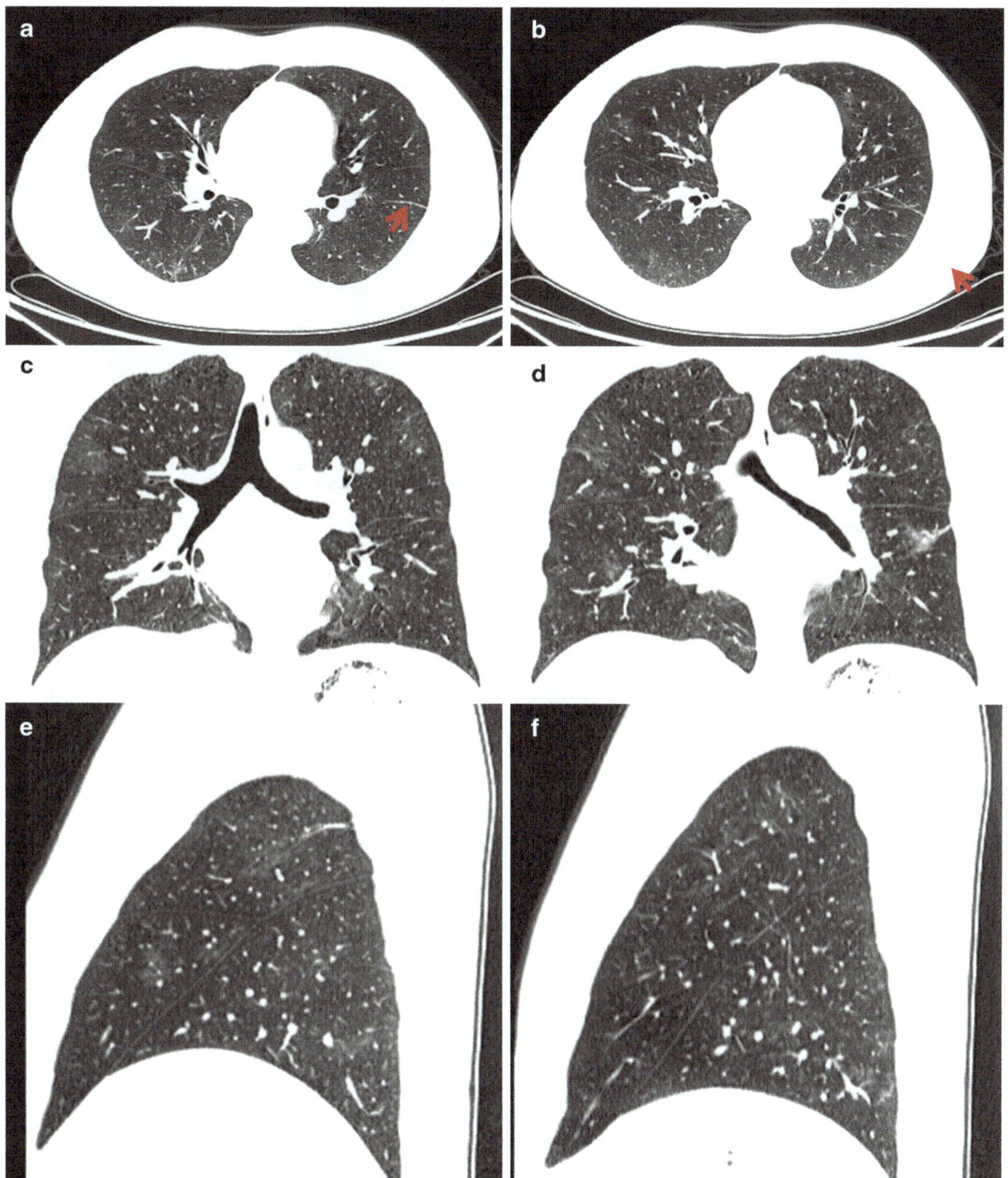

Fig. 4.18 Follow-up axial chest CT (**a**, **b**), reconstructed coronal (**c**, **d**) and sagittal (**e**, **f**) images 21 days after initial scan

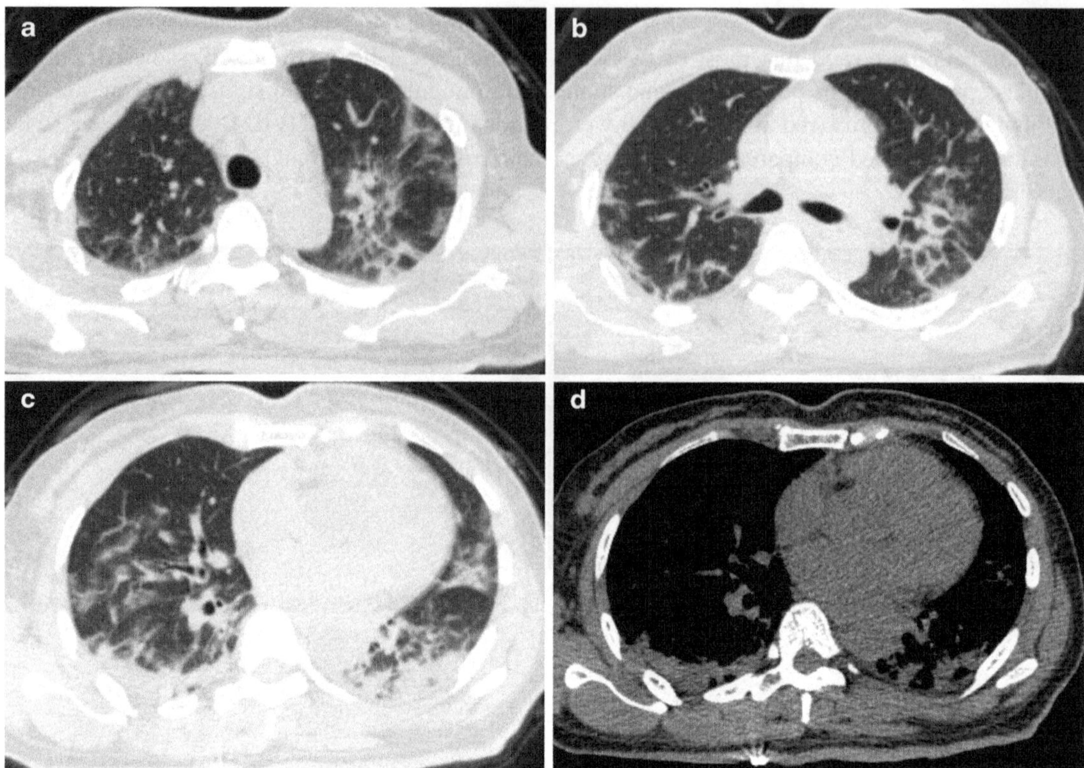

Fig. 4.19 Initial chest CT images

Case 6

Medical History and Clinical Manifestation

A 51-year-old female was admitted in the hospital for fever (highest body temperature: 38.5 °C) for 9 days, occasionally accompanied by dry cough, dizziness, and breathing difficulties. Laboratory test results indicated a normal white blood cell count of 3.98 × 10^9/L, 76.7% neutrophils, and decreased lymphocytes 14.4%. There were elevated blood levels for erythrocyte sedimentation rate (41 mm/h), C-reactive protein (63.93 mg/L), and PCT (0.064 ng/mL). Exposure history: The patient returned to hometown from Wuhan, China. Her SARS-CoV-2 nucleic acid test was positive during hospitalization.

Imaging Features

Initial chest CT showed multiple patchy GGOs, consolidations, and linear opacities in bilateral lungs. The posterior subpleural area of both lungs showed arc-shaped consolidation shadows, and no obvious effusion was seen in the bilateral thoracic cavity (Fig. 4.19).

Follow-up chest CT (6 days after initial CT examination) showed that the patchy inflammatory lesions in both lungs were absorbed than before, and fibrous cords (**a**: red arrows) appeared in the subpleural areas of both lungs (Fig. 4.20).

After 19 days of treatment, two times of SARS-CoV-2 nucleic acid test were negative. Follow-up chest CT showed further absorption of two pneumonia lesions, and more fibrous cords in the subpleural area of the lower lobe of both lungs (Fig. 4.21).

Comments: This case demonstrates the dynamic change process of chest CT in the SARS-CoV-2 nucleic acid test transformation process. It is suggested that the transformation of nucleic acid to negative may be earlier than the complete absorption of lung lesions in chest CT.

Case 7

Medical History and Clinical Manifestation

A 34-year-old female was admitted in the hospital for fever (highest body temperature: 38.5 °C) for 7 days, accompanied by cough,

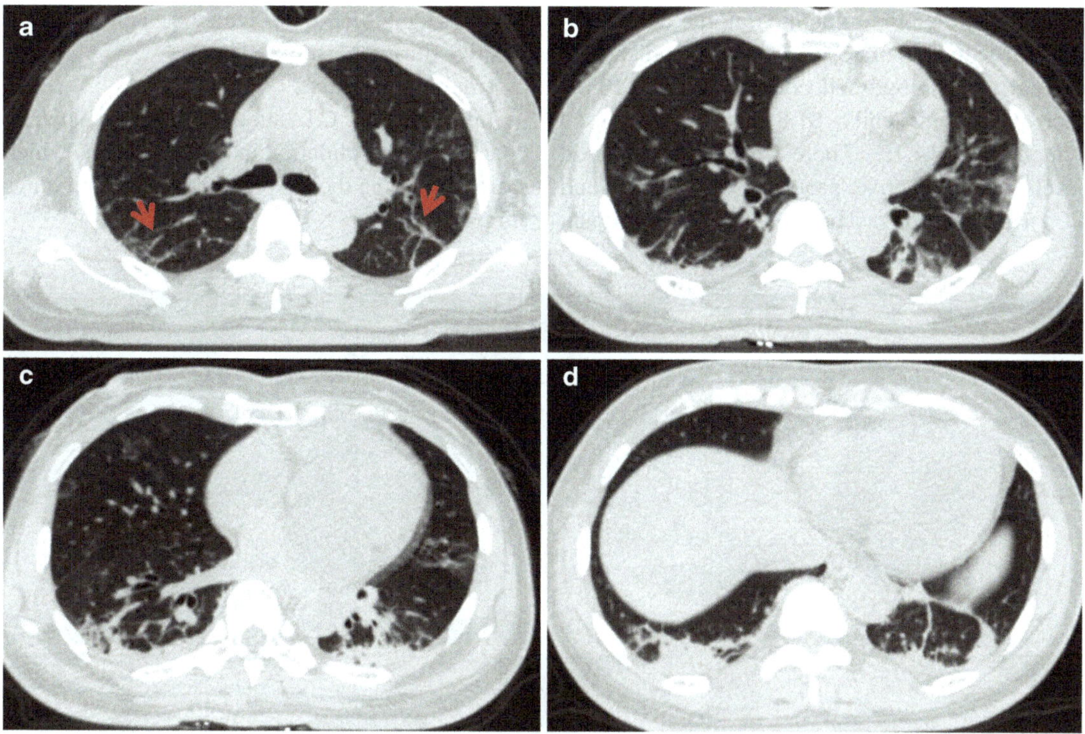

Fig. 4.20 Follow-up CT images 6 days after initial scan

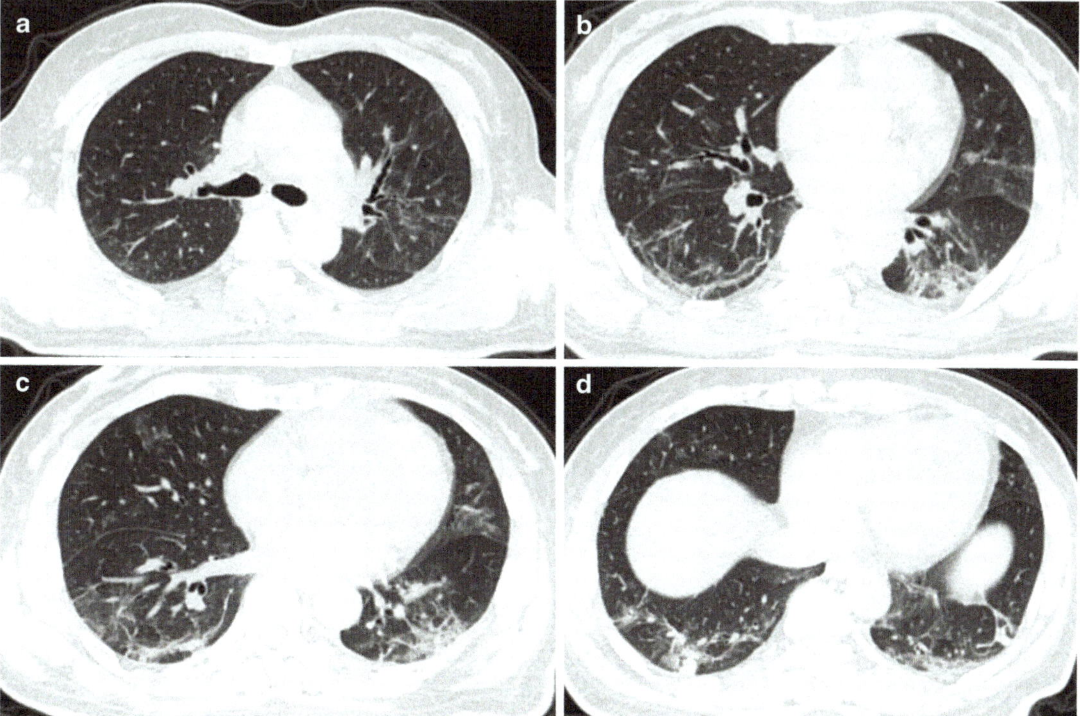

Fig. 4.21 Follow-up CT images 19 days after initial scan

mainly dry cough, systemic fatigue, and pharyngeal pain. Laboratory test results indicated a normal white blood cell count of 4.35 × 10^9/L, increased neutrophils 81.8%, and decreased lymphocytes 14.1%. There were elevated blood levels for C-reactive protein (36.8 mg/L) and PCT (0.058 ng/mL). The patient lived in Wuhan, China. Her SARS-CoV-2 nucleic acid test was positive during hospitalization.

Imaging Features

Initial chest CT showed multiple patchy GGOs and consolidation in bilateral lungs, which were obvious in the subpleural area of both lungs (Fig. 4.22).

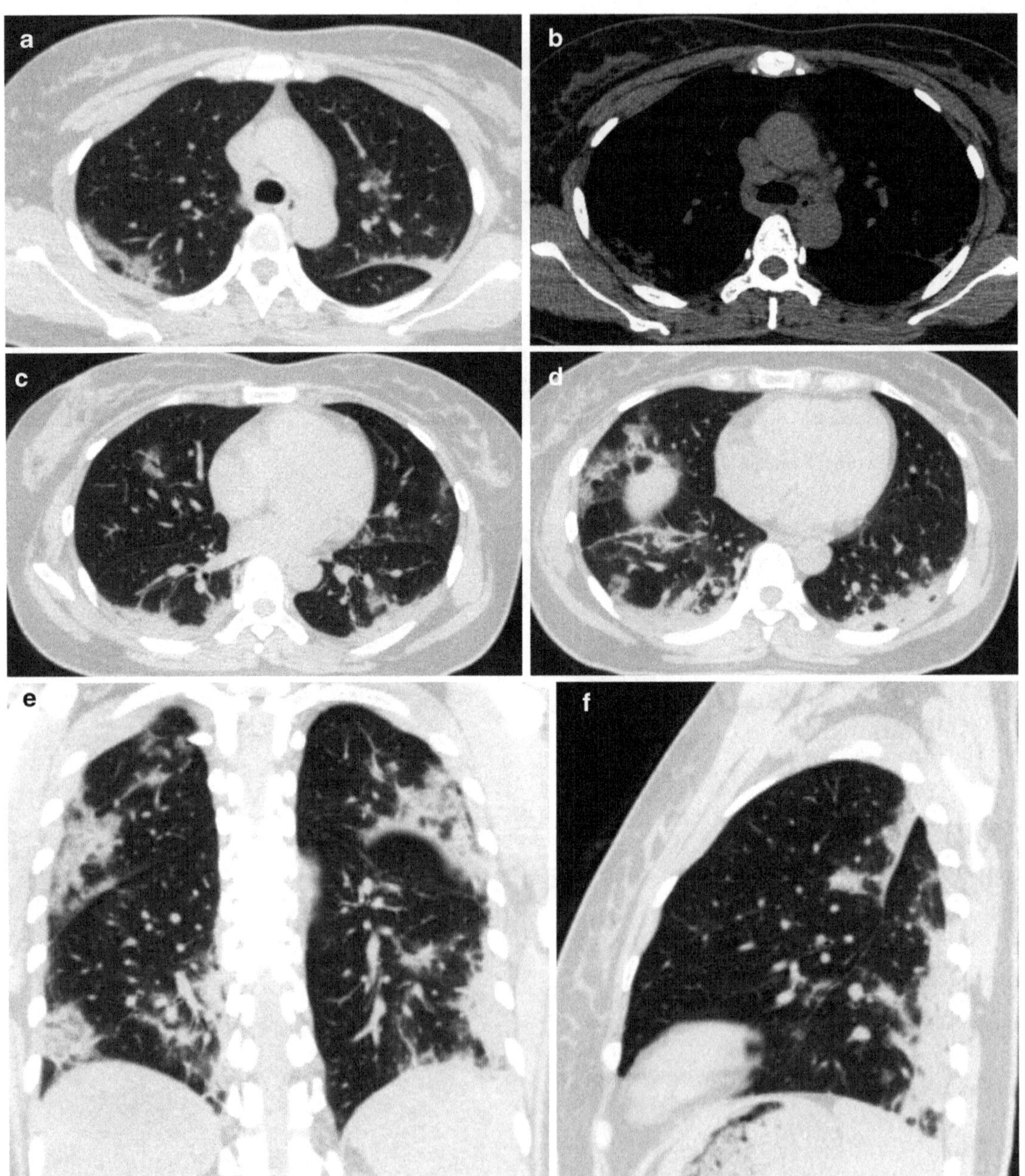

Fig. 4.22 Initial chest CT (**a–d**), reconstructed coronal (**e**) and sagittal (**f**) images of the patient

Follow-up chest CT (5 days after initial CT examination) showed that the patchy inflammatory lesions in both lungs were more absorbed than before, and fiber strip appeared in the subpleural area of both lungs (**c**, **d**: white arrow) (Fig. 4.23).

After 18 days of treatment, SARS-CoV-2 nucleic acid test was negative. Follow-up chest CT showed obvious absorption of exudative lesions in both lungs. There were less fibrous

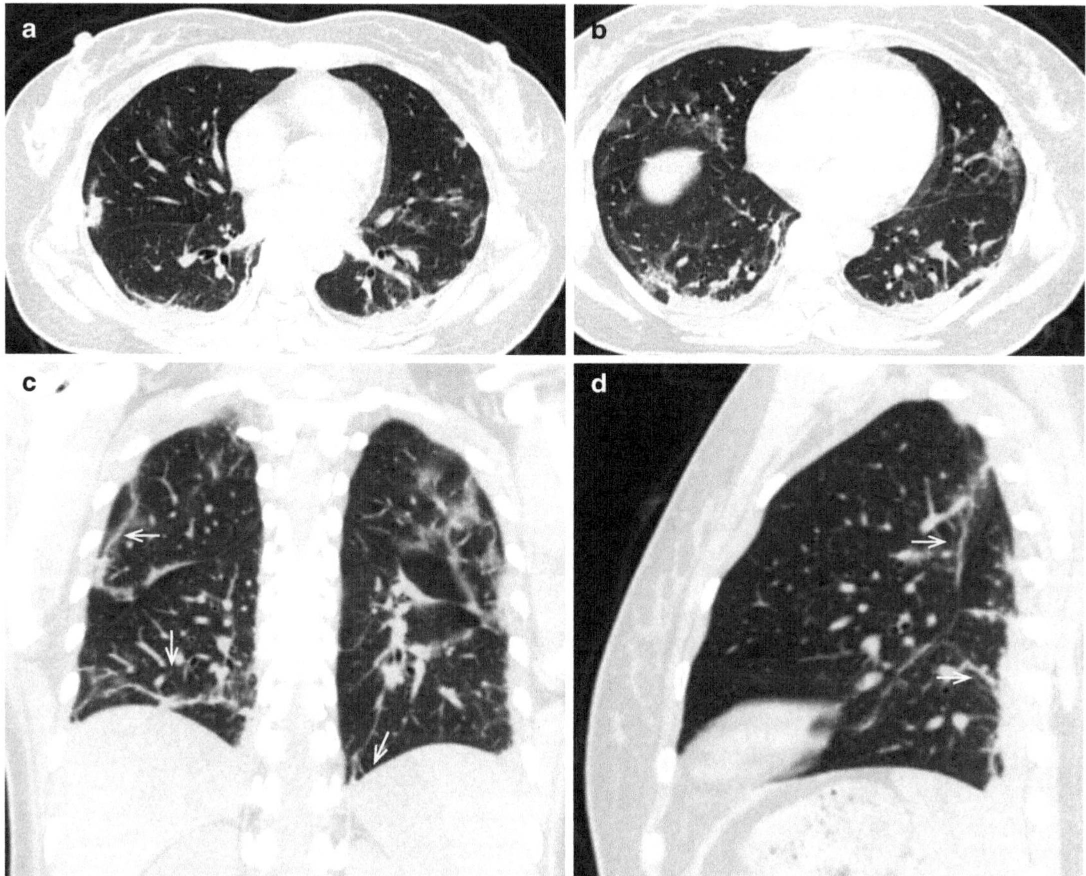

Fig. 4.23 Follow-up axial chest CT (**a–d**), reconstructed coronal and sagittal images 5 days after initial scan

cords in the subpleural area with clearer boundary (**a**, **b**: white arrow) (Fig. 4.24).

Comments: The imaging feature of this case is that there are significant fibrous bands in the process of improvement, and they could be absorbed dynamically, suggesting that some of the bands are not fibrosis, but atelectasis or local alveolar collapse.

Case 8

Medical History and Clinical Manifestation

A 42-year-old female was admitted in the hospital for 10 days with fever (highest body temperature: 38.5 °C), accompanied by cough, chilly, and slight pharyngeal pain. Laboratory test results indicated a normal white blood cell count of 7.36 × 10^9/L, 75.4% neutrophils, and decreased lymphocytes 15.8%. There were elevated blood levels for C-reactive protein (59.62 mg/L), erythrocyte sedimentation rate (39 mm/h), and PCT (0.106 ng/mL). Exposure history: The patient drove to Yueyang, China to attend the banquet and go shopping alone. Her SARS-CoV-2 nucleic acid test was positive during hospitalization. The patient has a history of scapula surgery.

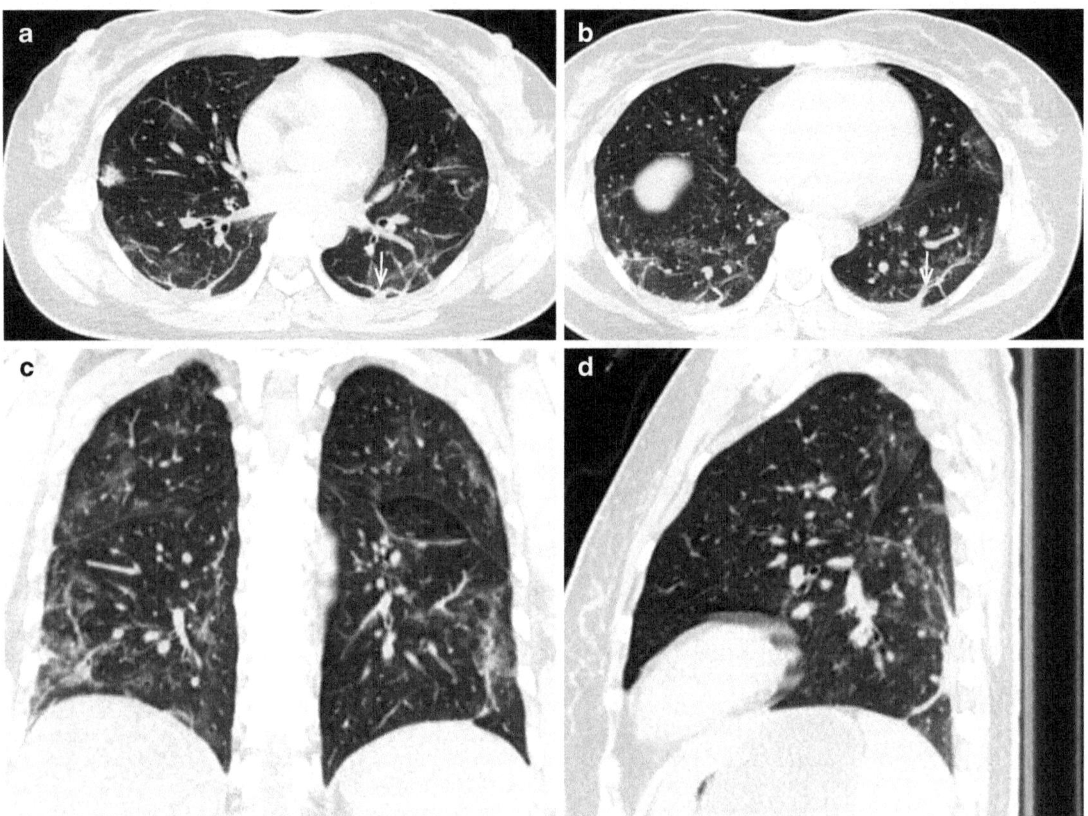

Fig. 4.24 Follow-up axial chest CT (**a–d**), reconstructed coronal and sagittal images 18 days after initial scan

Imaging Features

Initial chest CT scan showed the arc-shaped ground-glass opacities and consolidation in the subpleural area of the upper and lower lobes of the right lung, and the vascular thickening sign (**b**: fine white arrow), paving stone sign (**c**: thick white arrow), and air bronchi sign were seen in the lesion area (Fig. 4.25).

Follow-up chest CT (17 days after initial CT examination) showed that inflammatory lesions in the subpleural area of the right lung were more absorbed than before, and the scope of the lesions was smaller, with local changes like fibrous cords (Fig. 4.26).

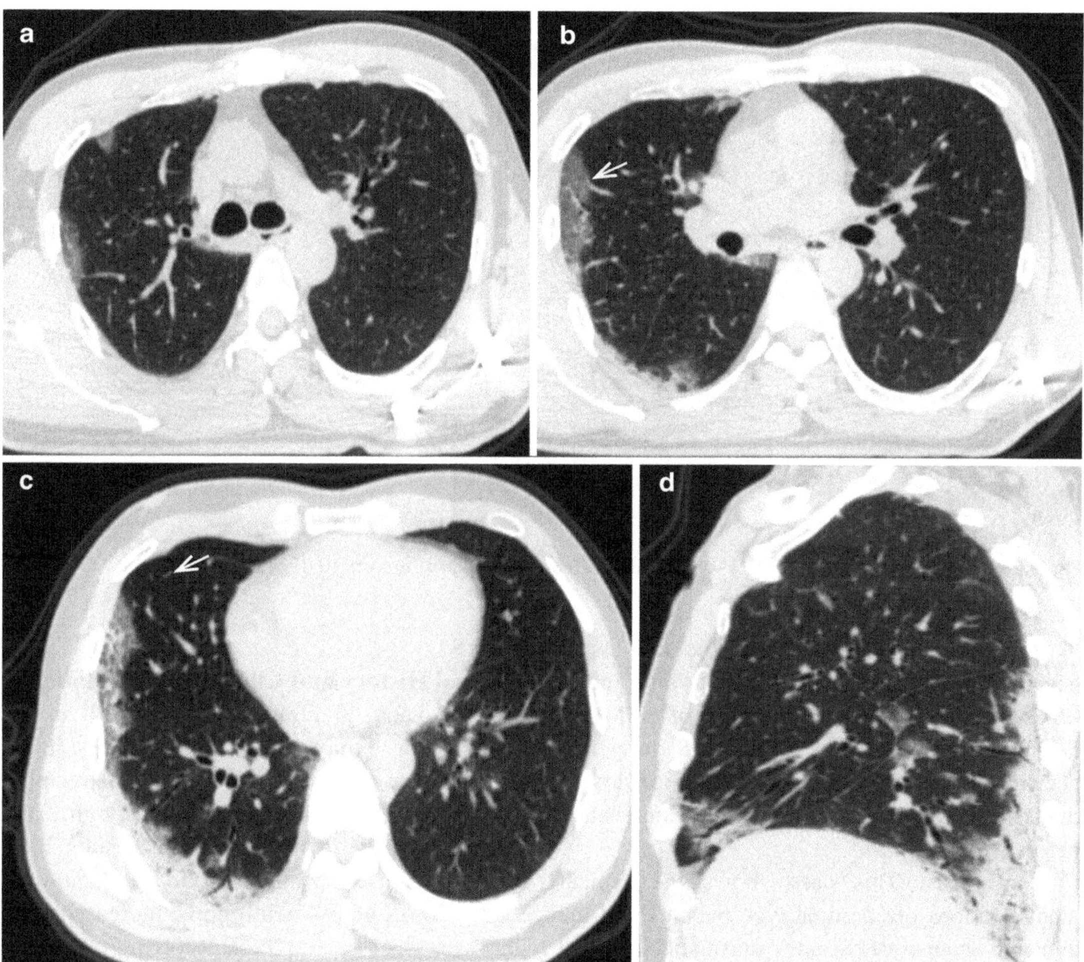

Fig. 4.25 Initial axial chest CT (**a–c**) and reconstructed sagittal (**d**) images of the patient

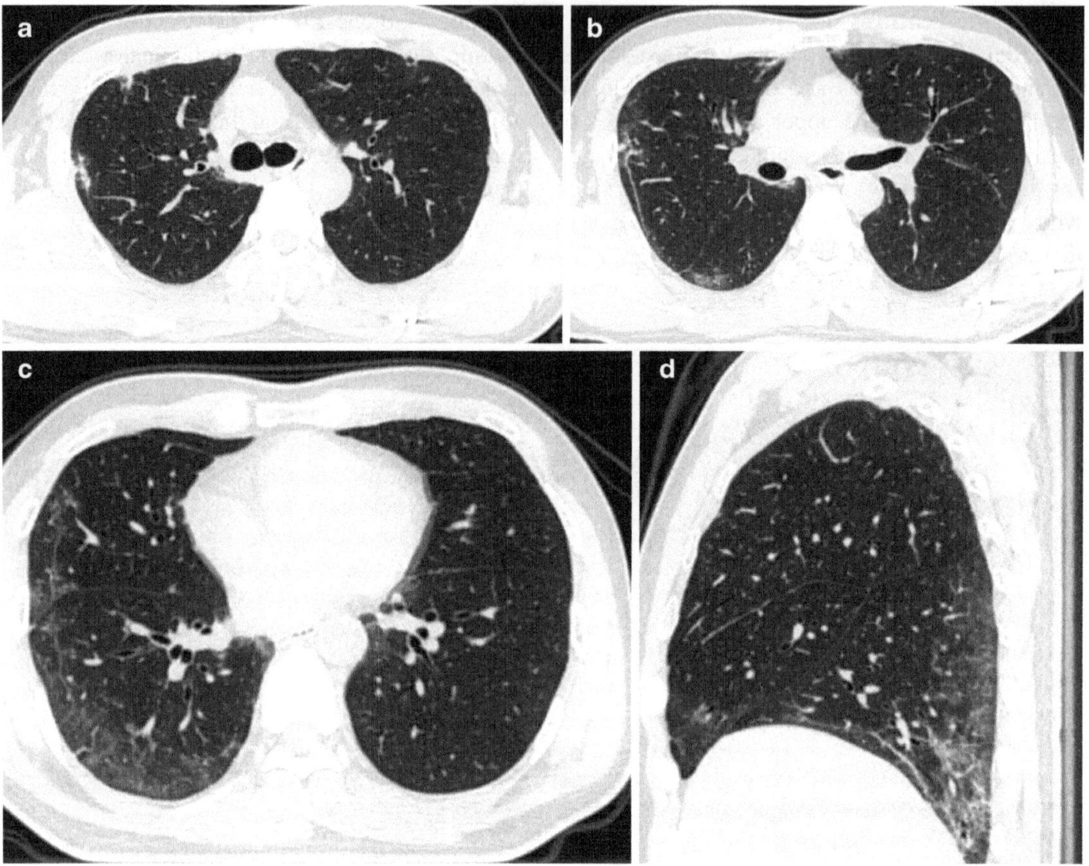

Fig. 4.26 Follow-up axial chest CT (**a–c**), and reconstructed sagittal (**d**) images 10 days after initial scan

After twice SARS-CoV-2 nucleic acid tested negative, follow-up chest CT (25 days after initial CT examination) showed that most of the original inflammatory lesions of the right lung had been absorbed, and the fibrous cord boundary of the lesion in the subpleural area was clearer than before (Fig. 4.27).

Comments: This case shows the typical manifestations of common type patients and the dynamic changes of chest CT during nucleic acid convert. The patient's SARS-CoV-2 nucleic acid test was twice negative, but there was still an unabsorbed lesion in the lung.

Case 9

Medical History and Clinical Manifestation

A 49-year-old female was admitted in the hospital for 3 days with fever (highest body temperature: 40 °C), accompanied by pharyngeal pain, cough (mainly dry cough), and systemic fatigue. Laboratory test results indicated decreased white blood cell count of 3.58×10^9/L, 46.6% neutrophils, increased lymphocytes 43.1%, and PCT (0.06 ng/mL). The patient worked in Wuhan, China for more than half a month. Her SARS-CoV-2 nucleic acid test was positive.

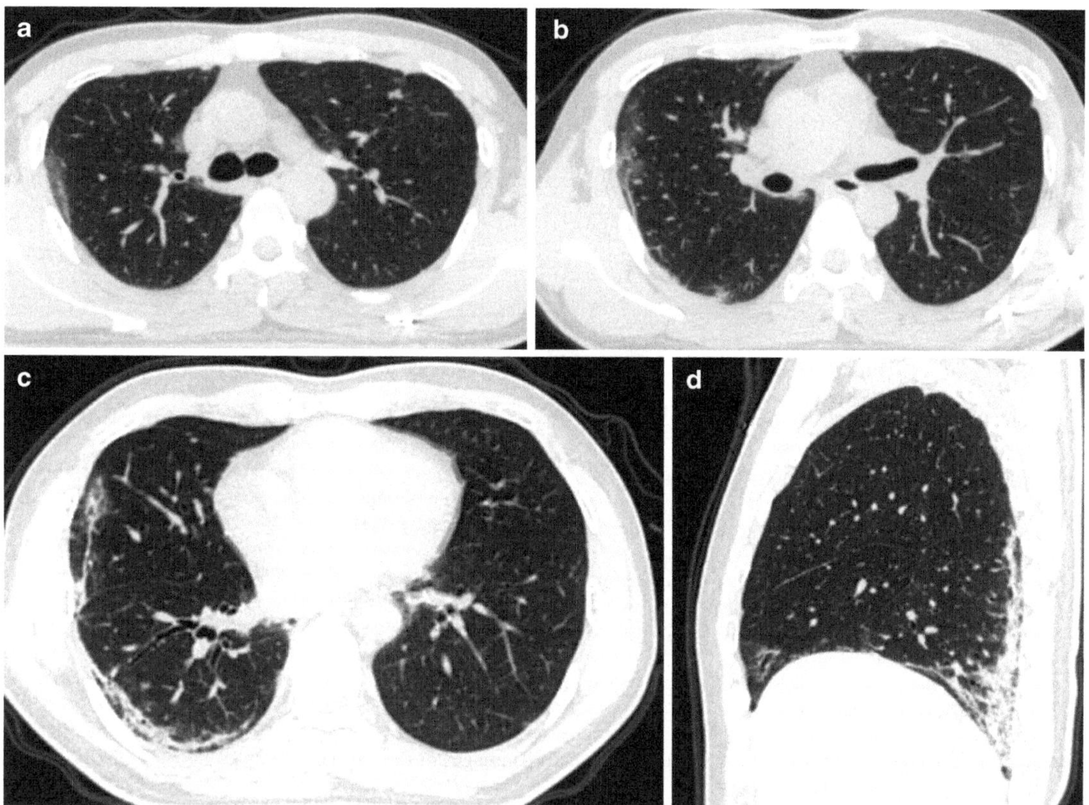

Fig. 4.27 Follow-up axial chest CT (**a–c**), and reconstructed sagittal (**d**) images 25 days after initial scan

Imaging Features

Initial chest CT showed multiple patchy GGOs in both lungs, some of which were grid-like changes. The lesions were mainly distributed in the subpleural area (Fig. 4.28).

Follow-up chest CT (3 days after initial CT examination) showed that the inflammatory lesion range in both lungs was larger and the density was higher than before, and the local vessel thickening signs in the lesion in the right upper lobe of the lung were clearer than before (Fig. 4.29).

Follow-up chest CT (25 days after initial CT examination) showed that the exudative lesions in both lungs were significantly absorbed, the consolidation shadow was reduced, and the lesions were diluted and dispersed. Fibrous cord foci (**b**, **c**: white arrows) appear in the subpleural areas of bilateral lungs. The patient's SARS-CoV-2 nucleic acid tests turned negative after 12 days after initial CT examination (Fig. 4.30).

Comments: This case demonstrates the dynamic changes of chest CT during nucleic acid turned negative in a common type patient. When

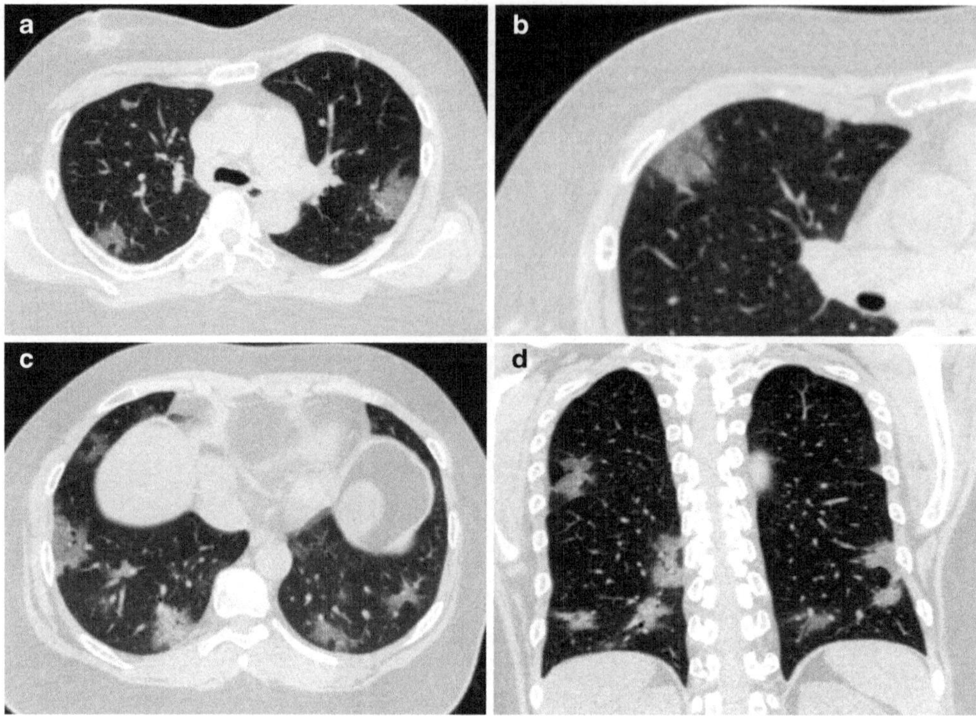

Fig. 4.28 Initial chest CT (**a–c**) and reconstructed coronal (**d**) images of the patient

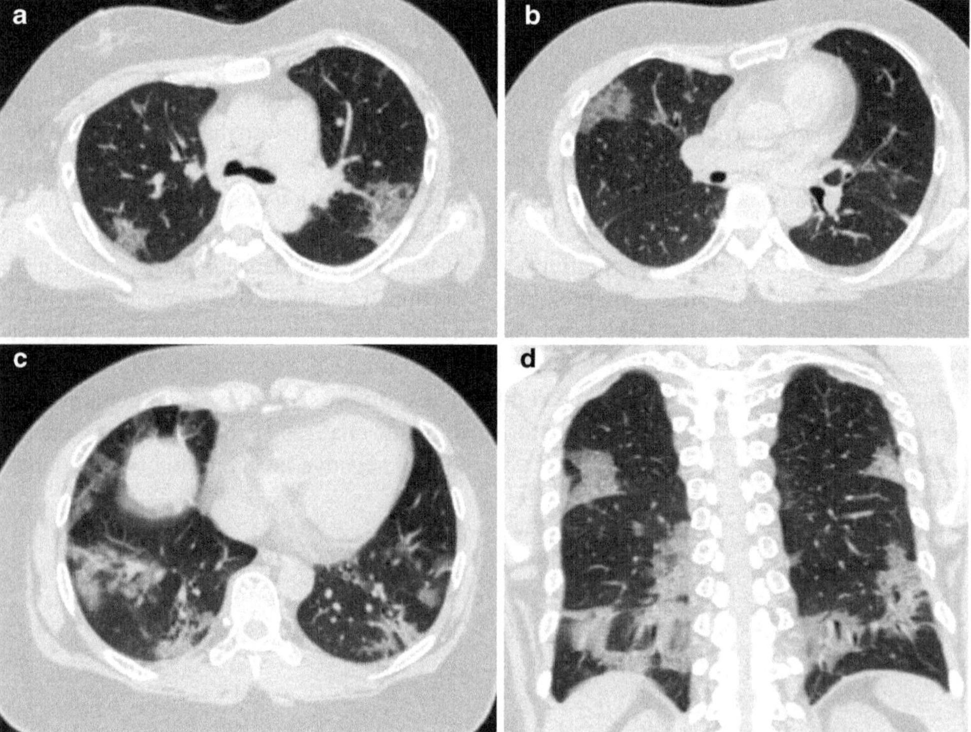

Fig. 4.29 Follow-up axial chest CT (**a–c**), and reconstructed coronal (**d**) images 3 days after initial scan

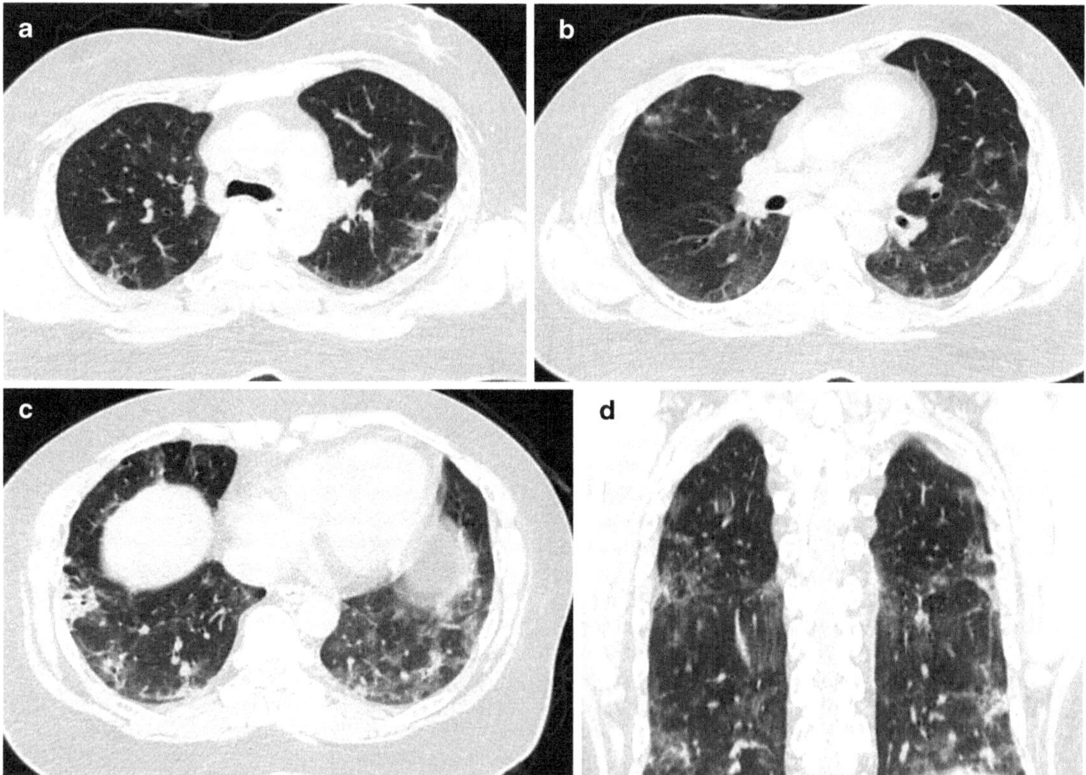

Fig. 4.30 Follow-up axial chest CT (**a–c**), and reconstructed coronal (**d**) images 25 days after initial scan

the patient was discharged, the SARS-CoV-2 nucleic acid test was negative, but the chest CT still showed lesions, which suggested continued isolation and vigilance against the possibility of recurrence.

Case 10

Medical History and Clinical Manifestation

A 41-year-old male was admitted in the hospital for dry cough for 3 days, fever (highest body temperature: 38.1 °C) for 5 h, accompanied by runny nose, sore throat, and systemic fatigue. Laboratory test results indicated a normal white blood cell count of 8.35×10^9/L, 71.2% neutrophils, and decreased lymphocytes 17.1%. There were elevated blood levels for PCT (0.09 ng/mL). The patient was tested positive for SARS-CoV-2 nucleic acid during hospitalization. He had 2 years history of hypertension.

Imaging Features

Initial chest CT showed multiple ground-glass nodules and some solid nodules scattered in both lungs, with slightly blurred edges (Fig. 4.31).

Follow-up chest CT (16 days after initial CT examination) showed multiple new cords and patchy high-density opacities in both lungs, multiple cords (white arrows) were still seen in the subpleural areas of both lungs. And the patient's SARS-CoV-2 nucleic acid test was still positive (Fig. 4.32).

After 34 days of treatment, SARS-CoV-2 nucleic acid test was negative for two times, and the follow-up chest CT (34 days after initial CT examination) showed that the original two pneumonia lesions were absorbed, and a few fibrous cords remained in the subpleural areas of both lungs. The patient was discharged and continued

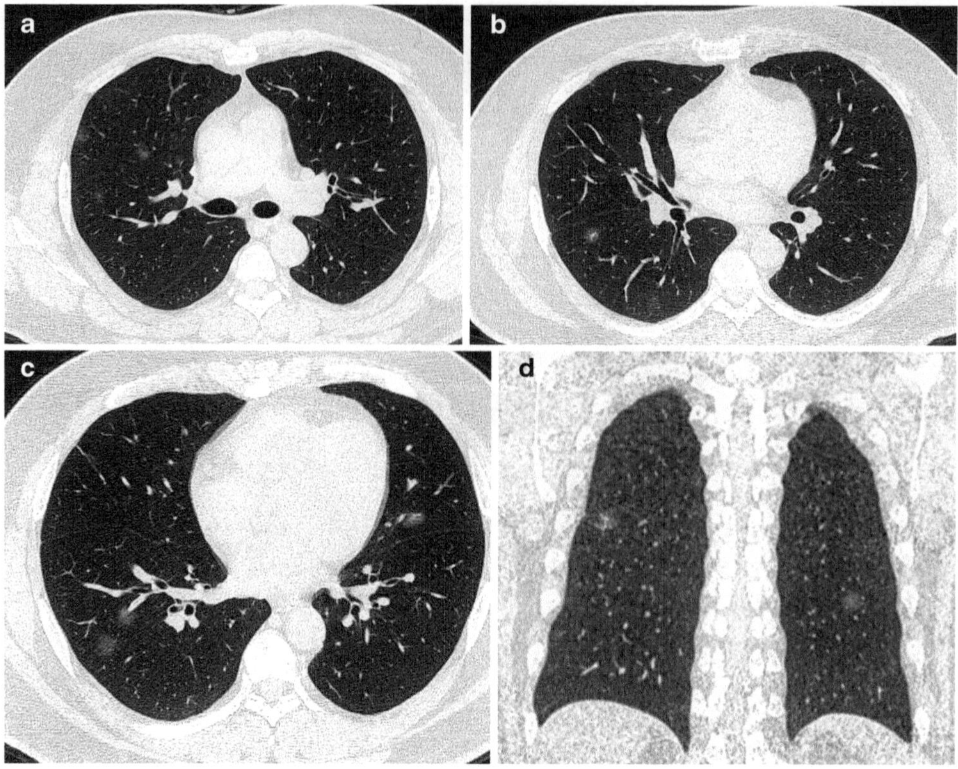

Fig. 4.31 Initial chest CT (**a–c**) and reconstructed coronal (**d**) images of the patient

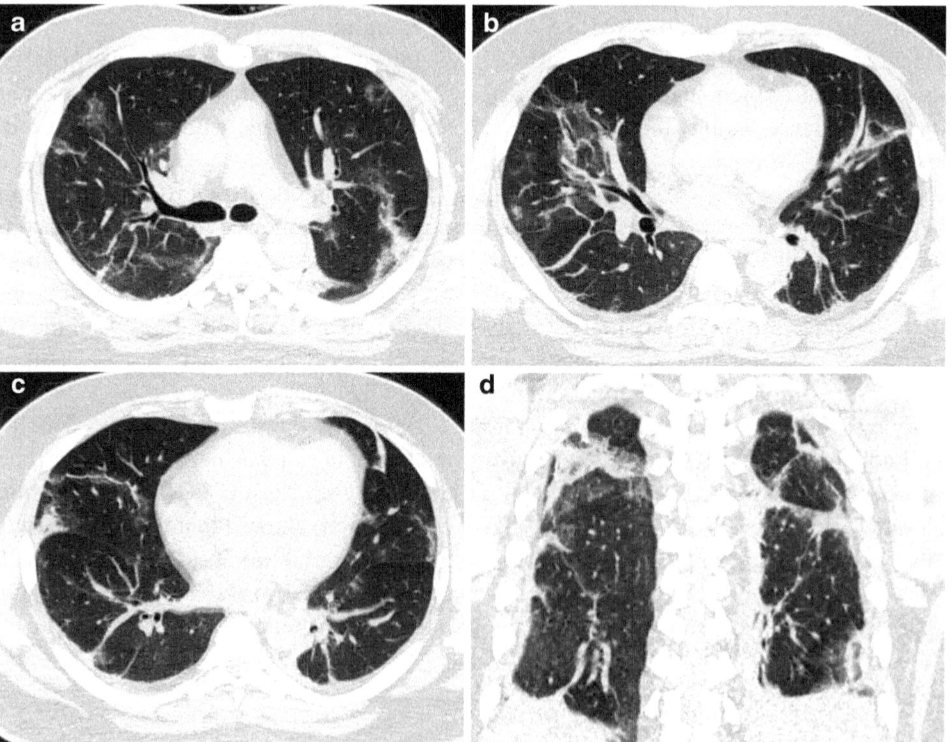

Fig. 4.32 Follow-up axial chest CT (**a–c**), and reconstructed coronal (**d**) images 16 days after initial scan

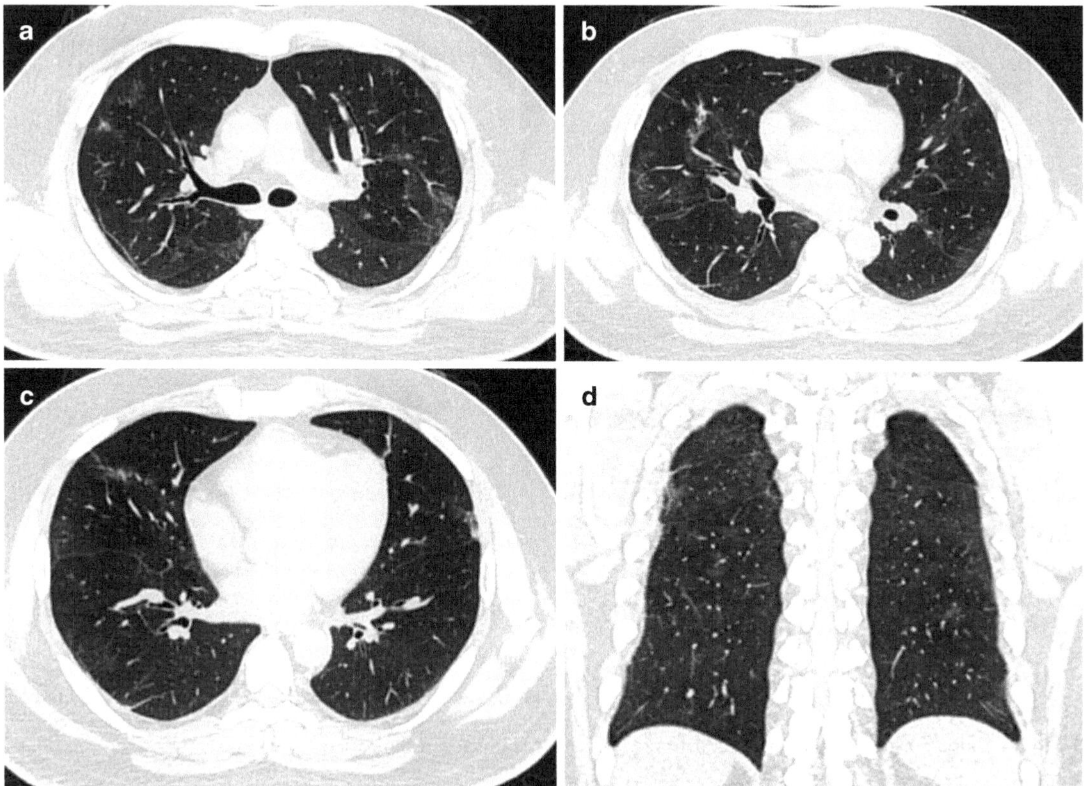

Fig. 4.33 Follow-up axial chest CT (**a–c**), and reconstructed coronal (**d**) images 34 days after initial scan

to be isolated in a local medical establishment for observation (Fig. 4.33).

Comments: The first chest CT findings of the patient were mild, only small ground-glass density nodules. But 16 days later, the lesions developed multiple cords and high density patches in both lungs, suggesting that COVID-19 changes rapidly, and chest CT could monitor the disease process.

Case 11

Medical History and Clinical Features

A 57-year-old female suffered from fever for 2 days, with the highest temperature of 38.5 °C, accompanied by intolerance of cold, shiver, cough, mainly dry cough, occasionally chest tightness, shortness of breath, abdominal swelling pain, and discomfort. Laboratory test results indicated a normal white blood cell count of 7.41×10^9/L, 72.9% neutrophils, and 20.4% lymphocytes. There were elevated blood levels for erythrocyte sedimentation rate (21 mm/h). Exposure history: The patient was in contact with a confirmed COVID-19 patient before symptom onset. The SARS-CoV-2 nucleic acid test was positive during hospitalization. The patient had recurrent abdominal pain and discomfort for 2 years.

Imaging Features

Initial chest CT showed circular ground-glass opacities in the upper lobe of the left lung and the lower lobe of the right lung, with a relatively increased marginal density and typical "reversed halo sign" appearance (**b**, **c**: white arrows) (Fig. 4.34).

Follow-up chest CT (5 days after initial CT examination) showed that the lesions in the left upper lobe and the right lower lobe of the lung were significantly larger and more progressed than before, and the lesions in the right lower lobe showed large flaps of ground glass with thickened interlobular septa and thickened microvascular (Fig. 4.35).

Follow-up chest CT (23 days after initial CT examination) showed that the multiple opacities of both lungs were resolved (Fig. 4.36).

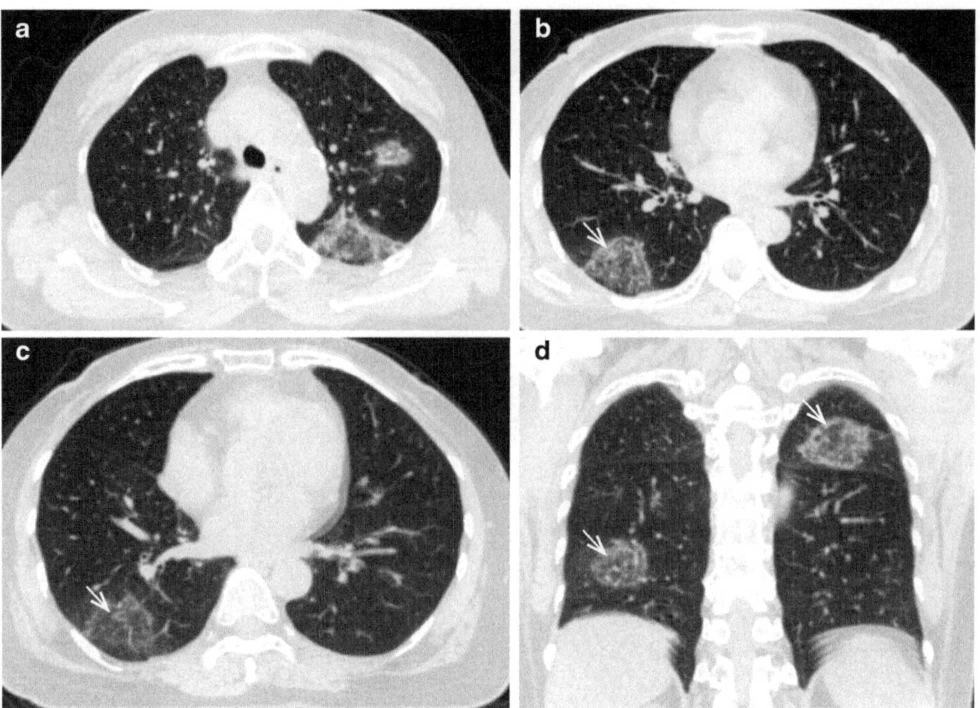

Fig. 4.34 Initial chest CT (**a–c**) and reconstructed coronal (**d**) images of the patient

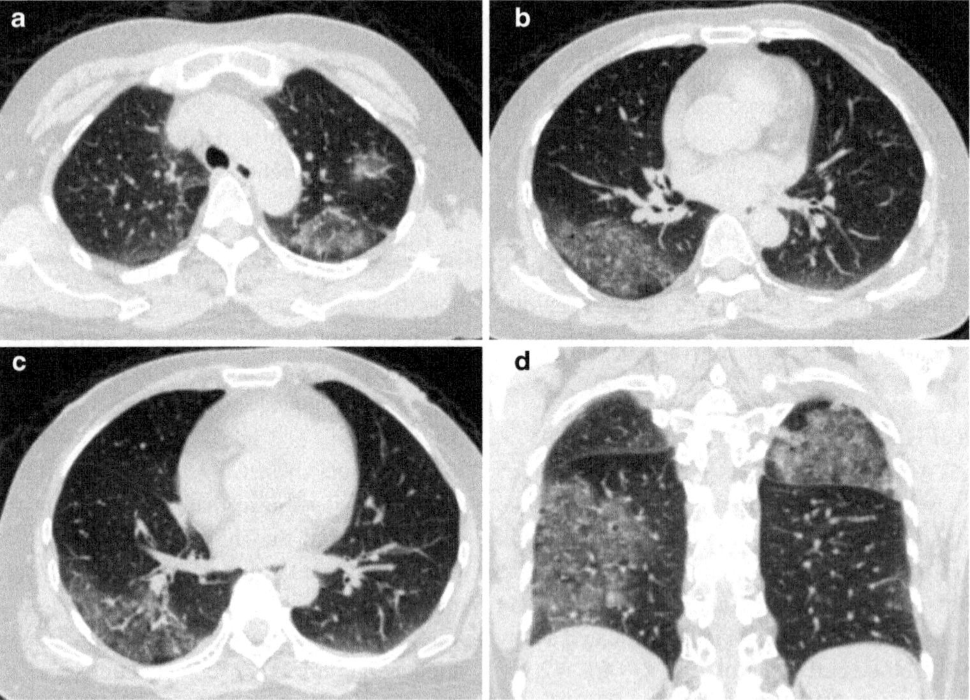

Fig. 4.35 Follow-up axial chest CT (**a–c**), and reconstructed coronal (**d**) images 5 days after initial scan

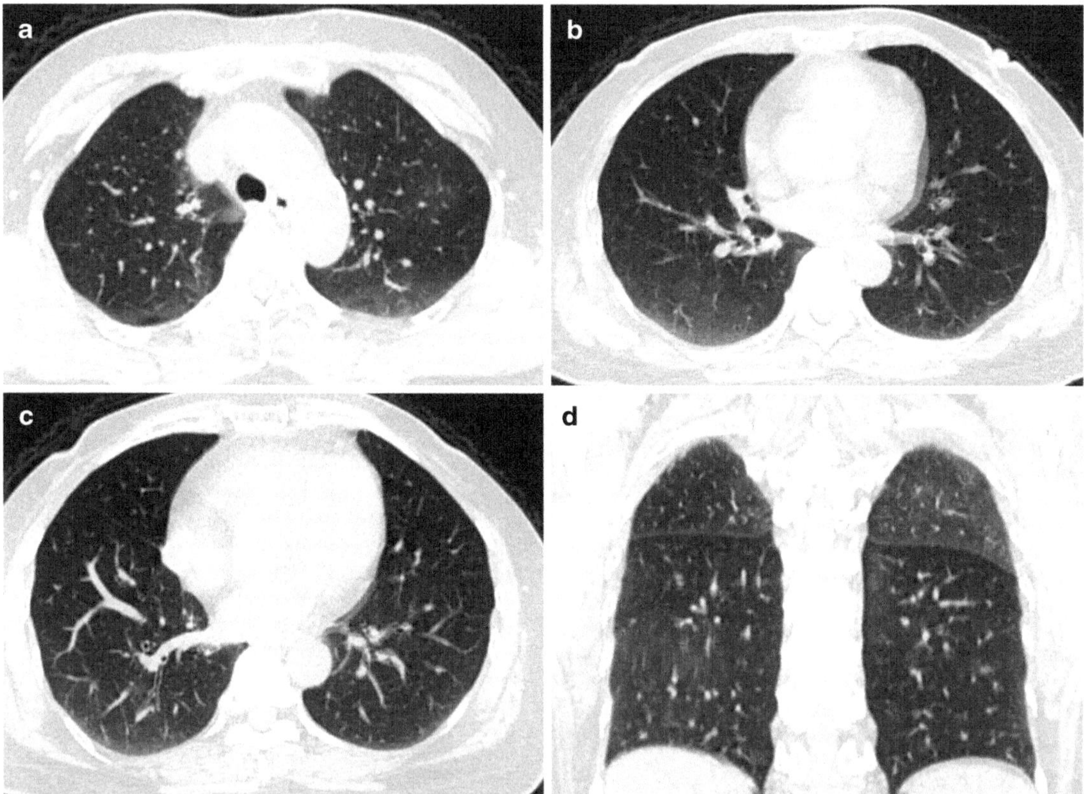

Fig. 4.36 Follow-up axial chest CT (**a–c**), and reconstructed coronal (**d**) images 23 days after initial scan

Comments: The chest CT of this case showed typical "reversed halo sign" which is unusual in COVID-19 patients. The pathological mechanism needs further explanation.

Case 12

Medical History and Clinical Features

A 54-year-old male suffered from fever for 8 h with low fever (highest body temperature: 37.5 °C), accompanied by headache, fatigue, muscle pain, and cough with a little white phlegm. Laboratory test results indicated a normal white blood cell count of $4 \times 10^9/L$, 61% neutrophils, and 23.6% lymphocytes. There were elevated blood levels for erythrocyte sedimentation rate (28 mm/h). Exposure history: The patient returned home from Wuhan, China before symptom onset. The SARS-CoV-2 nucleic acid test was positive during hospitalization.

Imaging Features

Initial chest CT showed multiple nodules and patchy high-density opacities in both lungs. The lesions in the upper lobe of the left lung were mainly solid components. "Reversed halo sign" (**c**: white arrows) was seen in the lesions in the right lower lobe (Fig. 4.37).

Follow-up chest CT (4 days after initial CT examination) showed that the nodules in both

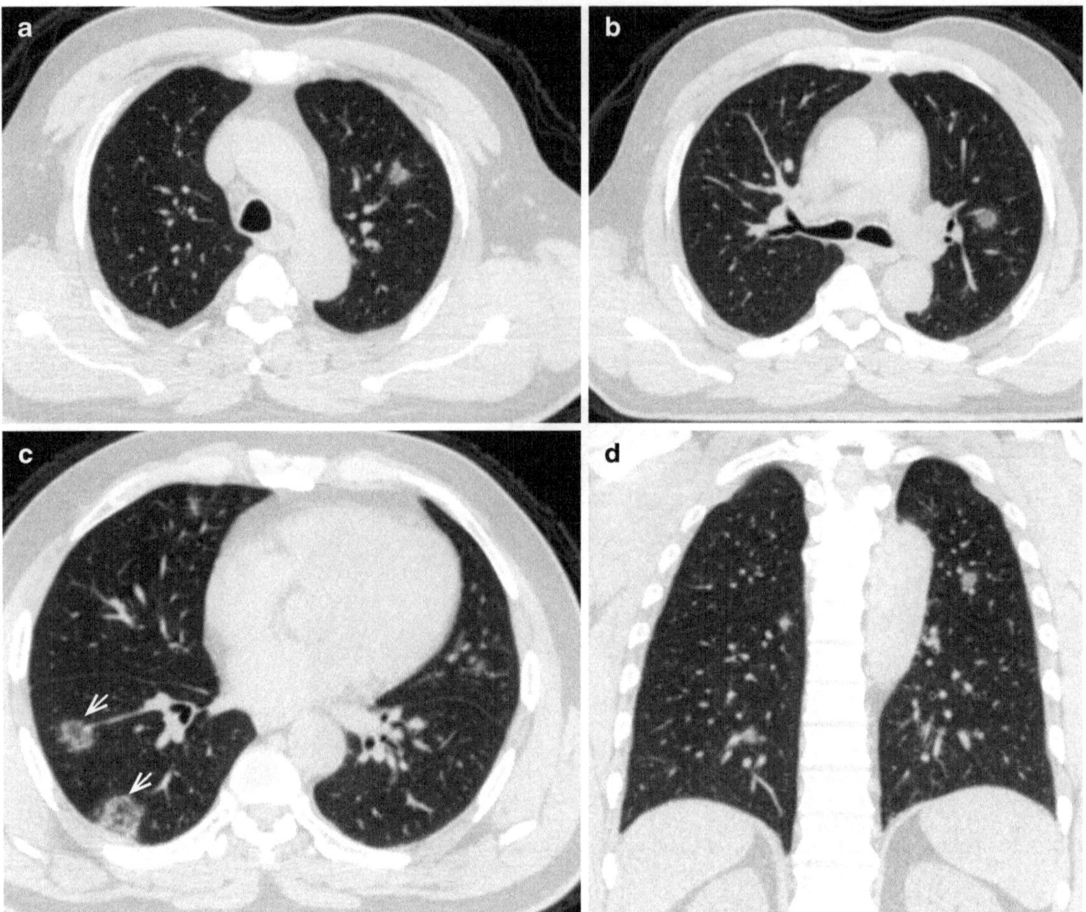

Fig. 4.37 Initial chest CT (**a–c**) and reconstructed coronal (**d**) images of the patient

lungs were significantly increased (>50%), and enlarged. Some lesions became solid (Fig. 4.38).

After treatment, the SARS-CoV-2 nucleic acid test was negative for two consecutive times. Follow-up chest CT (24 days after Initial CT examination) showed that the pneumonia lesions were almost absorbed. The patient was discharged and continued to be isolated in a local medical institution for observation (Fig. 4.39).

Comments: This case demonstrates the dynamic changes of chest CT in a common type patient. The lesions were first increased, enlarged, and consolidated, and the lesions were almost absorbed after 20 days of continuous treatment.

Case 13

Medical History and Clinical Manifestations

A 48-year-old male had no obvious symptoms. The laboratory test also showed normal results. Because the patient has lived in Wuhan, China for a long time, and recently returned home from Wuhan; he received SARS-CoV-2 nucleic acid test and was positive, so he was hospitalized.

Imaging Features

Initial chest CT showed thin patchy and nodular GGOs of the bilateral lungs (Fig. 4.40).

Follow-up chest CT (9 days after initial CT examination) showed the patchy ground-glass opacities in the subpleural area of both lungs with unclear boundary. The focus becomes more obvious compared with previous CT (Fig. 4.41).

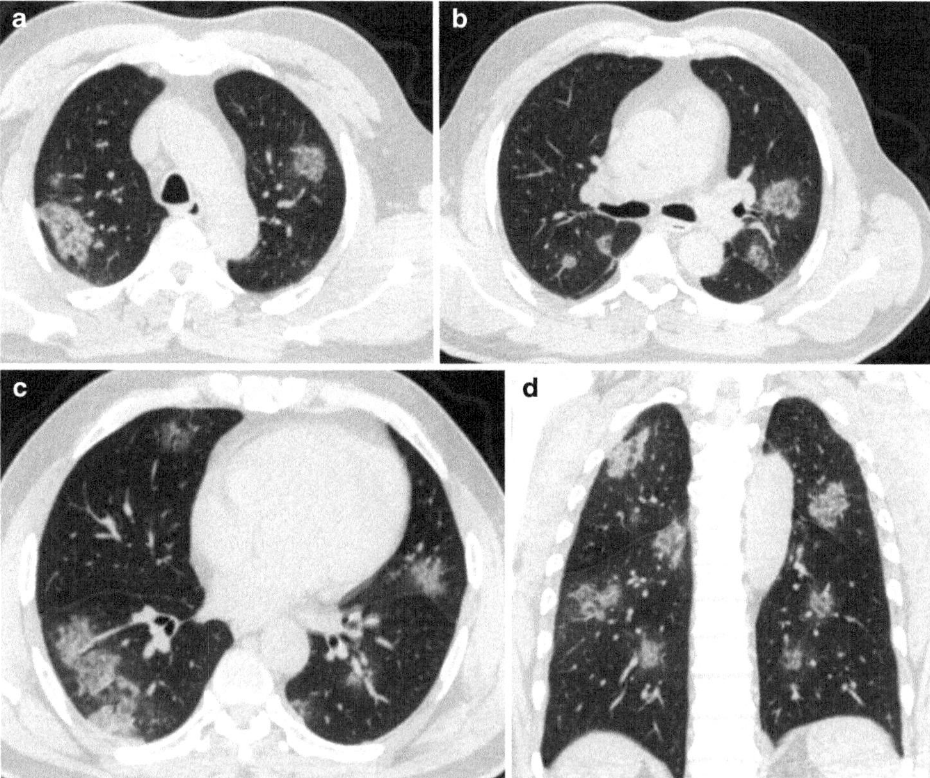

Fig. 4.38 Follow-up axial chest CT (**a–c**), and reconstructed coronal (**d**) images 4 days after initial scan

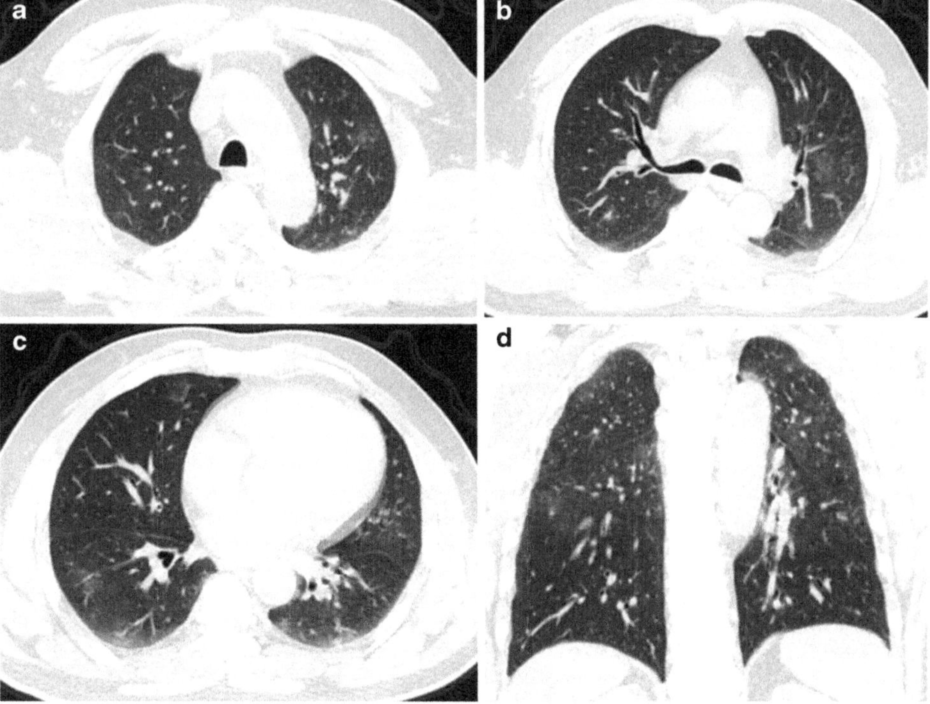

Fig. 4.39 Follow-up axial chest CT (**a–c**), and reconstructed coronal (**d**) images 24 days after initial scan

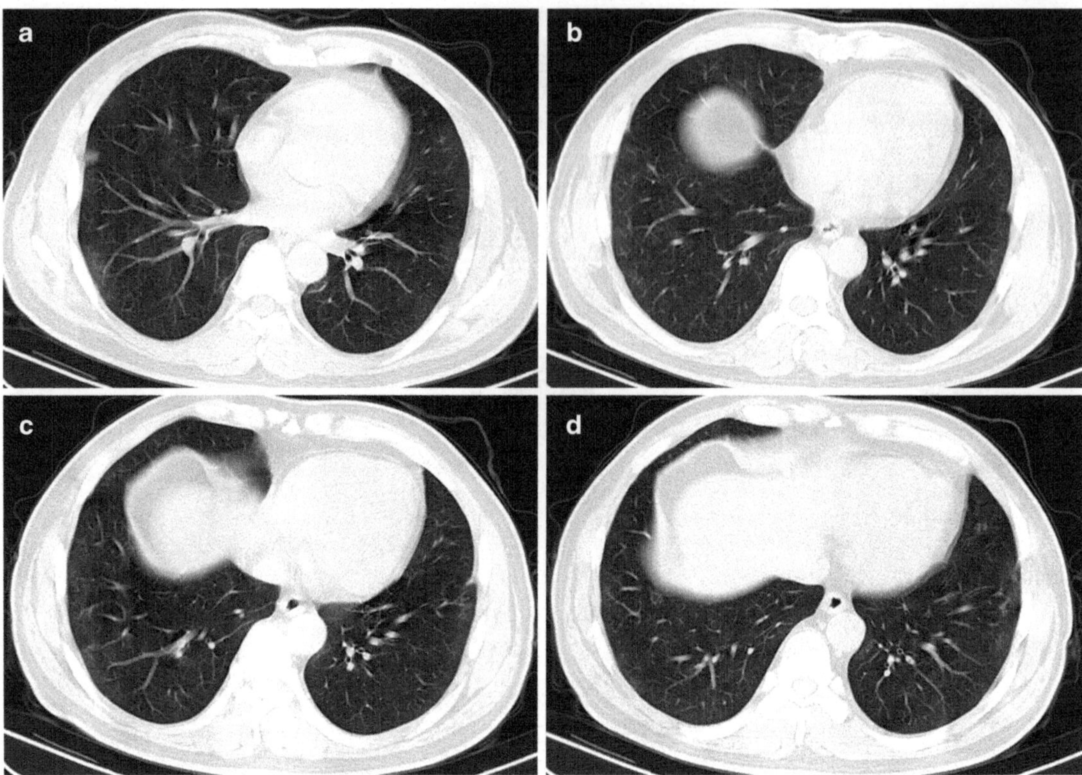

Fig. 4.40 Initial CT image

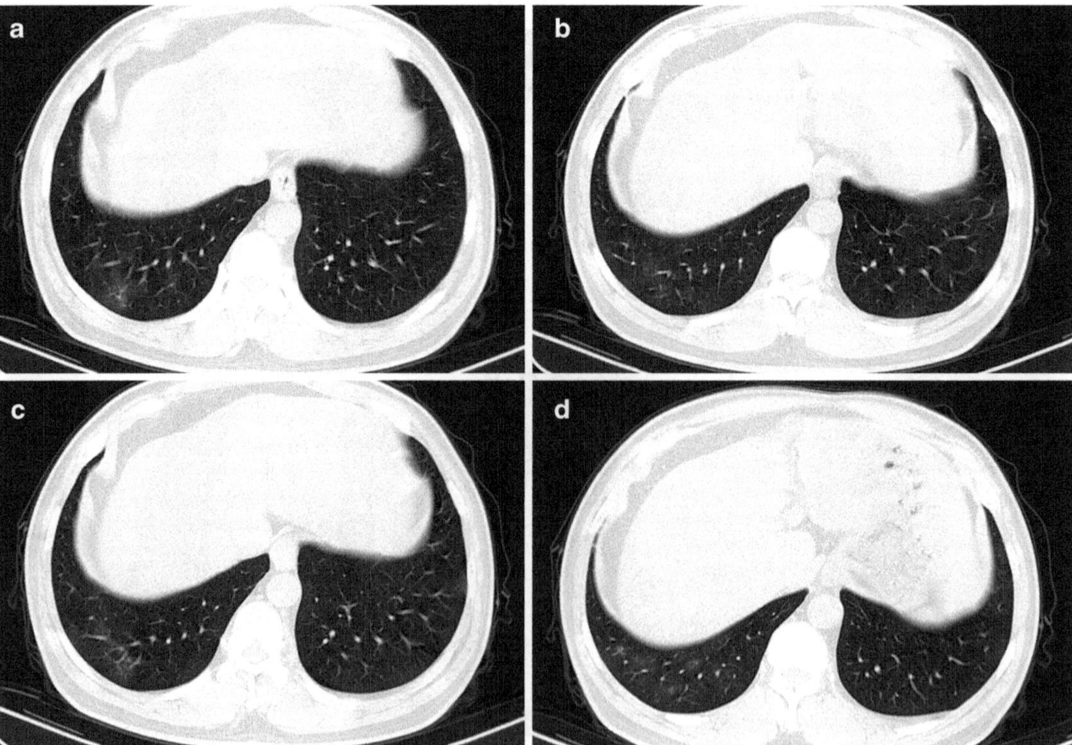

Fig. 4.41 Follow-up CT images 9 days after initial scan

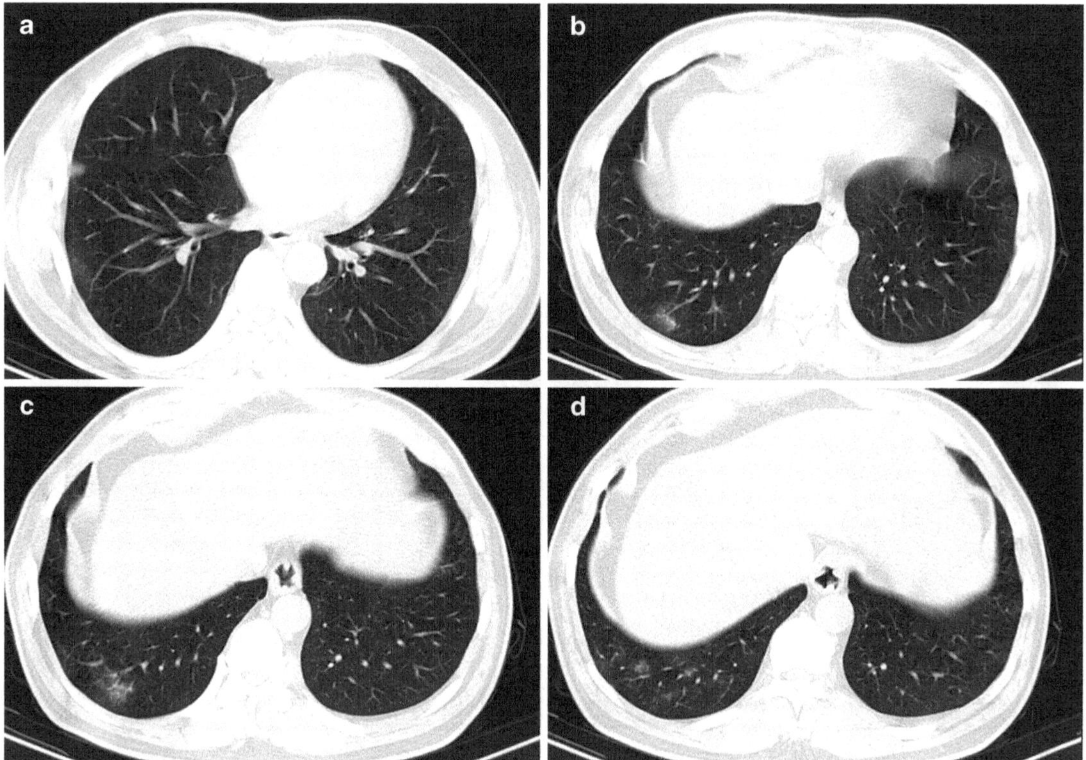

Fig. 4.42 Follow-up CT images 19 days after initial scan

After 19 days follow-up and reexamination, CT showed that patchy ground-glass opacities became slightly denser (Fig. 4.42).

Comments: This patient seems to be a healthy virus carrier clinically, but CT showed slight lung lesions.

Case 14

Medical History and Clinical Manifestations

A 28-year-old male was admitted in the hospital for 7 days with cough. Laboratory test results indicated an increased white blood cell count of 10.51×10^9/L. Exposure history: He had been contacted his mother who returned home from Wuhan, China. The SARS-CoV-2 nucleic acid test was positive on the day of admission.

Imaging Features

Initial chest CT showed a small partial solid nodules in the right lower lobe (Fig. 4.43).

Follow-up chest CT (9 days after initial CT examination) showed multiple patchy high-density opacities in both lungs with blurred boundaries, which were significantly increased and enlarged compared with the previous lesions (Fig. 4.44).

After 23 days follow-up and reexamination, CT showed almost normal (Fig. 4.45).

Comments: This is a case with mild clinical and imaging manifestations.

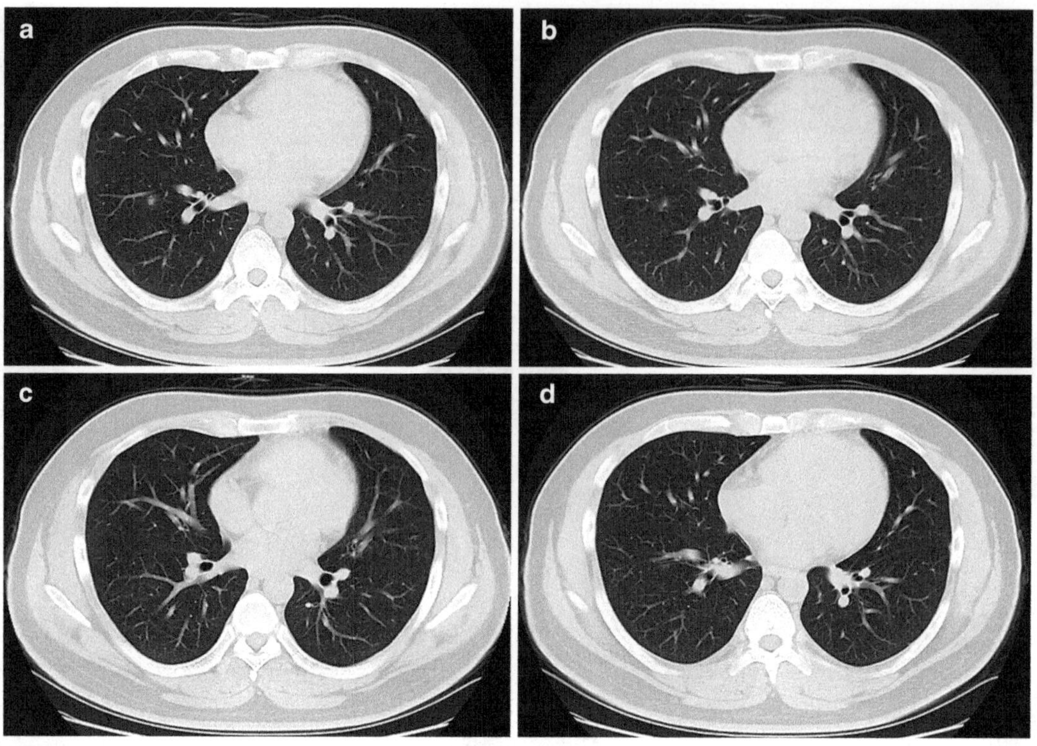

Fig. 4.43 Initial CT image

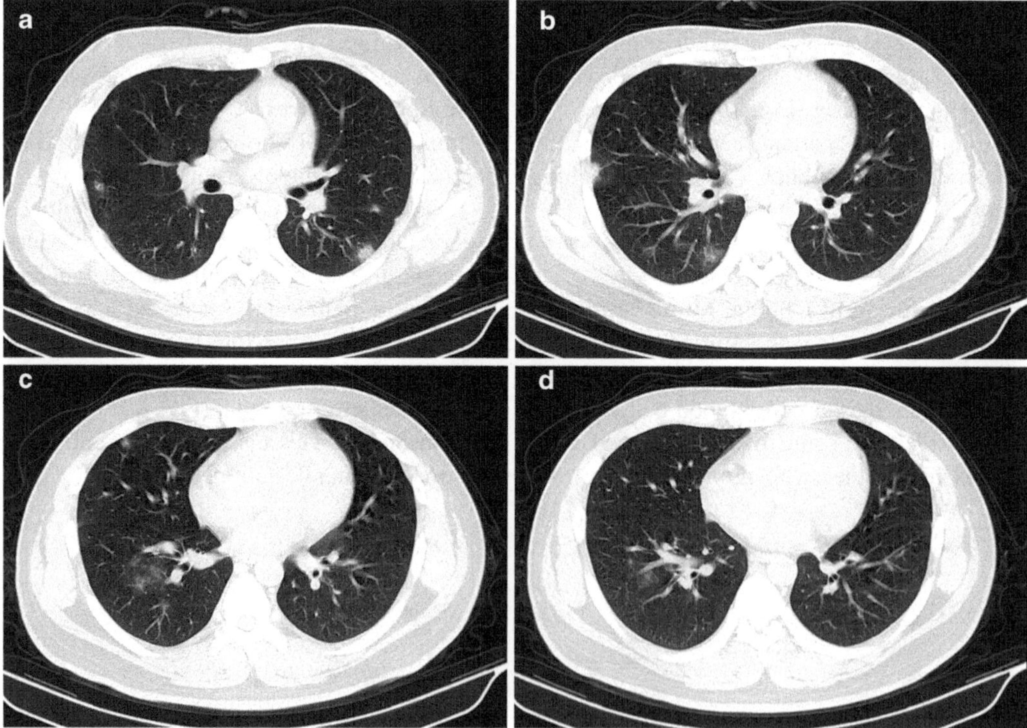

Fig. 4.44 Follow-up CT images 9 days after initial scan

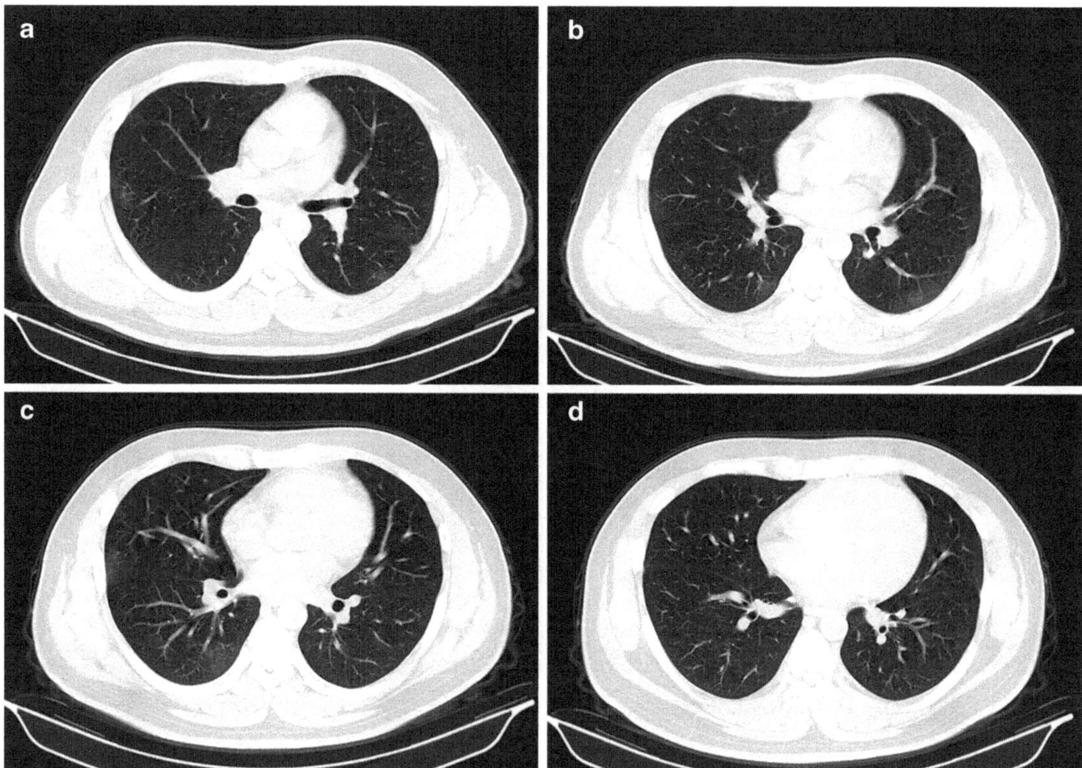

Fig. 4.45 Follow-up CT images 23 days after initial scan

Case 15

Medical History and Clinical Manifestations

A 35-year-old female was admitted in the hospital for 7 days with fever (highest body temperature: 37.6 °C), cough, and sputum. Laboratory test results indicated a decreased white blood cell count of 3.69×10^9/L. The patient lived in Wuhan, China for a long time. He drove back to home from Wuhan before symptom onset. The SARS-CoV-2 nucleic acid test was positive during hospitalization.

Imaging Features

Initial chest CT showed patchy GGOs in the subpleural area of the left lower lobe of the lung (Fig. 4.46).

Follow-up chest CT (8 days after initial CT examination) showed the small flaps of ground-glass opacities under pleura in the lower lobe of both lungs. The lesion extends to the contralateral side, while the original lesion decreased in size and density, and fibrosis formed in the adjacent area (Fig. 4.47).

After 25 days follow-up and reexamination, CT showed that most of the lesions were absorbed (Fig. 4.48).

Comments: This is a case with mild clinical and imaging manifestations.

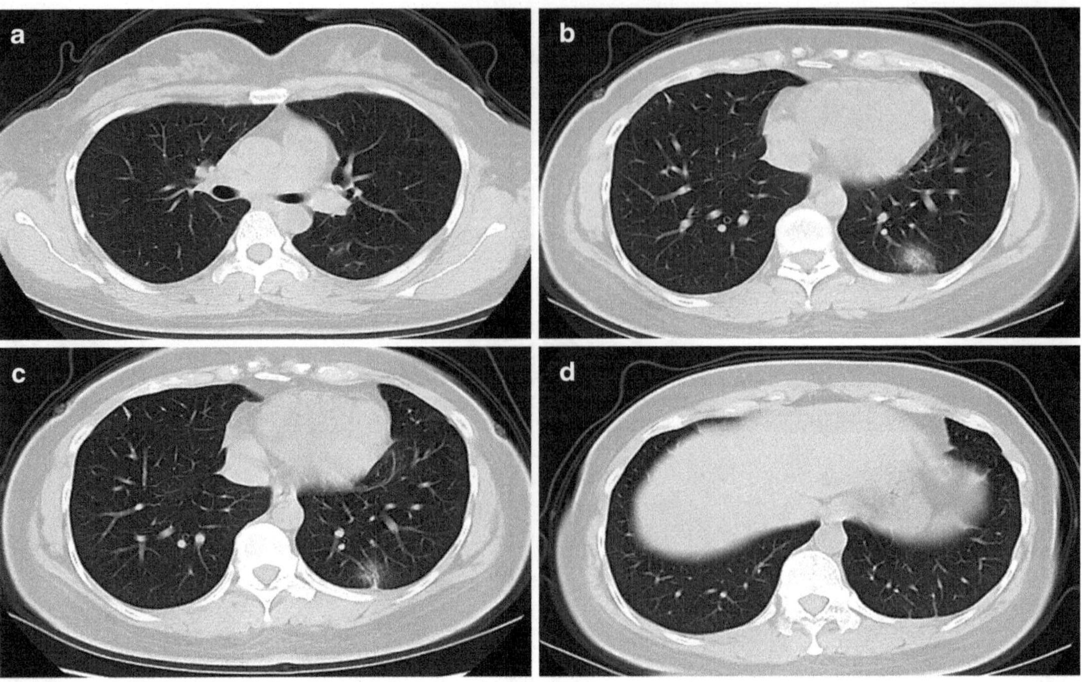

Fig. 4.46 Initial CT image

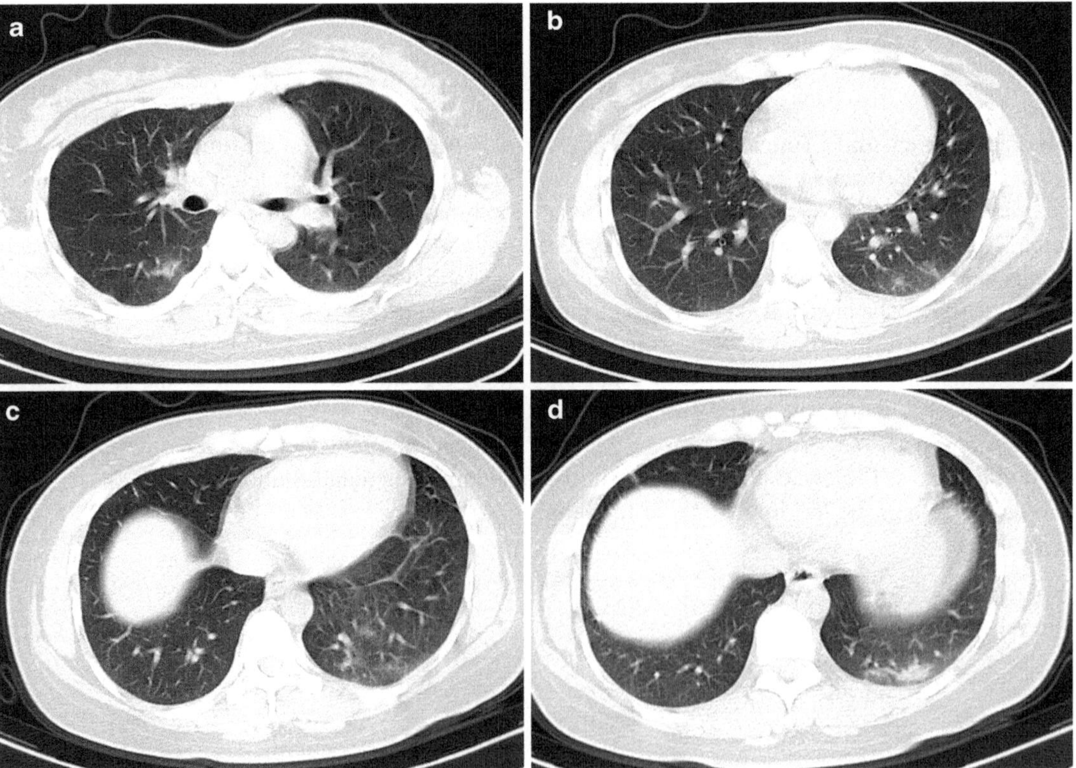

Fig. 4.47 Follow-up CT images 8 days after initial scan

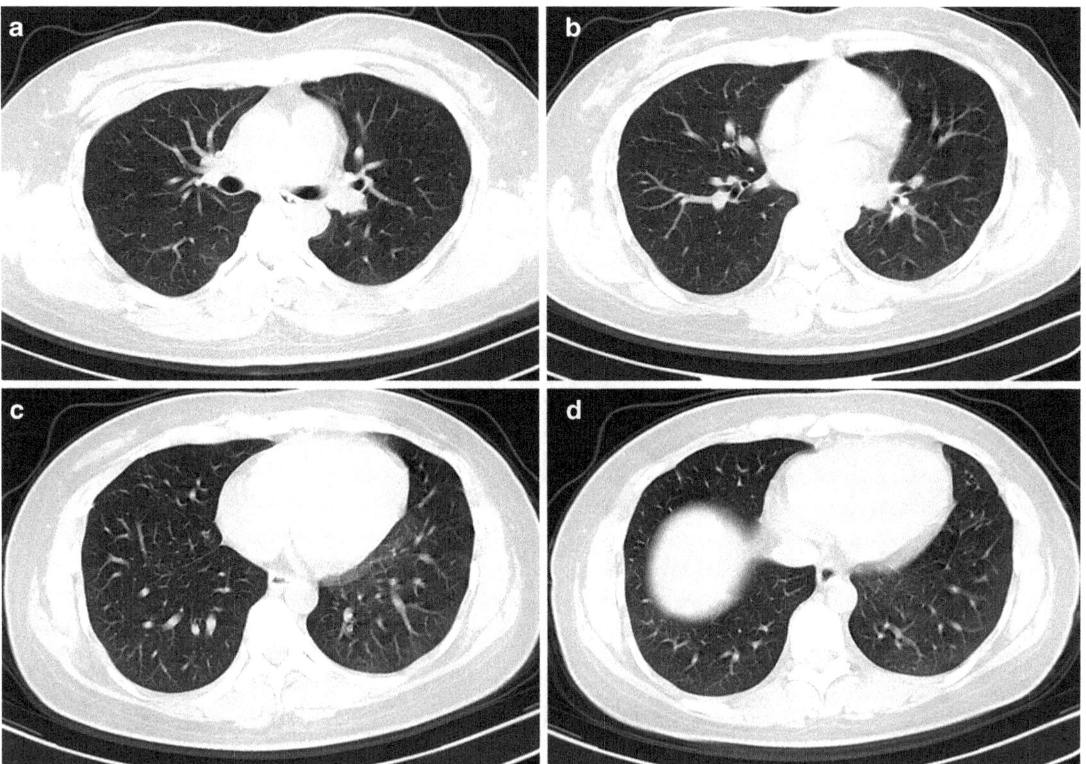

Fig. 4.48 Follow-up CT images 25 days after initial scan

Case 16

Medical History and Clinical Manifestations

A 56-year-old female suffered from cough and sputum for 16 days. Laboratory test results indicated a decreased white blood cell count of $3.89 \times 10^9/L$. The patient lived in Wuhan, China and contacted with a COVID-19 patient before the symptom onset. The SARS-CoV-2 nucleic acid test was positive during hospitalization.

Imaging Features

Initial chest CT showed multiple subpleural cords with small flaky dense consolidation, mainly in the lower lobes of bilateral lungs (Fig. 4.49).

Follow-up chest CT (24 days after initial CT examination) showed that the lesion was nearly absorbed and showed fibrous cord opacities (Fig. 4.50).

Comments: This is a patient with mild disease. He was admitted to the hospital 16 days after the onset of the disease. The first CT examination showed multiple subpleural cords, which can indicate that the patient has been in the image staging of absorption.

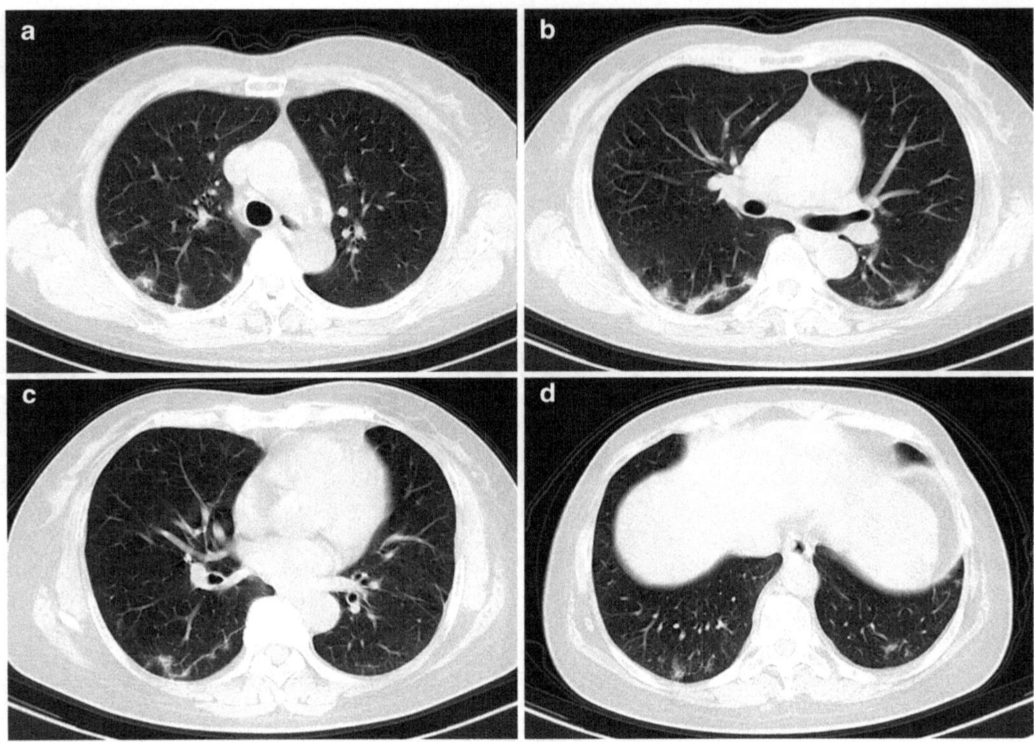

Fig. 4.49 Initial CT image

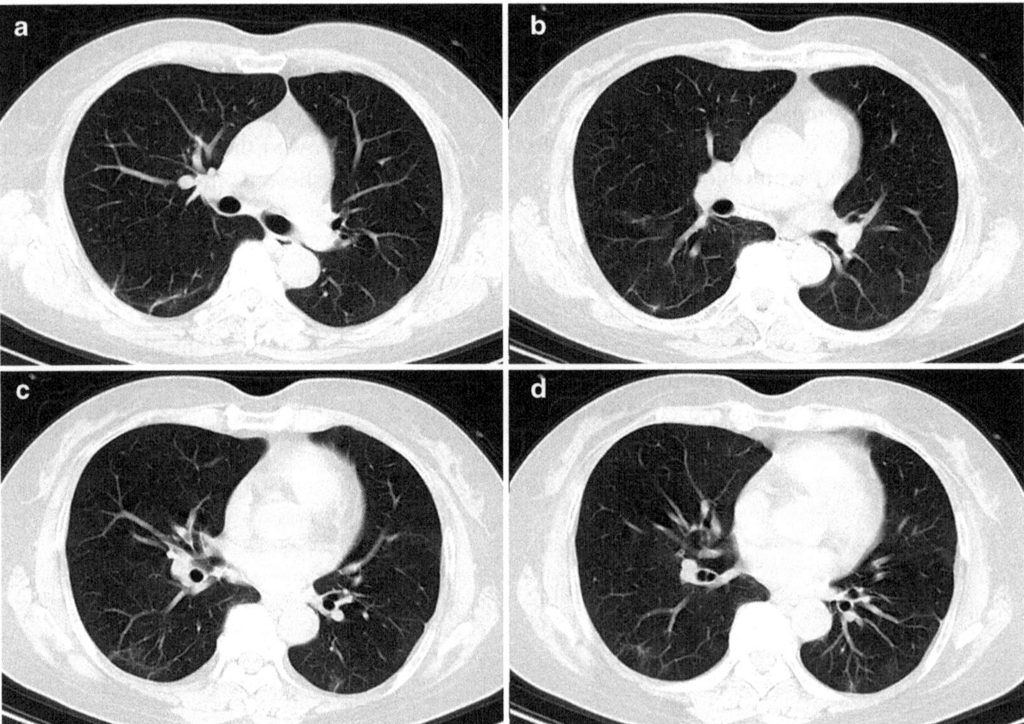

Fig. 4.50 Follow-up CT images 24 days after initial scan

Case 17

Medical History and Clinical Manifestations

A 50-year-old female suffered from cough, expectoration for 9 days, and fever (highest body temperature: 38 °C) for 7 days. Laboratory test results indicated a normal white blood cell count of 6.45×10^9/L. There were elevated blood levels for erythrocyte sedimentation rate (78 mm/h) and C-reactive protein (40.3 mg/L). The patient returned home from Wuhan, China. The SARS-CoV-2 nucleic acid test was positive during hospitalization.

Imaging Features

Initial chest CT showed consolidation mainly in the subpleural regions and parts of them surrounding the bronchovascular bundles in both lungs (Fig. 4.51).

Follow-up chest CT (4 days after initial CT examination) showed that the consolidated lesions changed to GGOs (Fig. 4.52).

After 23 days follow-up and reexamination, CT showed that the two lung lesions were attenuated and the scope was reduced, mainly ground glass, and fibrosis was observed inside (Fig. 4.53).

Comments: The chest CT manifestations of the patient were typical. The first chest CT findings of this patient were subpleural consolidation and nodular, and the lesion gradually absorbed as a ground-glass opacity.

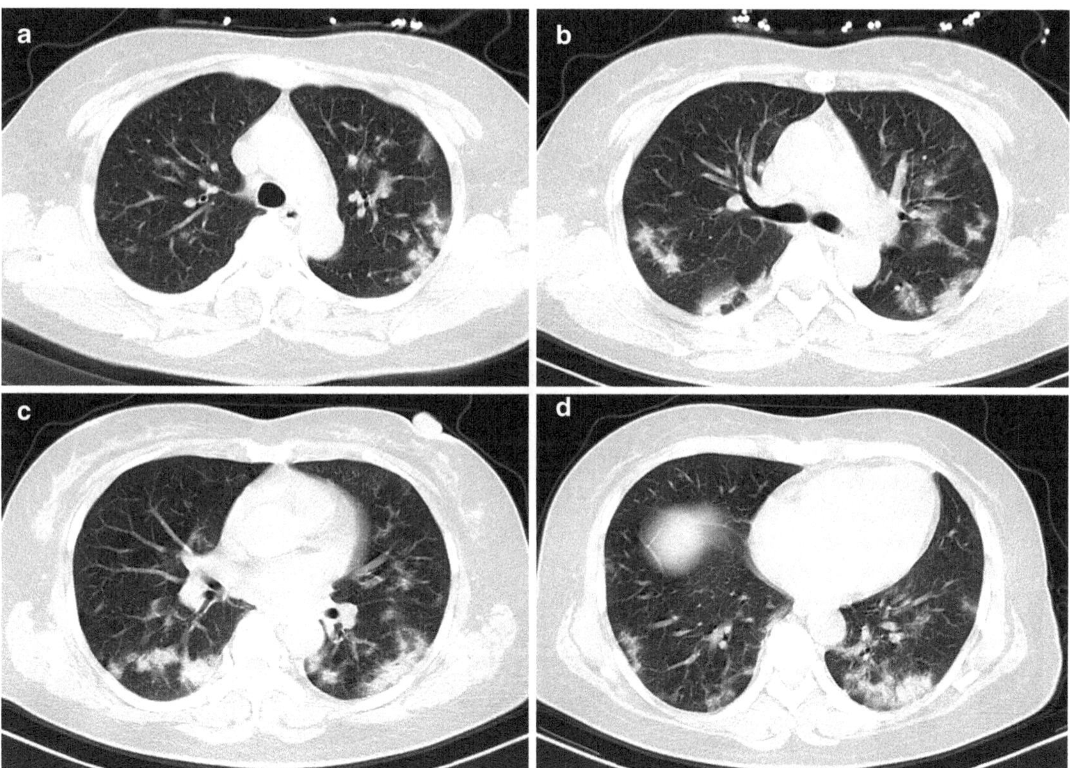

Fig. 4.51 Initial CT image

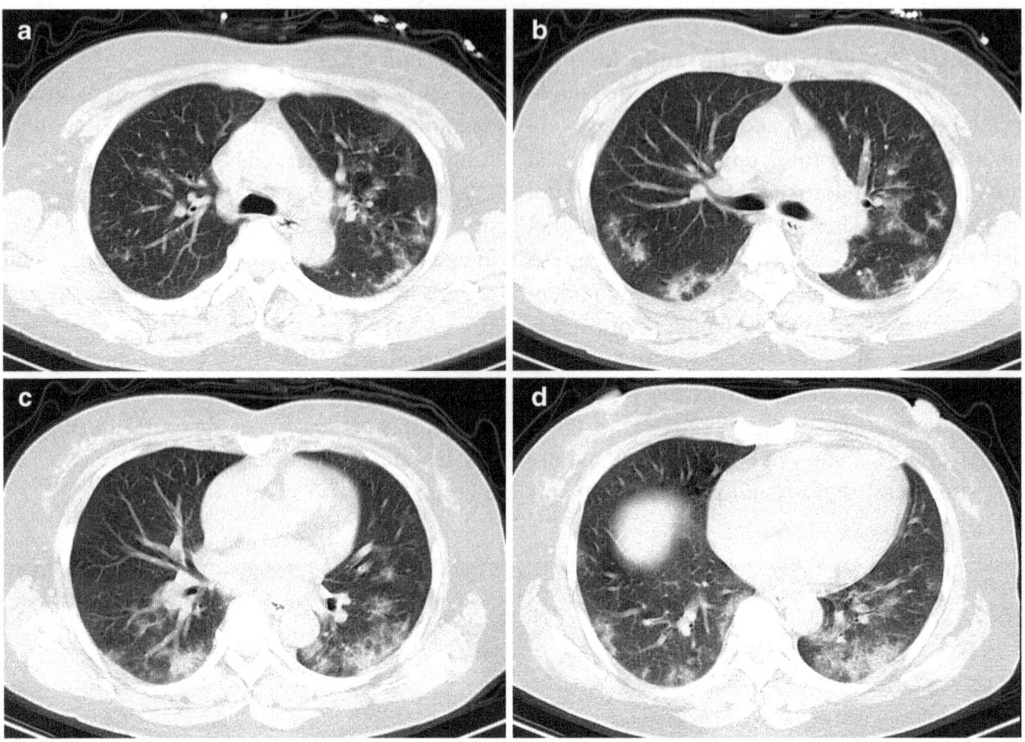

Fig. 4.52 Follow-up CT images 4 days after initial scan

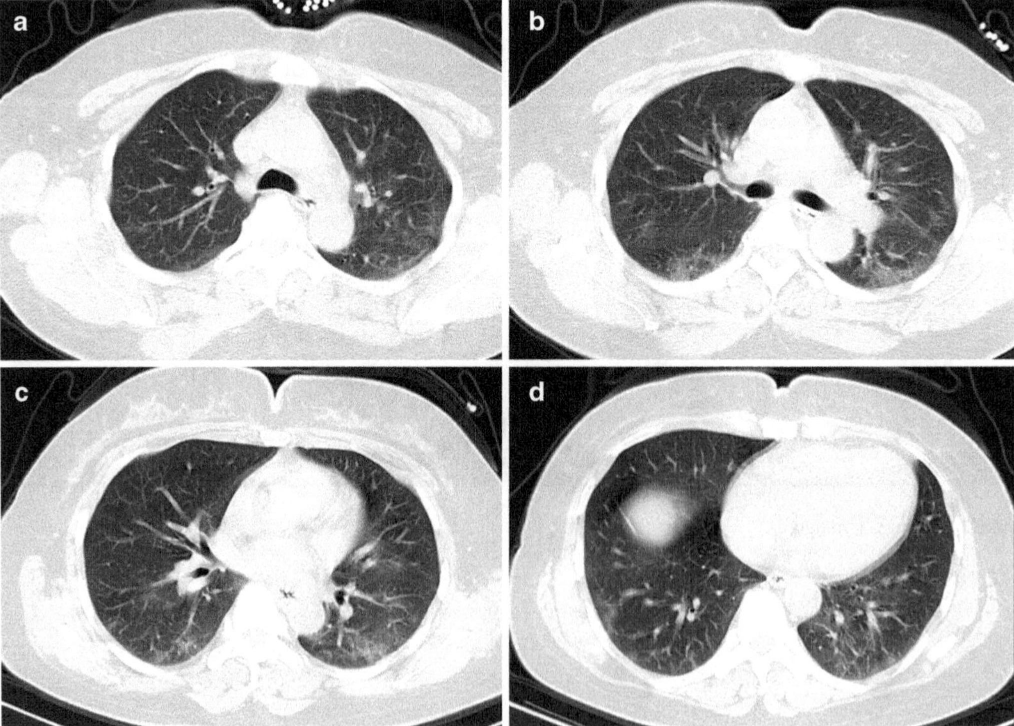

Fig. 4.53 Follow-up CT images 23 days after initial scan

Case 18

Medical History and Clinical Manifestations

A 28-year-old male was admitted in the hospital for 7 days with fever (highest body temperature: 38.5 °C) accompanied by cough and sputum, with mild headache. Laboratory test results indicated a decreased white blood cell count of 3.81×10^9/L and 44.1% neutrophils. Exposure history: The patient came from Wuhan, China to home by high-speed train. The SARS-CoV-2 nucleic acid test was positive during hospitalization.

Imaging Features

Initial chest CT showed ground-glass nodules in the left upper and lower lobes with halo changes (Fig. 4.54).

Follow-up chest CT (8 days after initial CT examination) showed increased lung lesions and increased density. Some nodules showed changes of halo, and small blood vessels in the lesions of the left lower lobe were thickened (Fig. 4.55).

Follow-up chest CT (26 days after initial CT examination) showed that the primary lesion changed to pure GGOs (Fig. 4.56).

Comments: The imaging and clinical manifestations of this patient were mild, mainly small pieces of ground glass. After 26 days of treatment, the lesions were completely absorbed.

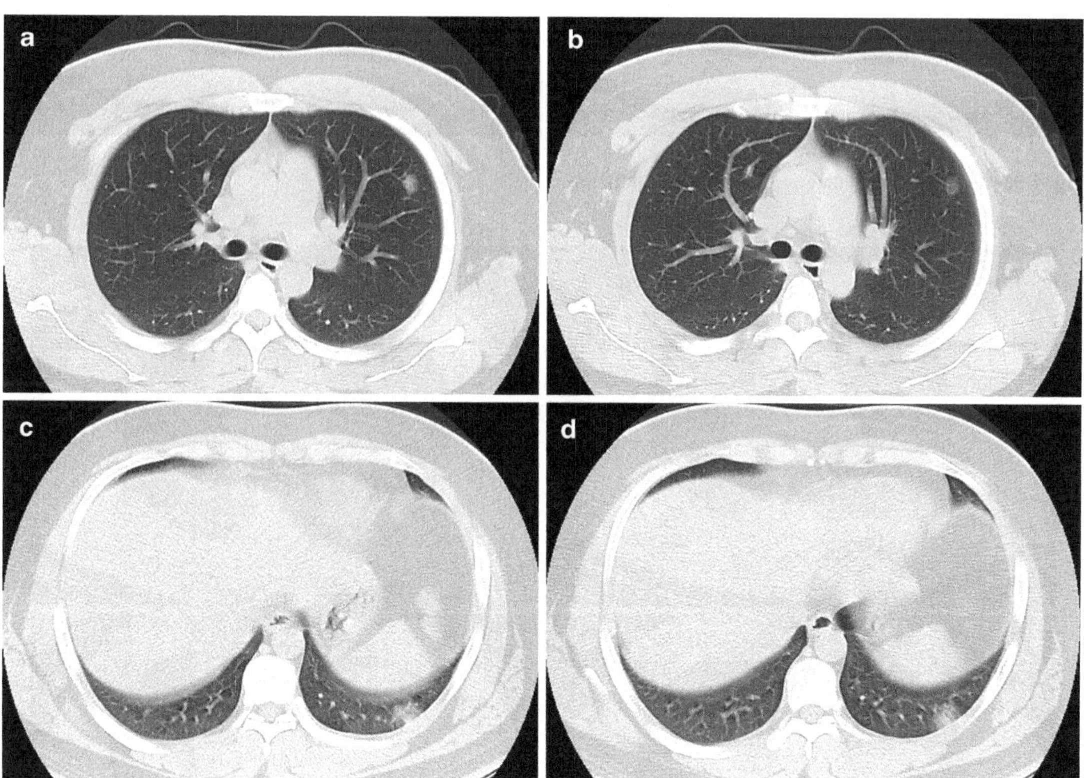

Fig. 4.54 Initial CT image

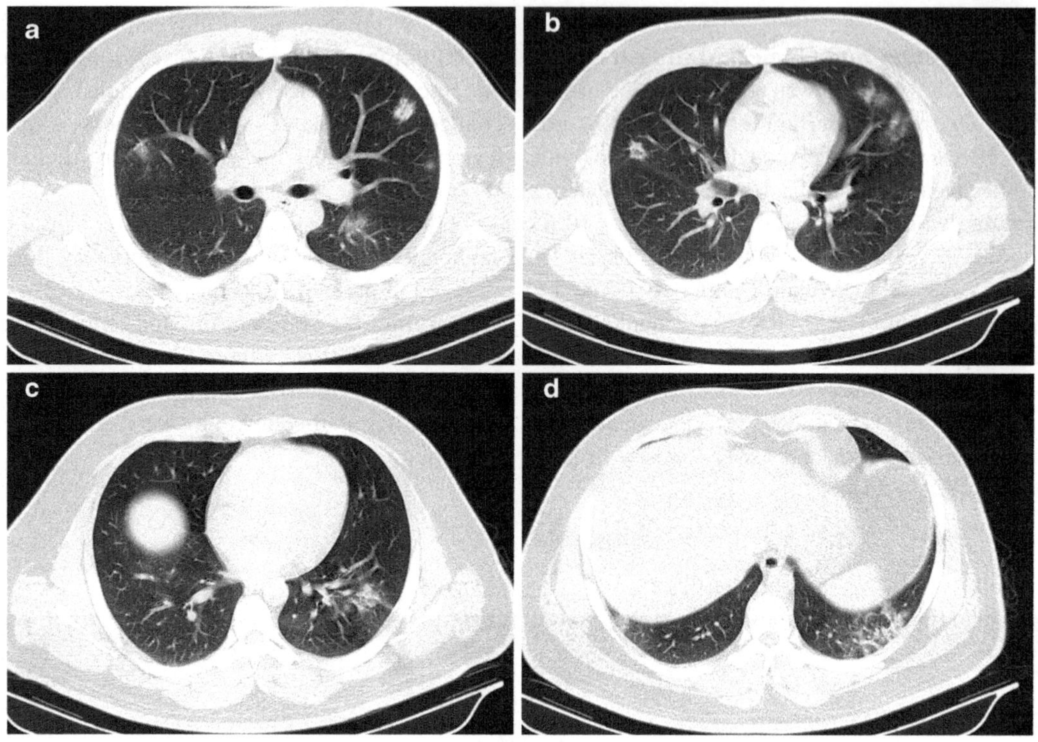

Fig. 4.55 Follow-up CT images 8 days after initial scan

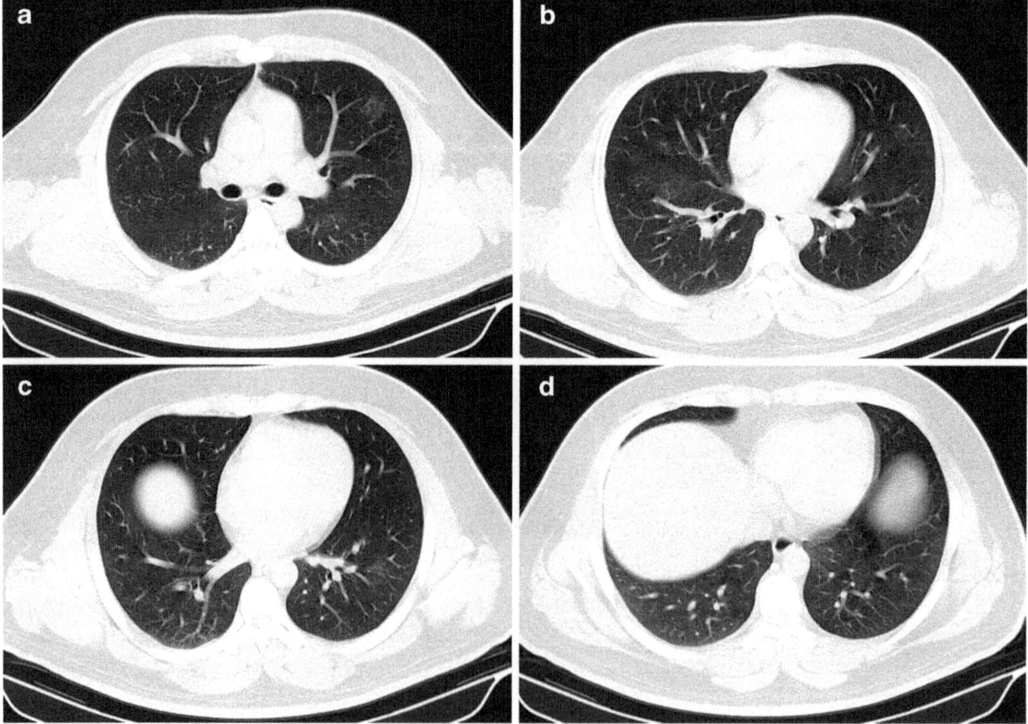

Fig. 4.56 Follow-up CT images 26 days after initial scan

Case 19

Medical History and Clinical Manifestations

A 59-year-old male suffered from cough for 7 days. Laboratory test results indicated a decreased white blood cell count of 3.29×10^9/L. The patient had close contact with the spouse returned to home from Wuhan, China. The SARS-CoV-2 nucleic acid test was positive on the day of admission. The patient has a history of type 2 diabetes for more than 2 years.

Imaging Features

Initial chest CT showed patchy consolidation in middle lobe of right lung; the boundary of the lesions was not clear (Fig. 4.57).

Follow-up chest CT (10 days after initial CT examination) showed that the lesion in the middle lobe of the right lung was attenuated, appeared as GGOs with a few fibrosis (Fig. 4.58).

Follow-up chest CT (23 days after initial CT examination) appeared normal (Fig. 4.59).

Comments: This was a patient with type 2 diabetes, COVID-19 of him appeared as a typical common type, not affected by his underlying diseases.

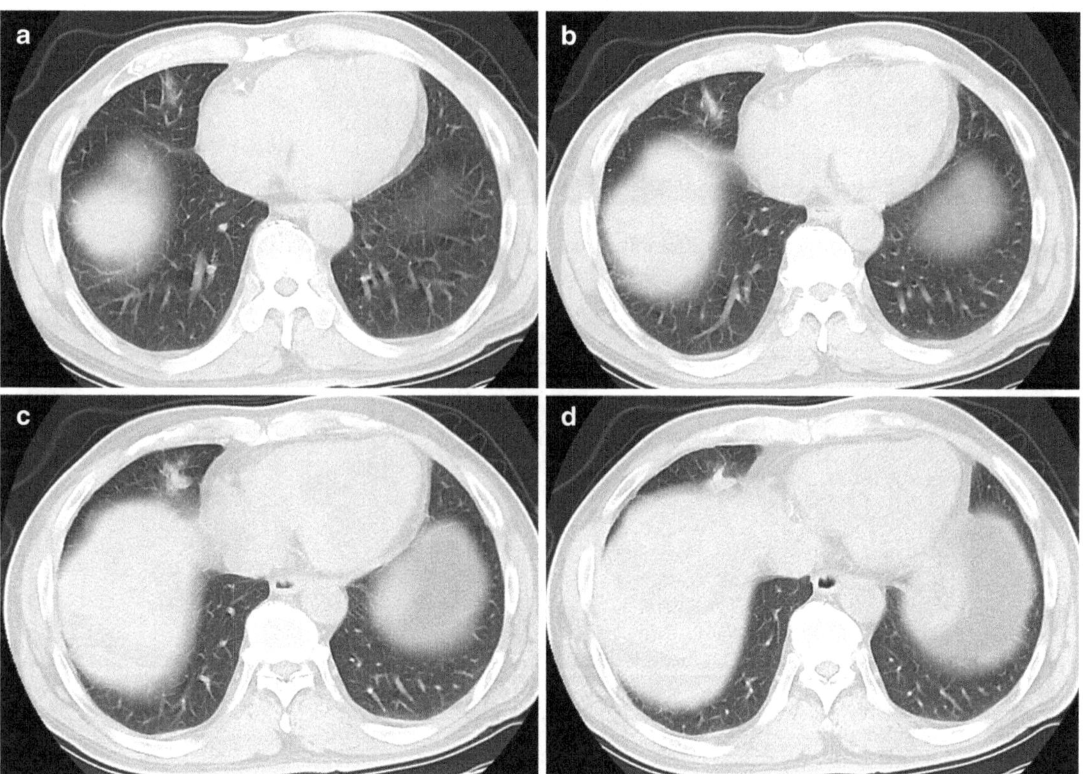

Fig. 4.57 Initial CT image

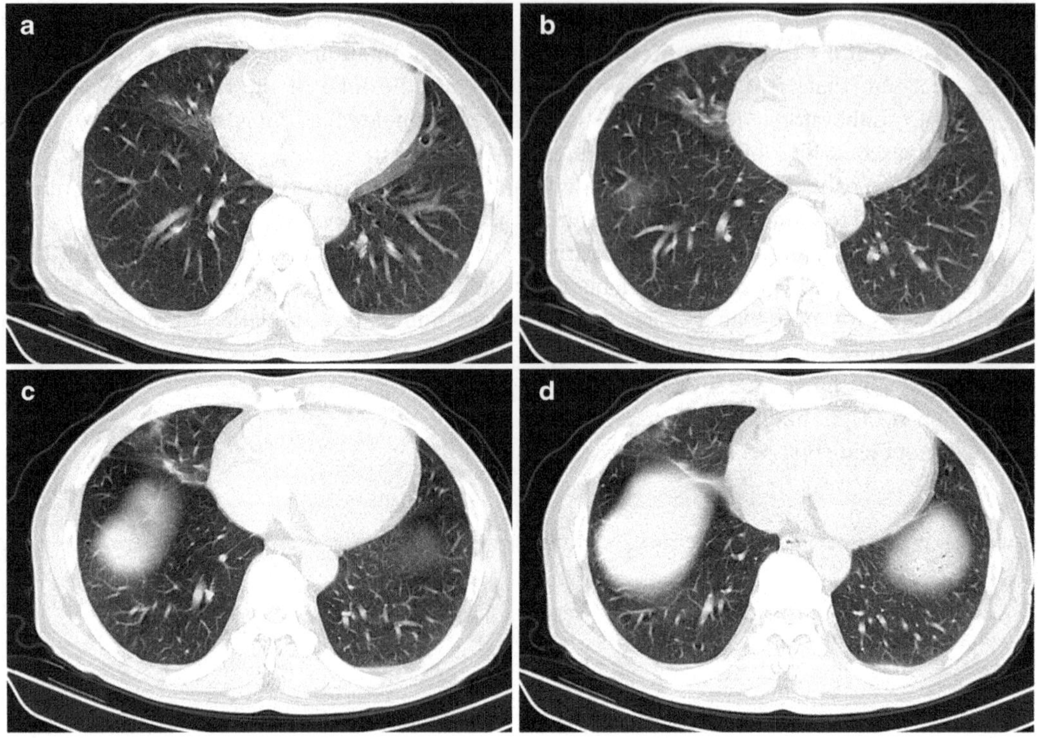

Fig. 4.58 Follow-up CT images 10 days after initial scan

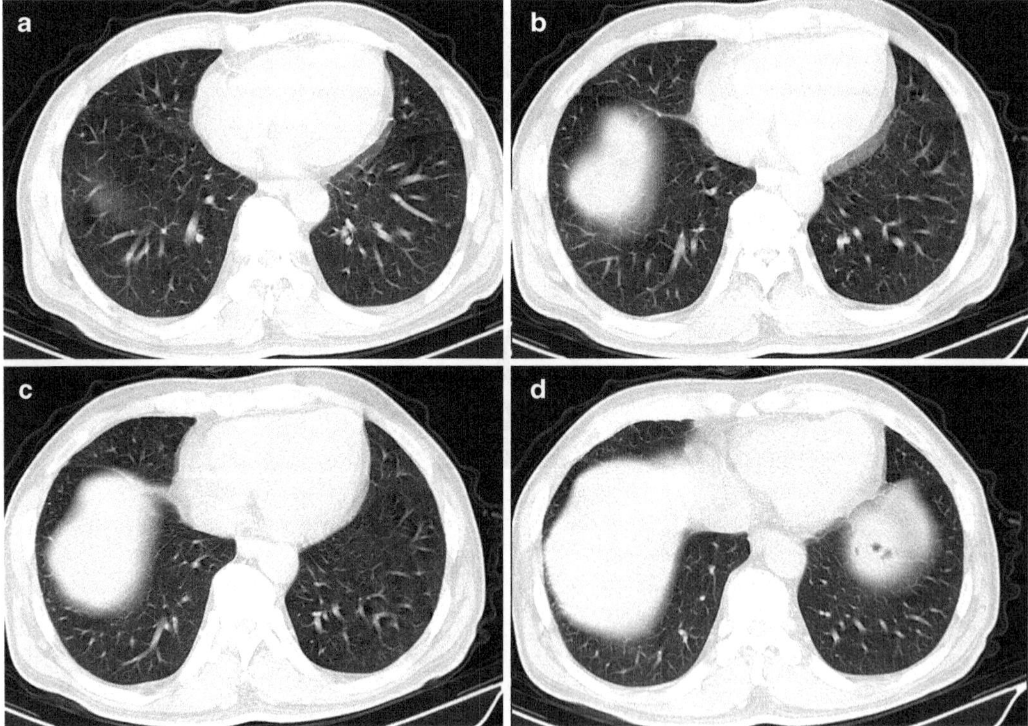

Fig. 4.59 Follow-up CT images 23 days after initial scan

Case 20

Medical History and Clinical Manifestations

A 57-year-old female suffered from fever (highest body temperature: 39 °C) for 6 days, paroxysmal cough for 2 days. Laboratory test results indicated a normal white blood cell count of 4.18 × 10^9/L. There was elevated blood level for C-reactive protein (47.9 mg/L). The patient only attended a banquet before the onset of the disease, and the epidemiological history was not clear. Her SARS-CoV-2 nucleic acid test was positive on the day of admission.

Imaging Features

Initial chest CT showed the patchy pure ground-glass opacities under the pleura of both lungs, the lesions in the lower lobe showed reversed halo sign (**c**, **d**: white arrows), and the nodules in the upper lobe showed halo changes, with the thickened vascular (Fig. 4.60).

Follow-up chest CT (8 days after initial CT examination) showed that the subpleural GGOs of both lungs became consolidation. The density was increased with the formation of fibrous foci, the upper lobe nodules were enlarged, and the edges were ground glass with fibrosis (Fig. 4.61).

Follow-up chest CT (29 days after initial CT examination) showed that most of the GGOs and consolidation lesions were absorbed, remaining a few fibrous lesions (**c**: white arrow) (Fig. 4.62).

Comments: The first chest CT image of the patient presented typical manifestations, with reversed halo sign and thickened vascular in the subpleural area of both lungs. After 29 days of treatment, the lesion was gradually absorbed.

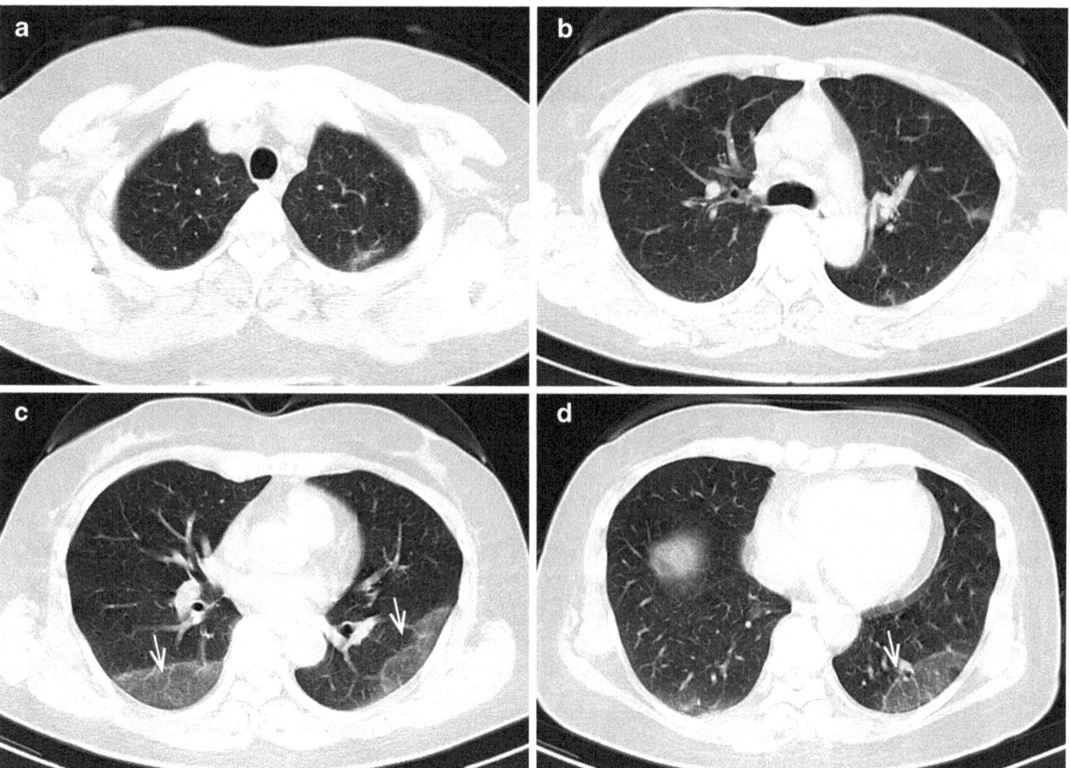

Fig. 4.60 Initial CT image

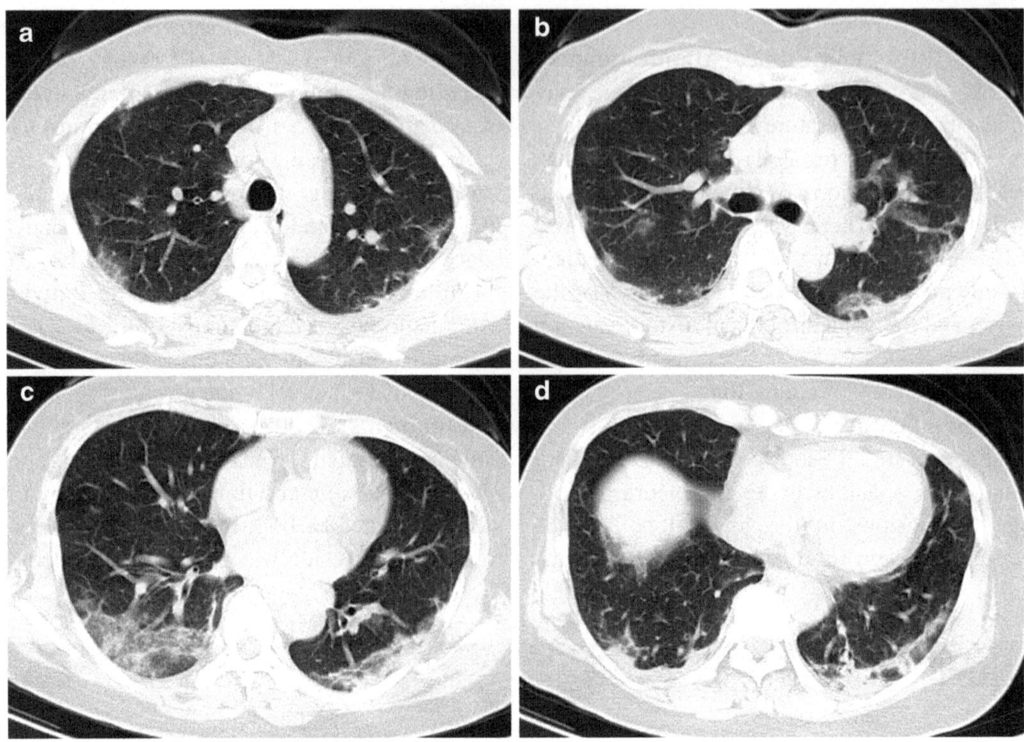

Fig. 4.61 Follow-up CT images 8 days after initial scan

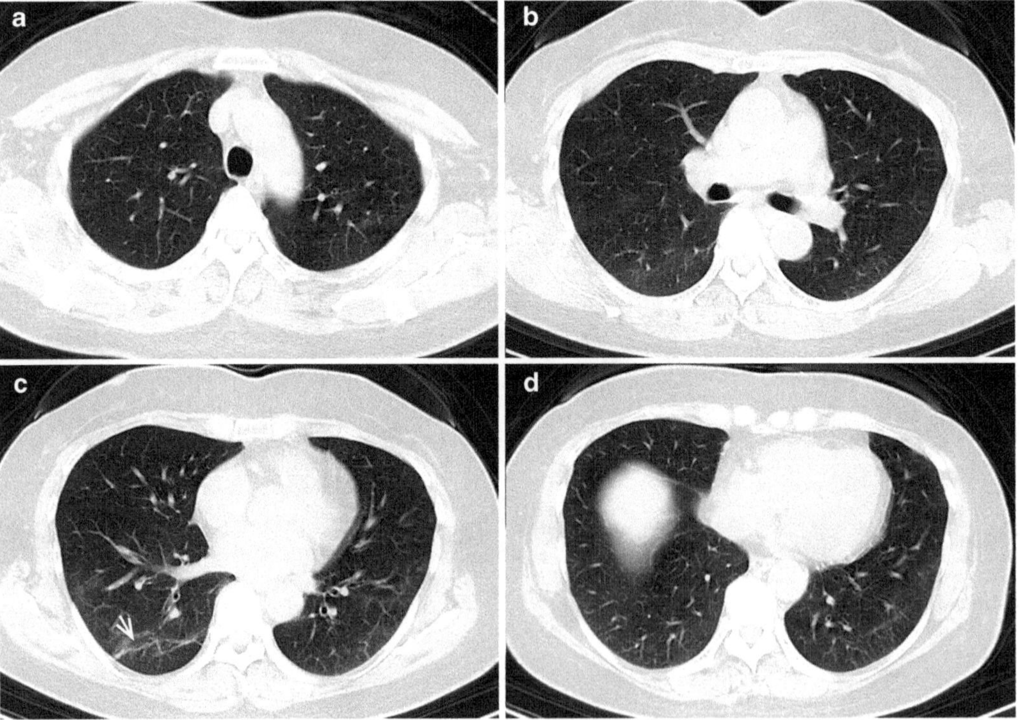

Fig. 4.62 Follow-up CT images 29 days after initial scan

Case 21

Medical History and Clinical Manifestations

A 54-year-old female was admitted in the hospital for 3 days with fever (highest body temperature: 37.4 °C), accompanied by chills and dizziness, no rigor and muscle soreness. Laboratory test results indicated a normal D-dimer of 0.35 mg/L, creatinine of 49 mol/L, ALT of 16 U/L, and potassium of 3.9 mmol/L. There were elevated blood levels for creatine kinase isoenzyme (29 U/L) and lactate dehydrogenase (243 U/L). She denied any contact with persons from Wuhan, China. The SARS-CoV-2 nucleic acid test was positive during hospitalization.

Imaging Features

Initial chest CT showed patchy consolidation in the subpleural region of the left upper lobe with ill-defined borders and air bronchograms (Fig. 4.63).

Follow-up chest CT (5 days after initial CT examination) showed the progression of lesions, including the enlarged consolidation in the left upper lobe and multiple patchy consolidation in both lungs, some with crazy-paving signs and thickening of blood vessels (Fig. 4.64).

Follow-up chest CT (17 days after initial CT examination) showed that the multiple consolidations in both lungs resolved, showing GGOs and fibrosis (Fig. 4.65).

Comments: This case showed the dynamic progressive pattern of chest CT in a COVID-19 patient. The image findings of the patient were typical.

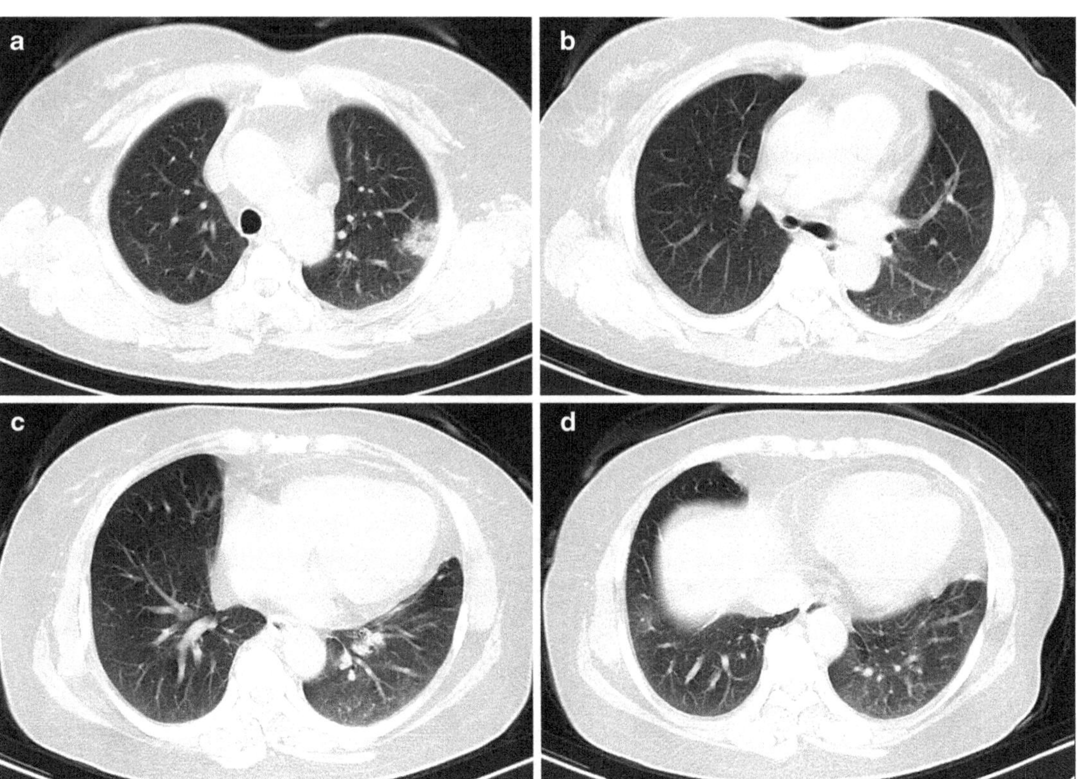

Fig. 4.63 Initial CT image

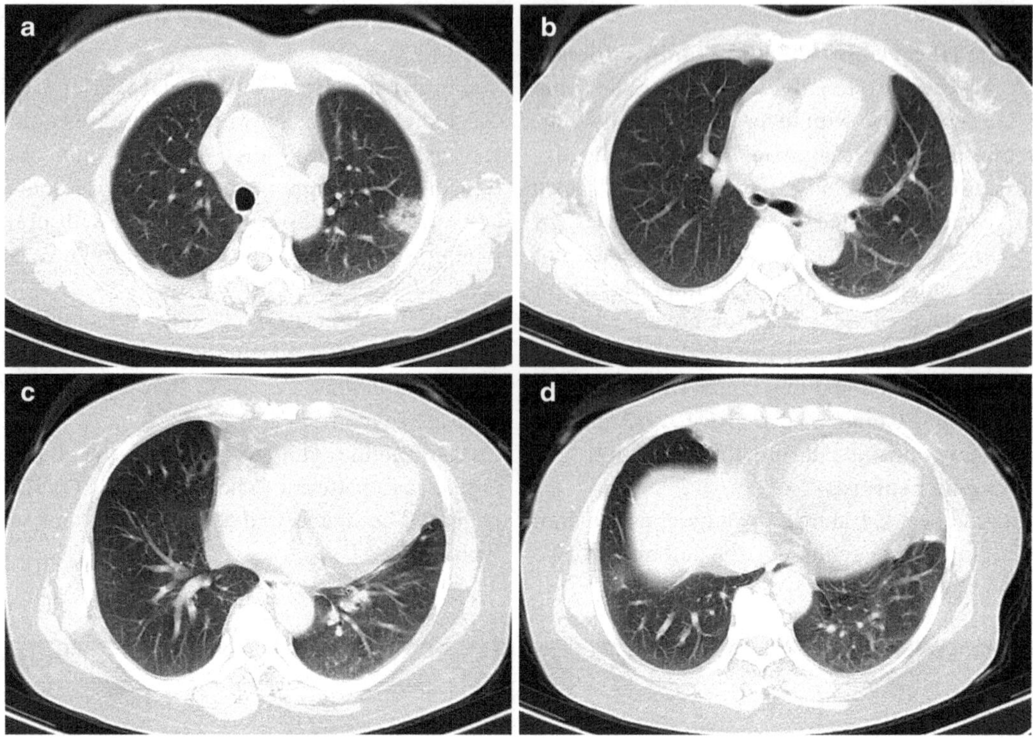

Fig. 4.64 Follow-up CT images 5 days after initial scan

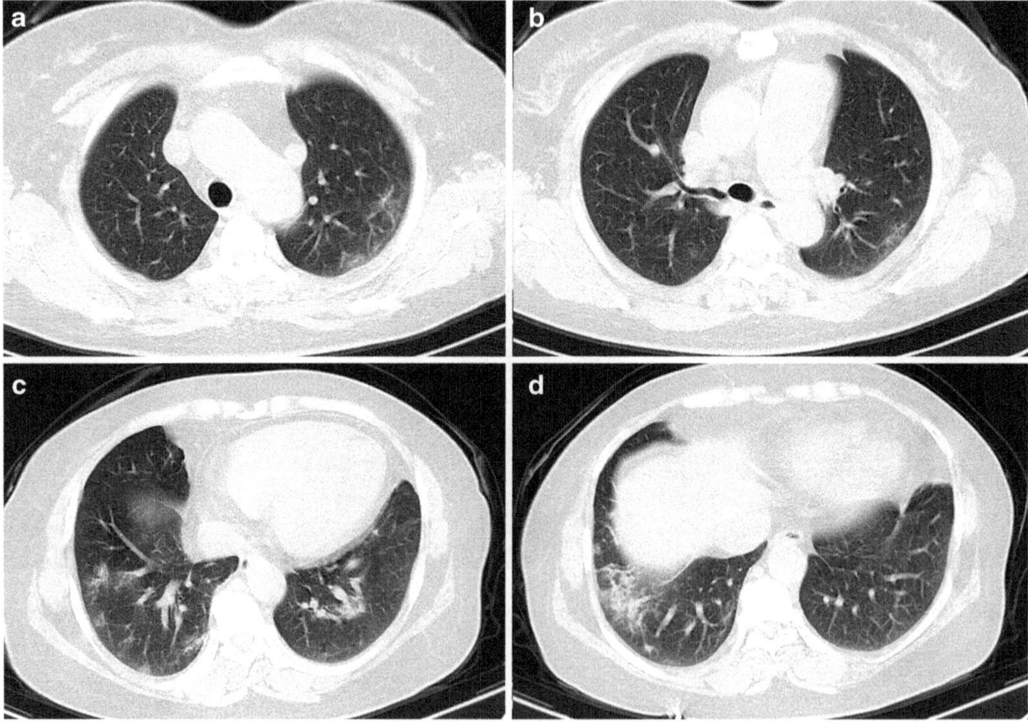

Fig. 4.65 Follow-up CT images 17 days after initial scan

Case 22

Medical History and Clinical Manifestations

A 26-year-old male was admitted in the hospital for 3 days with cough (paroxysms dry cough), without chills and fever. Laboratory test results indicated a decreased white blood cell count of 3.25×10^9/L, neutrophil count of 1.76×10^9/L, and platelet count of 98×10^9/L. There was an elevated blood level for C-reactive protein (11.4 mg/L). He contacted workers returning from Wuhan, China in the days prior to symptom onset. The SARS-CoV-2 nucleic acid test was positive during hospitalization.

Imaging Features

Initial chest CT showed ground-glass nodules in the left upper lobe and the right lower lobe, with vascular thickening (Fig. 4.66).

Follow-up chest CT (5 days after initial CT examination) showed the progression of the lesions, involving multiple lobes, showing a subpleural distribution of GGOs with thickening of blood vessels (Fig. 4.67).

On the tenth day, reexamination of chest CT showed that that the multiple ground-glass opacities turned to be consolidated, with twisted and dilated bronchi (Fig. 4.68).

After 14 days follow-up and reexamination, CT showed the multiple consolidations of both lungs resolved, showing ground-glass opacities (Fig. 4.69).

Comments: The initial chest CT of this patient showed ground-glass nodules, which were atypical in COVID-19. Five days later, it showed typical subpleural ground-glass opacities. Most lesions resolved after 23 days' treatment.

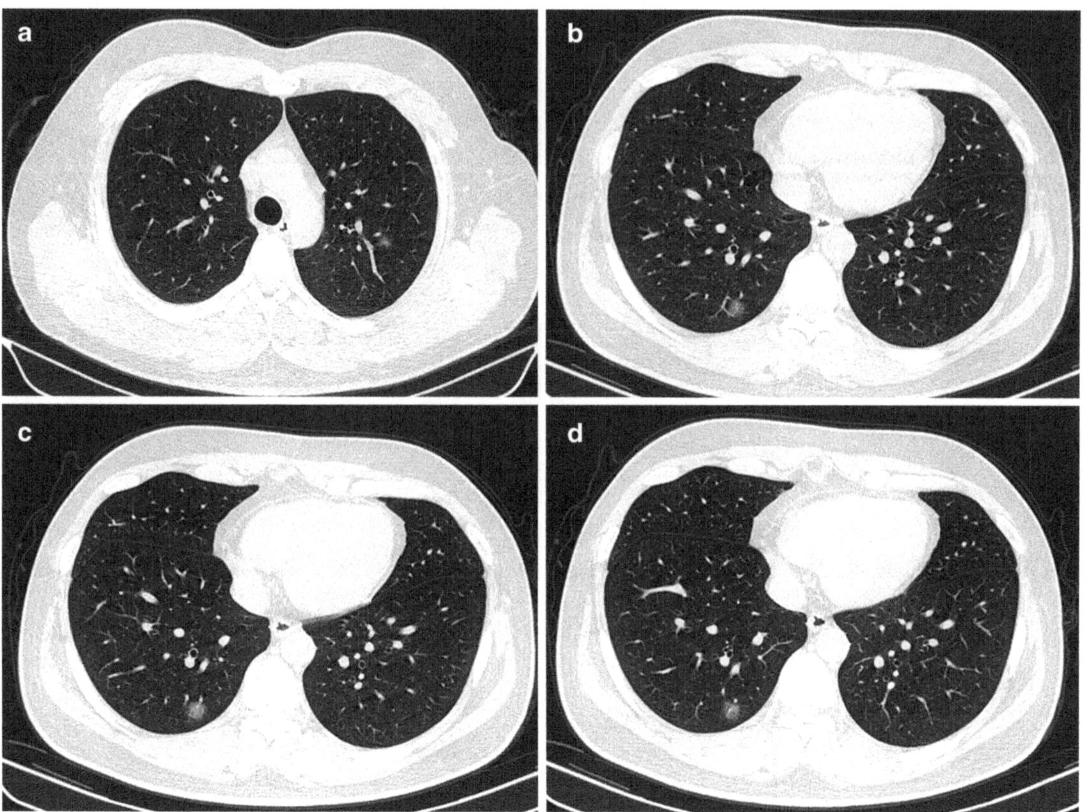

Fig. 4.66 Initial CT image

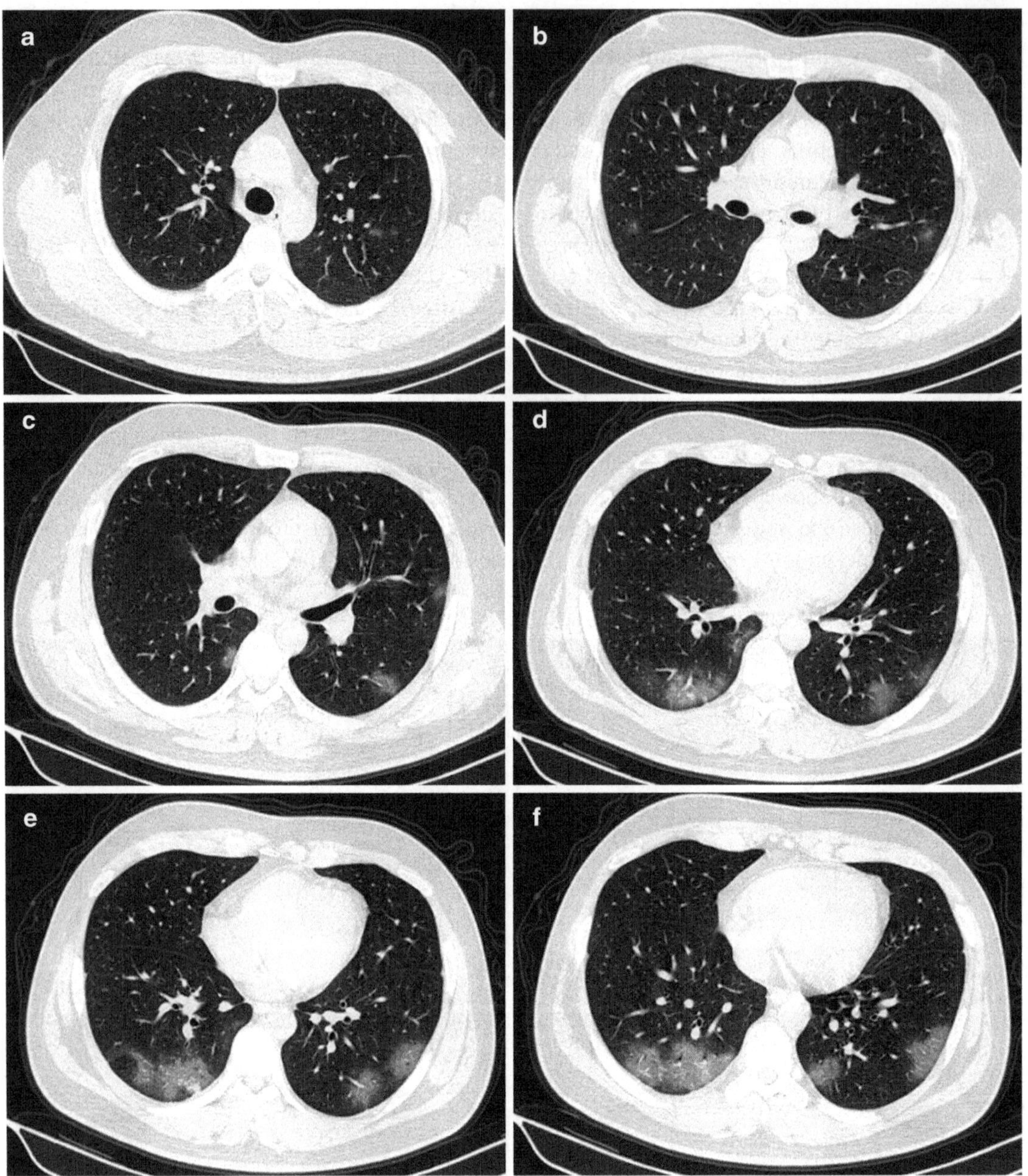

Fig. 4.67 Follow-up CT images 5 days after initial scan

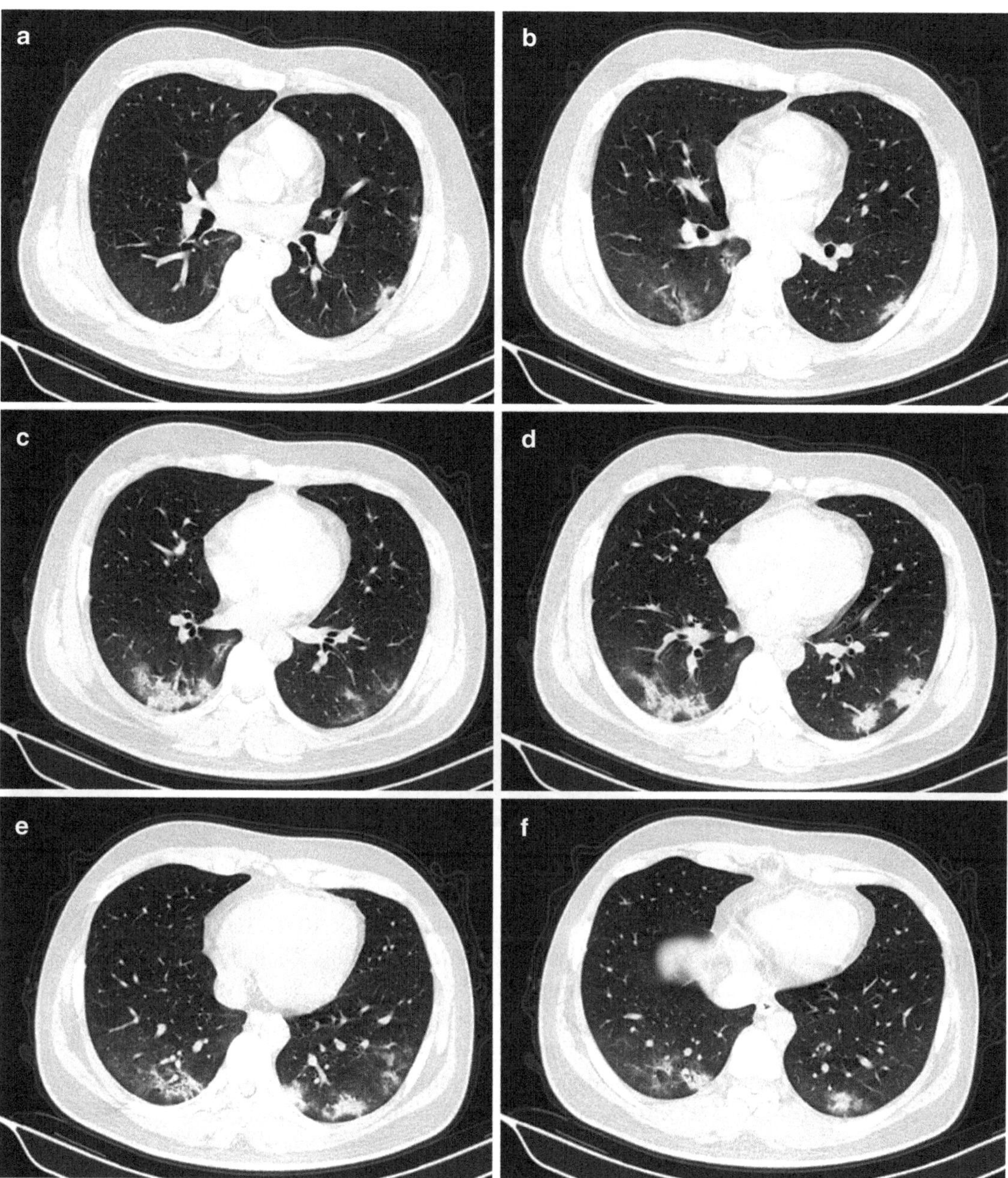

Fig. 4.68 Follow-up CT images 10 days after initial scan

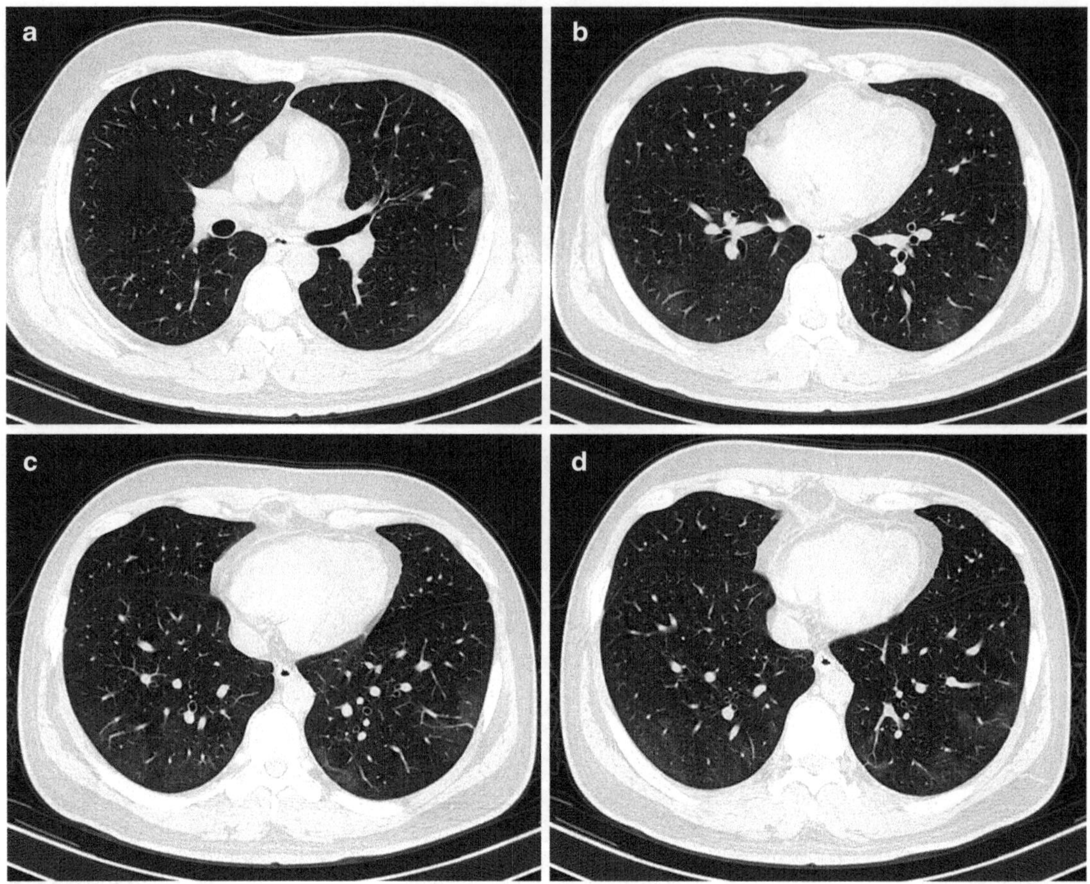

Fig. 4.69 Follow-up CT images 23 days after initial scan

Case 23
Medical History and Clinical Manifestations

A 28-year-old male was admitted in the hospital for 1 week with fever (highest body temperature: 37.8 °C), accompanied by sore throat and headache. Laboratory test results indicated a normal white blood cell count of 5.95×10^9/L, neutrophil count of 4.88×10^9/L, and C-reactive protein of 4.0 mg/L. There was a decreased lymphocytic count of 0.56×10^9/L. He traveled from Wuhan, China to Yueqing, Zhejiang Province, China prior to symptom onset. The SARS-CoV-2 nucleic acid test was positive during hospitalization.

Imaging Features

Initial chest CT showed a subpleural ground-glass nodule with "halo sign" (**a**: white arrow) in the posterior basal segment of the right lower lobe (Fig. 4.70).

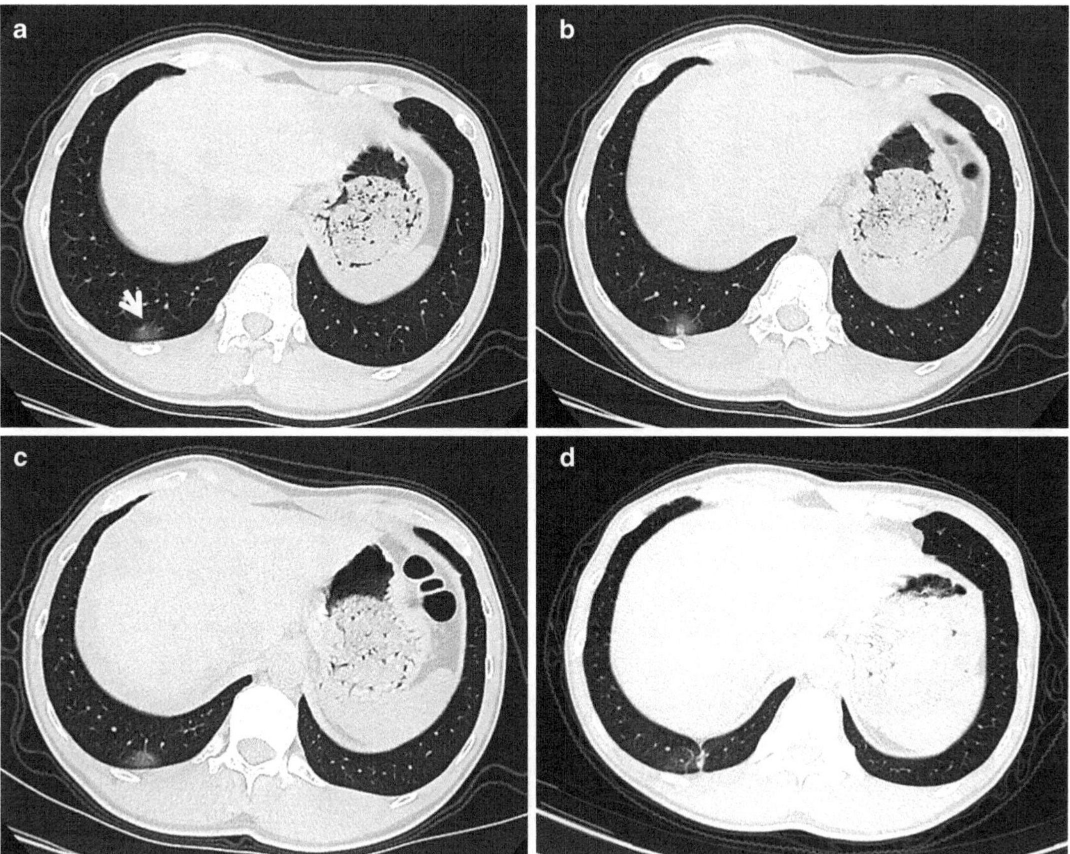

Fig. 4.70 Initial CT image

Follow-up chest CT (10 days after initial CT examination) showed patchy consolidation in the right lower lobe, with a ground-glass edge and air bronchograms (Fig. 4.71).

On the 33th day, reexamination of chest CT showed that the consolidations in the right lower lobe resolved, showing ground-glass opacities and fibrosis (Fig. 4.72).

Comments: The chest CT of this young male showed the typical progressive pattern of COVID-19. The initial CT showed a subpleural ground-glass nodule in the right lower lobe. The lesion was enlarged, consolidated, and gradually resolved.

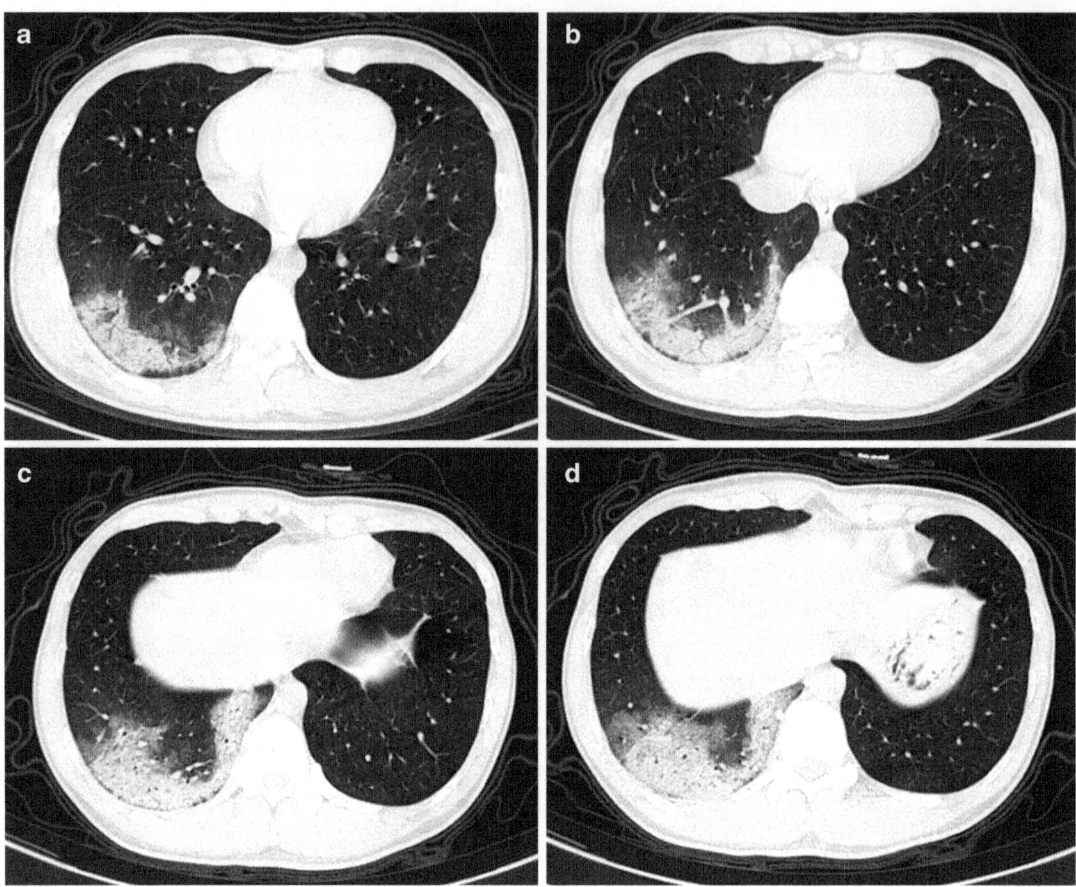

Fig. 4.71 Follow-up CT images 10 days after initial scan

Case 24

Medical History and Clinical Manifestations

A 35-year-old female was admitted in the hospital for 6 days with lung infection in CT, without any symptoms. Laboratory test result indicated a normal blood level of C-reactive protein (8.0 mg/L). She contacted returnees from Wuhan, China. The SARS-CoV-2 nucleic acid test was positive during hospitalization.

Imaging Features

Initial chest CT showed subpleural consolidation in the right lower lobe, with a ground-glass border and air bronchograms (Fig. 4.73).

Follow-up chest CT (8 days after initial CT examination) showed that the consolidation resolved completely and newly developed ground-glass opacities were in the right lower lobe, with air bronchograms (Fig. 4.74).

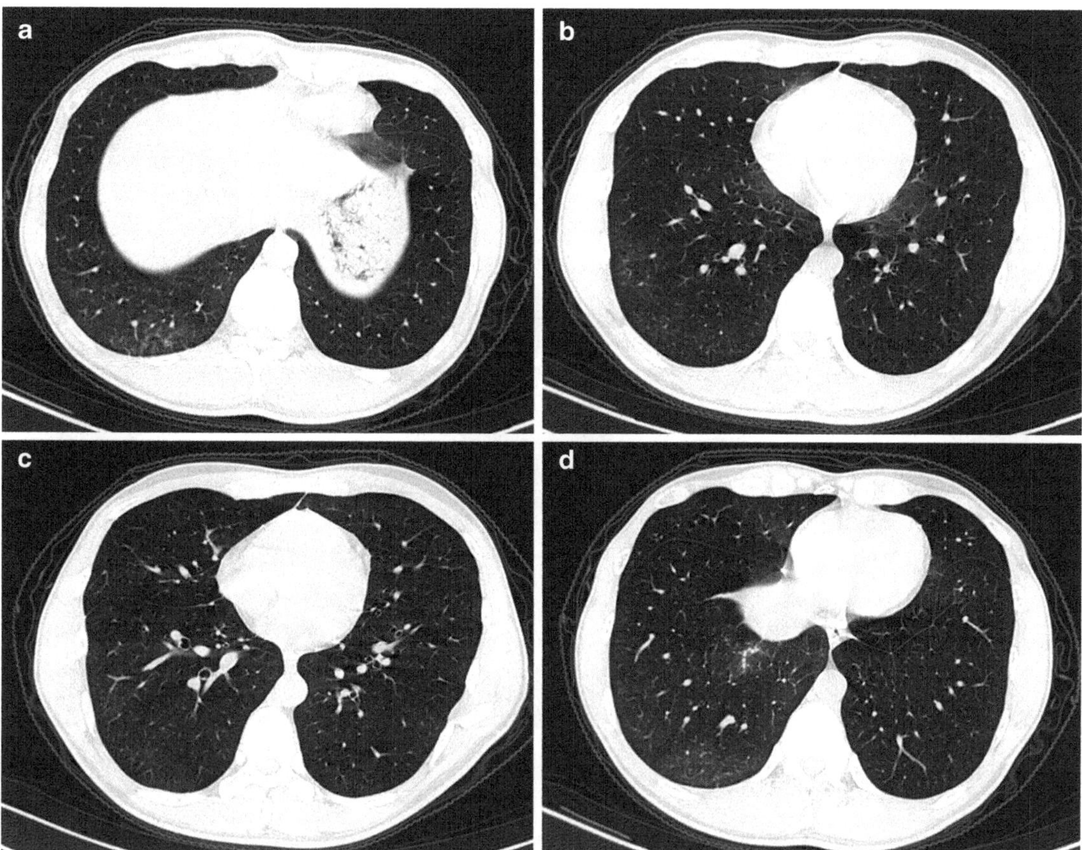

Fig. 4.72 Follow-up CT images 33 days after initial scan

After 14 days follow-up and reexamination, CT showed that the patchy ground-glass opacities resolved, showing patchy consolidation, with "reticular pattern" and parenchymal bands (Fig. 4.75).

On the 29th day, reexamination of chest CT showed that the lesions were almost resolved (Fig. 4.76).

Comments: This patient had no clinical symptoms at the beginning. The imaging features were that the focus was located in the axial region of the lung, dissipated rapidly, and then typical focus appeared in the subpleural region.

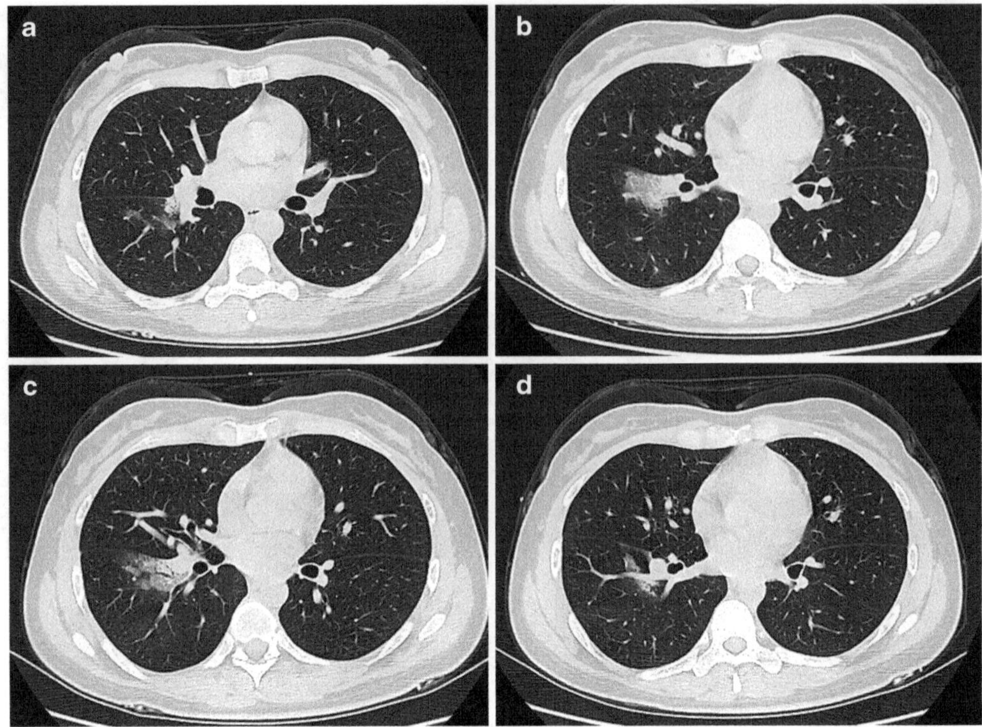

Fig. 4.73 Initial CT image

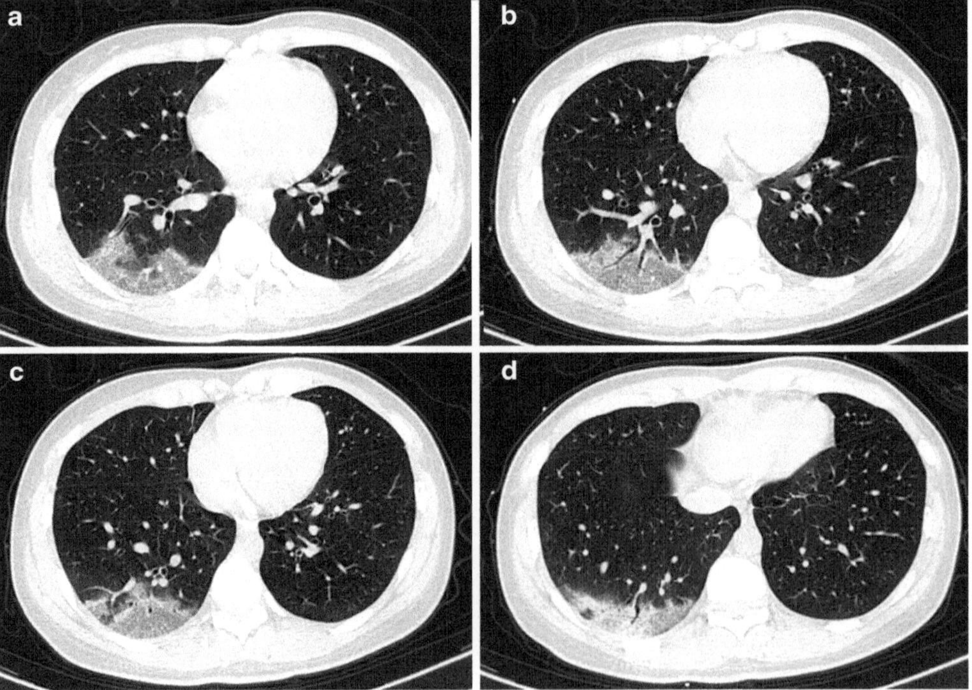

Fig. 4.74 Follow-up CT images 8 days after initial scan

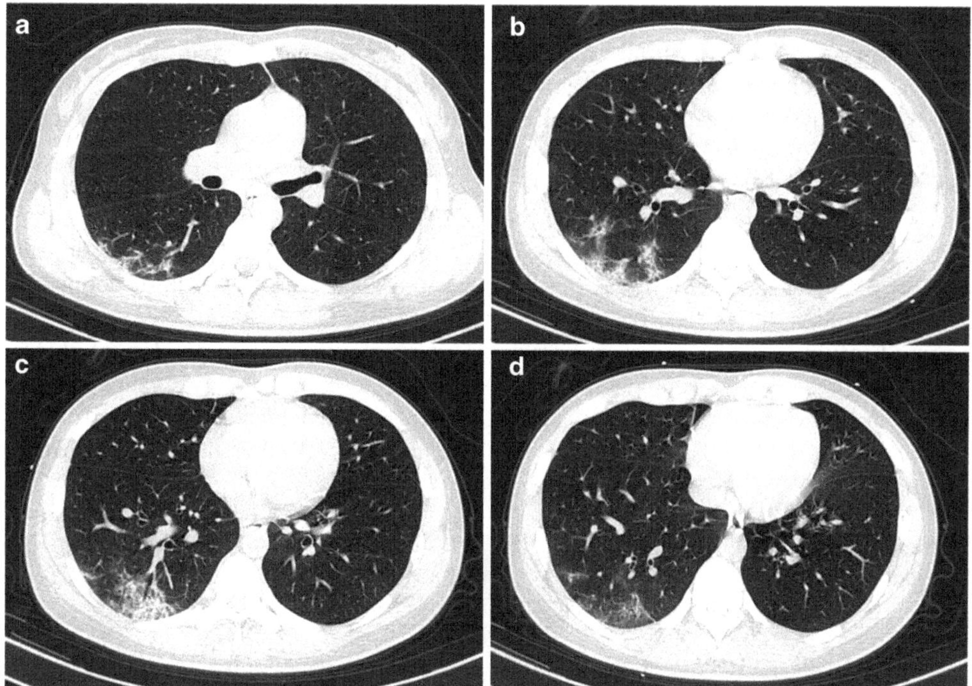

Fig. 4.75 Follow-up CT images 14 days after initial scan

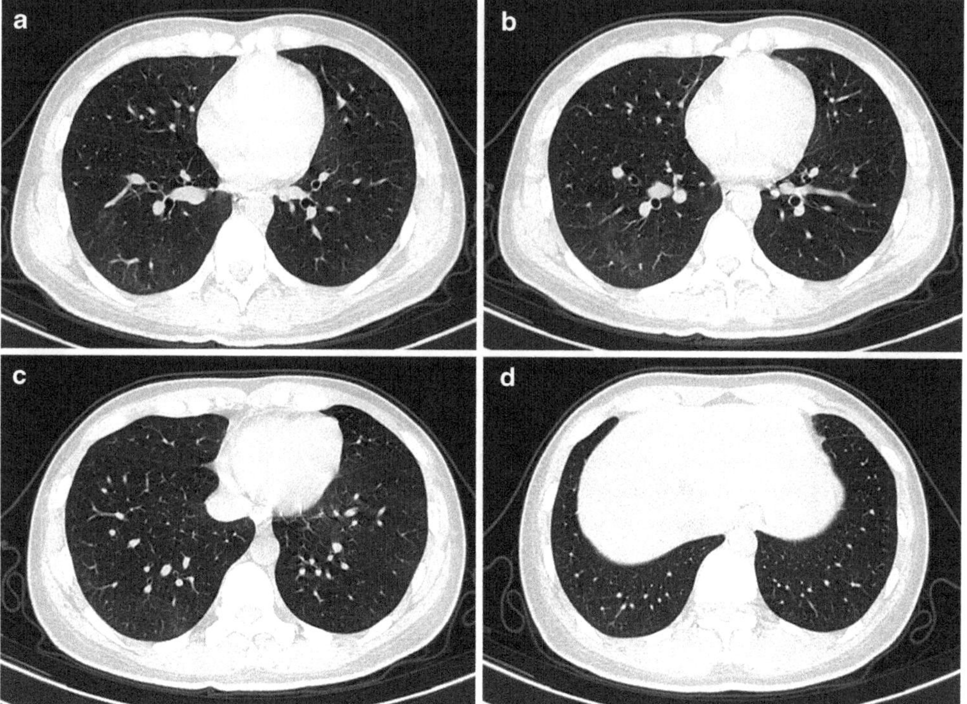

Fig. 4.76 Follow-up CT images 29 days after initial scan

Case 25

Medical History and Clinical Manifestations

A 54-year-old female was admitted in the hospital for 15 days with cough and sputum production, without fever and chills. Laboratory test result indicated an elevated blood level for C-reactive protein (48.7 mg/L). She returned to home from Wuhan, China before symptom onset. The SARS-CoV-2 nucleic acid test was positive during hospitalization.

Imaging Features

Initial chest CT showed subpleural patchy GGOs of both lungs with "reversed halo signs" (white arrows) (Fig. 4.77).

Follow-up chest CT (10 days after initial CT examination) showed that the subpleural lesions of both lungs resolved slightly, with ill-defined borders and thickening of blood vessels (Fig. 4.78).

Follow-up chest CT (19 days after initial CT examination) showed that the subpleural lesions of both lungs resolved, appeared as ground-glass opacities with ill-defined borders (Fig. 4.79).

Comments: The initial CT of this patient showed "reversed halo signs," suggesting that the patient had been infected for a period of time. And the lesions resolved gradually after treatment.

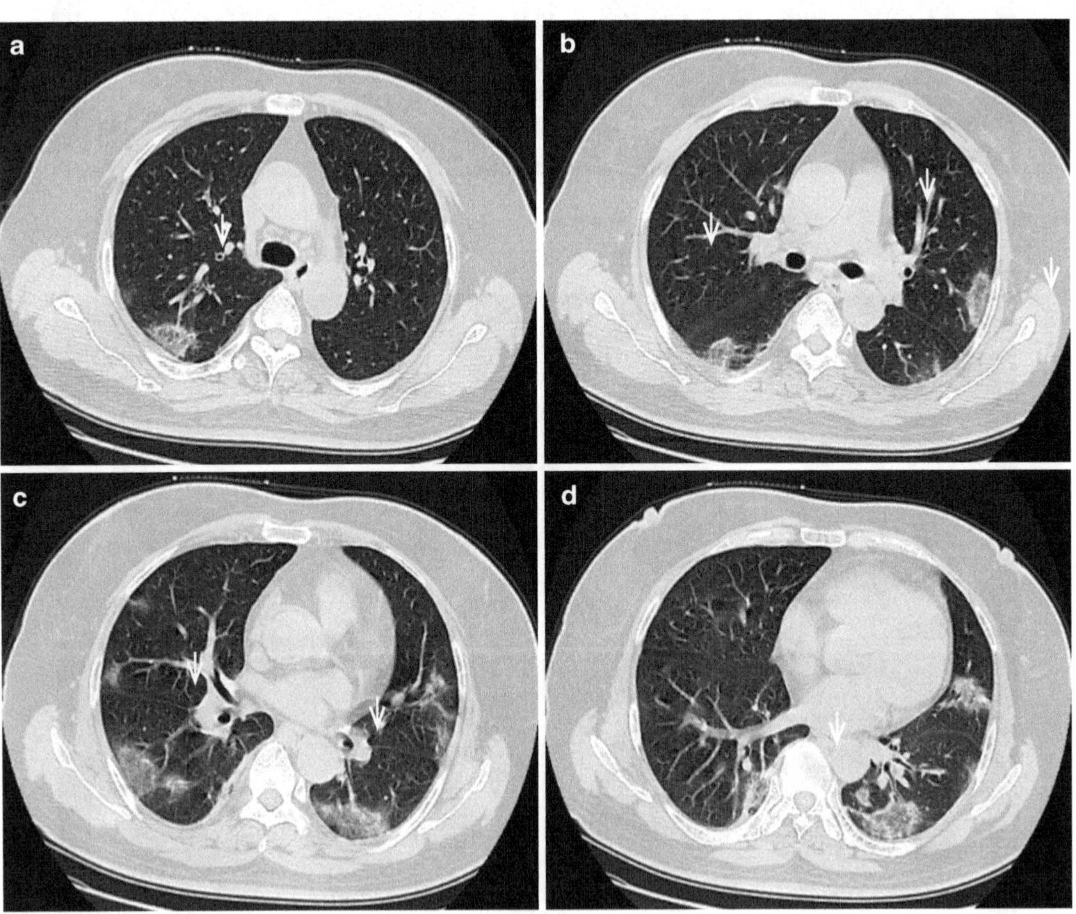

Fig. 4.77 Initial CT image

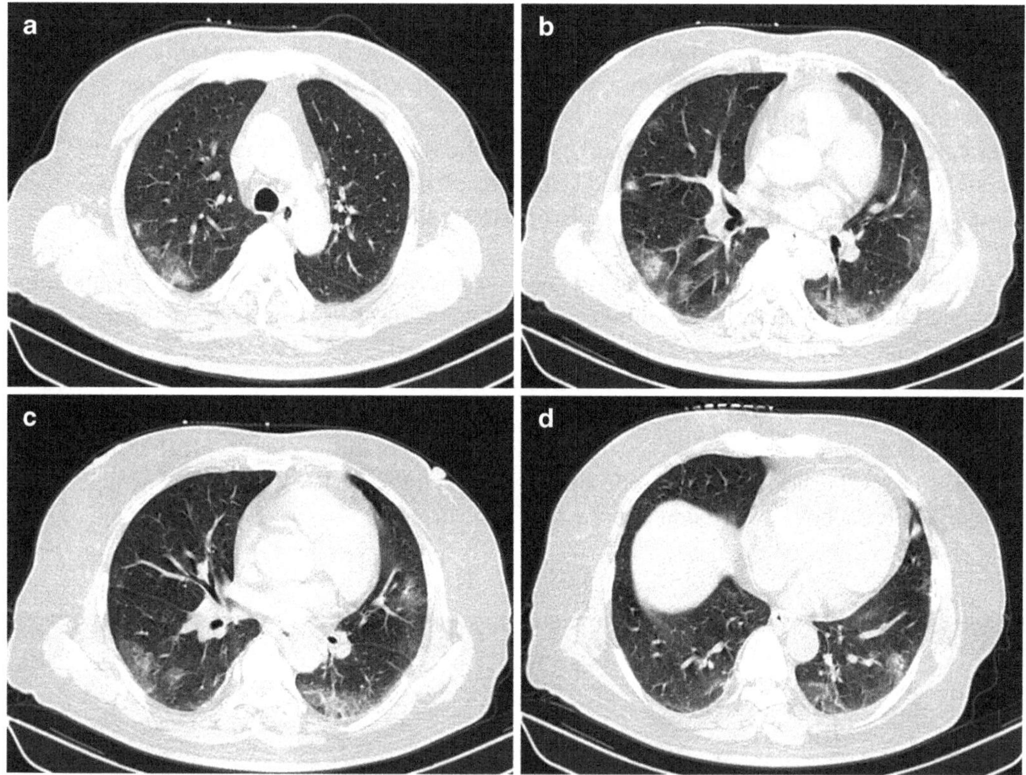

Fig. 4.78 Follow-up CT images 10 days after initial scan

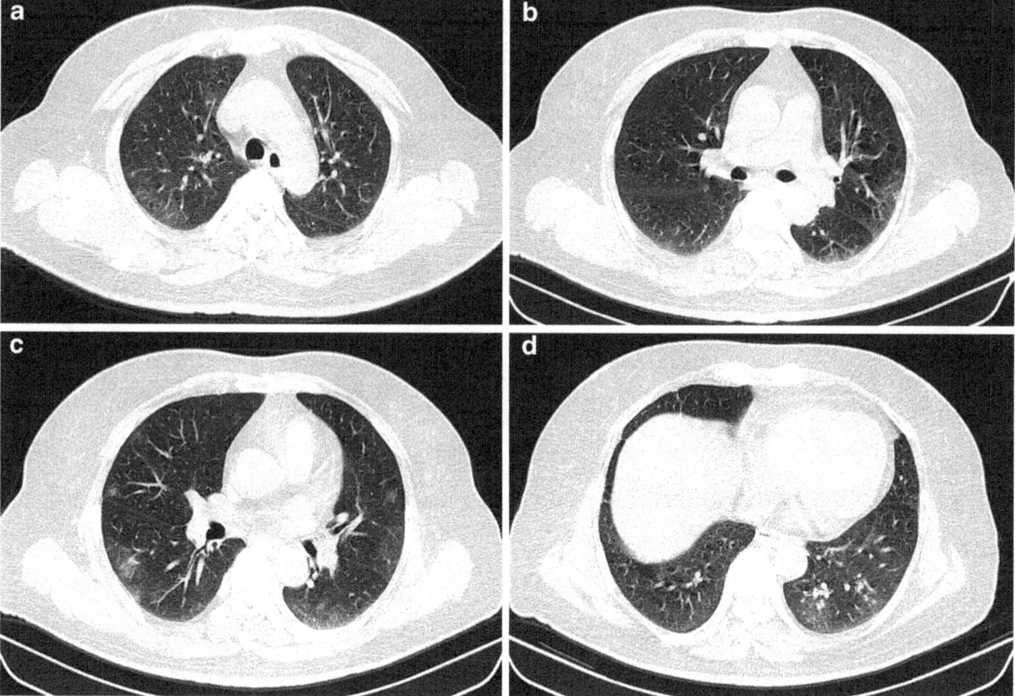

Fig. 4.79 Follow-up CT images 19 days after initial scan

Case 26

Medical History and Clinical Manifestations

A 46-year-old female was admitted in the hospital for 4 days with fever (highest body temperature: 39.5 °C), without chills and rigor. Laboratory test results indicated decreased lymphocytes of 19.9% and increased neutrophils of 73.0%. There were normal blood levels for eosinophils (0.3%), C-reactive protein (5.9 mg/L), and erythrocyte sedimentation rate (28.0 mm/h). She denied any contact with people in Wuhan, China. The SARS-CoV-2 nucleic acid test was positive during hospitalization.

Imaging Features

Initial chest CT showed patchy consolidation along the bronchovascular bundle in the left lower lobe, with ill-defined borders and air bronchograms (**a**, **b**: red arrows) (Fig. 4.80).

Follow-up chest CT (12 days after initial CT examination) showed that the consolidation lesion in the left lower lobe partly resolved, showing mixed ground-glass shadows (Fig. 4.81).

Follow-up chest CT (28 days after initial CT examination) showed that the consolidation in the left lower lobe resolved completely, showing ill-defined GGOs (Fig. 4.82).

Comments: This patient had no clear epidemiological history, but the clinical and imaging features were typical of the COVID-19, and the SARS-CoV-2 nucleic acid test was confirmed.

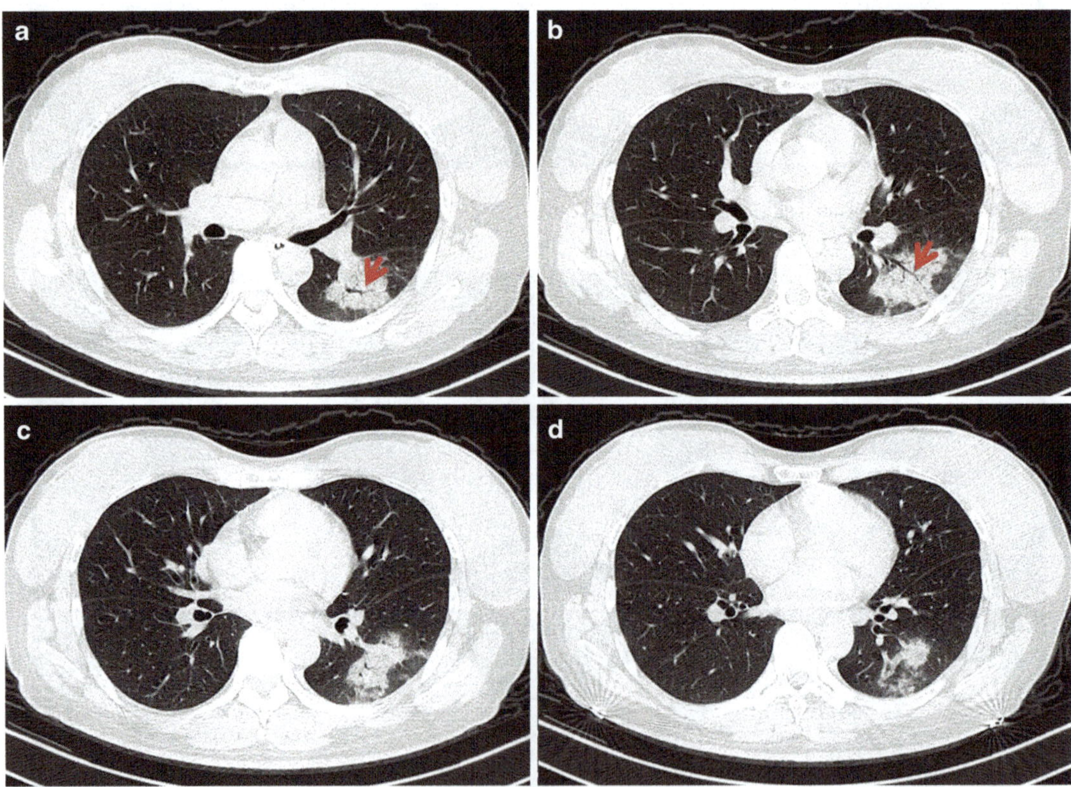

Fig. 4.80 Initial CT image

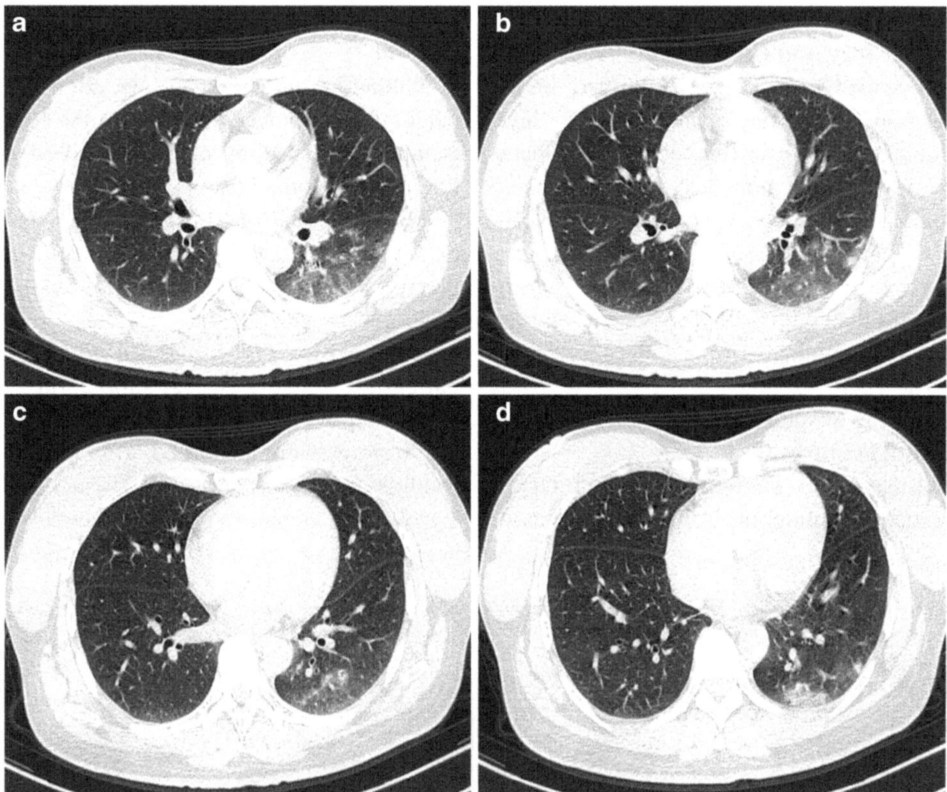

Fig. 4.81 Follow-up CT images 12 days after initial scan

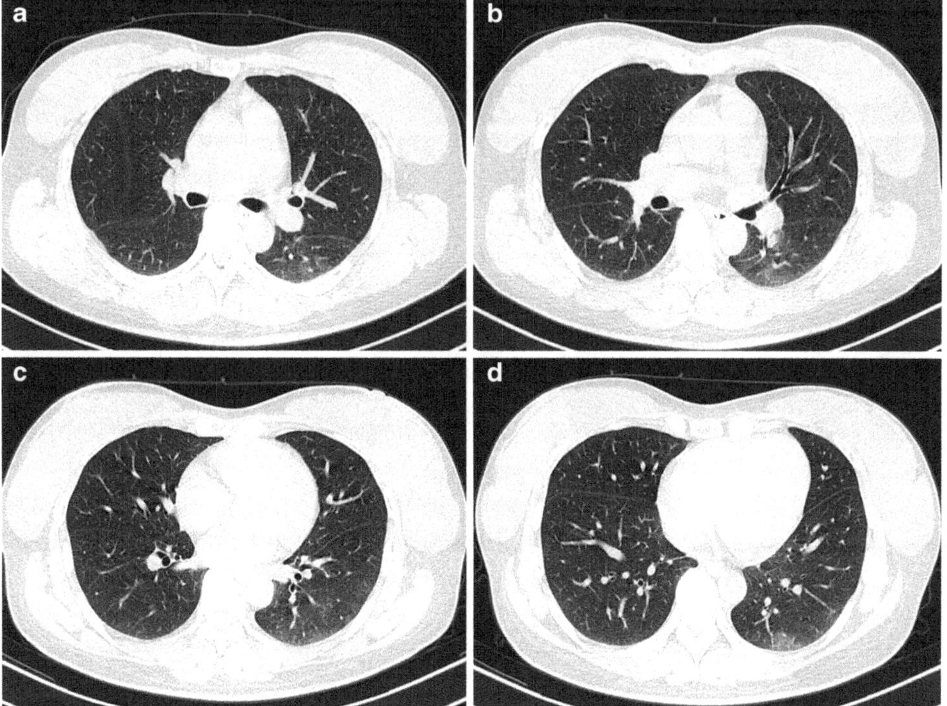

Fig. 4.82 Follow-up CT images 28 days after initial scan

Case 27

Medical History and Clinical Manifestations

A 56-year-old female was admitted in the hospital with cough and sputum for 15 days, and relatively early fever (highest body temperature: 37.5 °C). Laboratory test results indicated a normal white blood cell count of 4.04×10^9 /L, 38.0% neutrophils, 49.0% lymphocytes, and platelet count of 352×10^9/L. The C-reactive protein was less than 5.0 mg/L. The patient returned to home from Wuhan, China before symptom onset. The SARS-CoV-2 nucleic acid test was positive during hospitalization.

Imaging Features

Initial chest CT showed subpleural GGOs with partial consolidation in the lower lobes of both lungs. A few small vessels were thickened (Fig. 4.83).

Follow-up chest CT (9 days after initial CT examination) showed that most of the subpleural ground-glass shadow in the lower lobe of both lungs was absorbed (Fig. 4.84).

Follow-up chest CT (26 days after initial CT examination) showed that the subpleural ground-glass shadow of the lower lobe of both lungs was almost absorbed (Fig. 4.85).

Comments: The initial CT images of the patient presented a typical subpleural ground-glass shadow with a grid shape change, and the lesions were absorbed after 26 days of treatment.

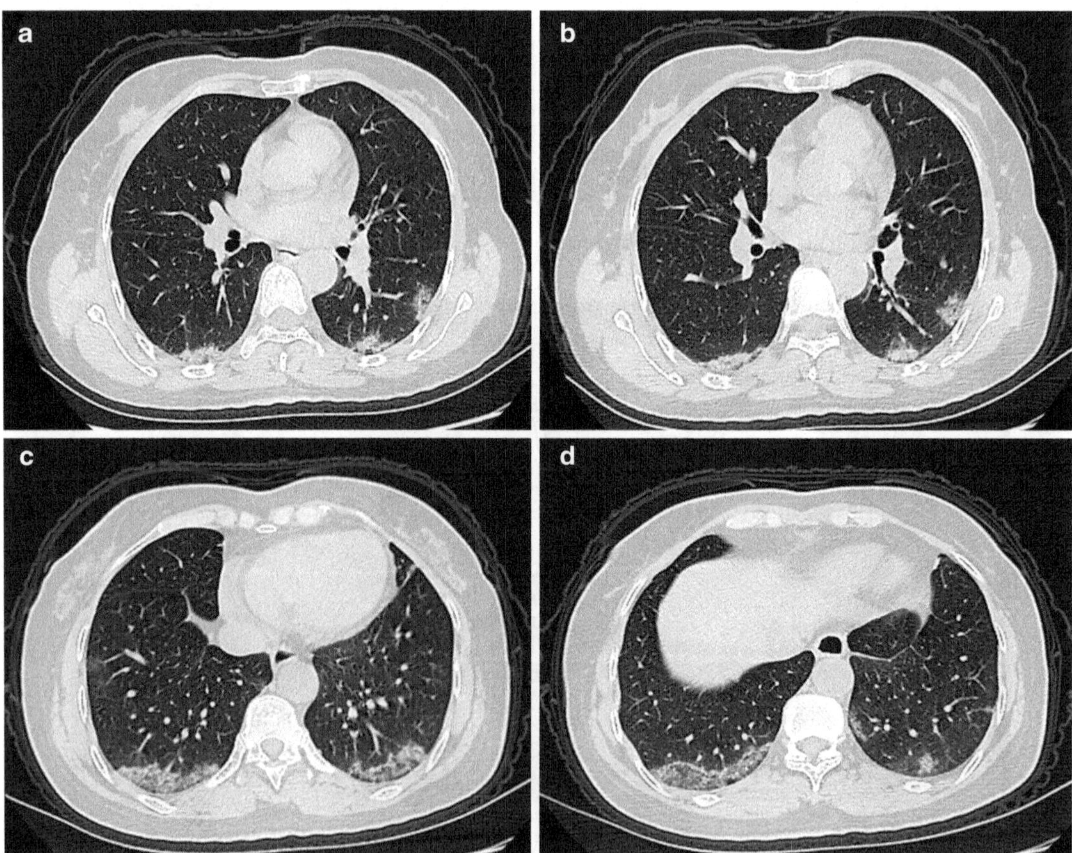

Fig. 4.83 Initial CT images

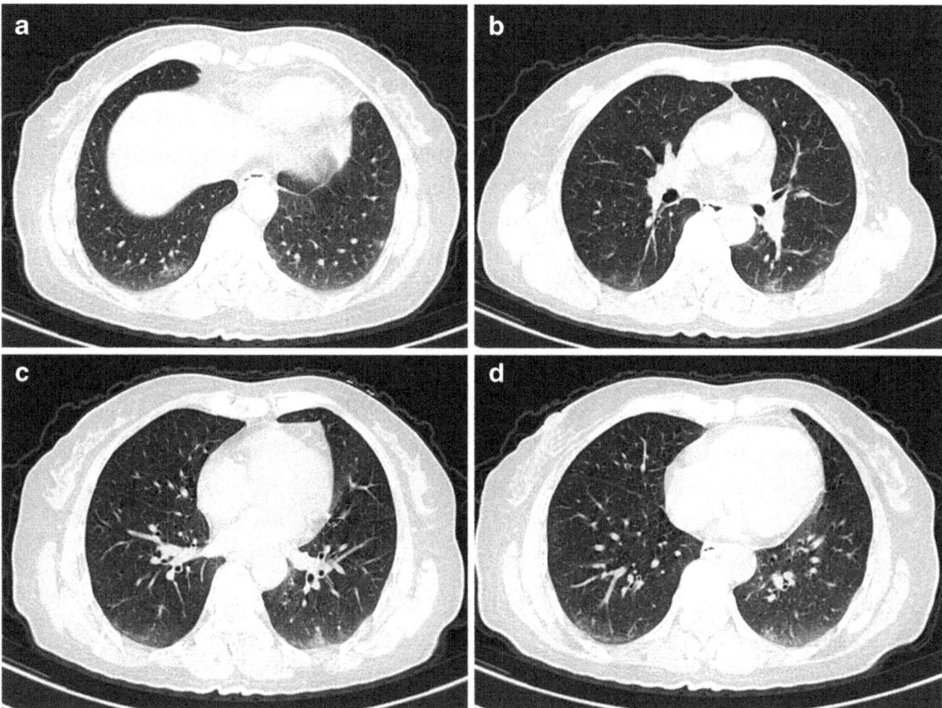

Fig. 4.84 Follow-up CT images 9 days after initial scan

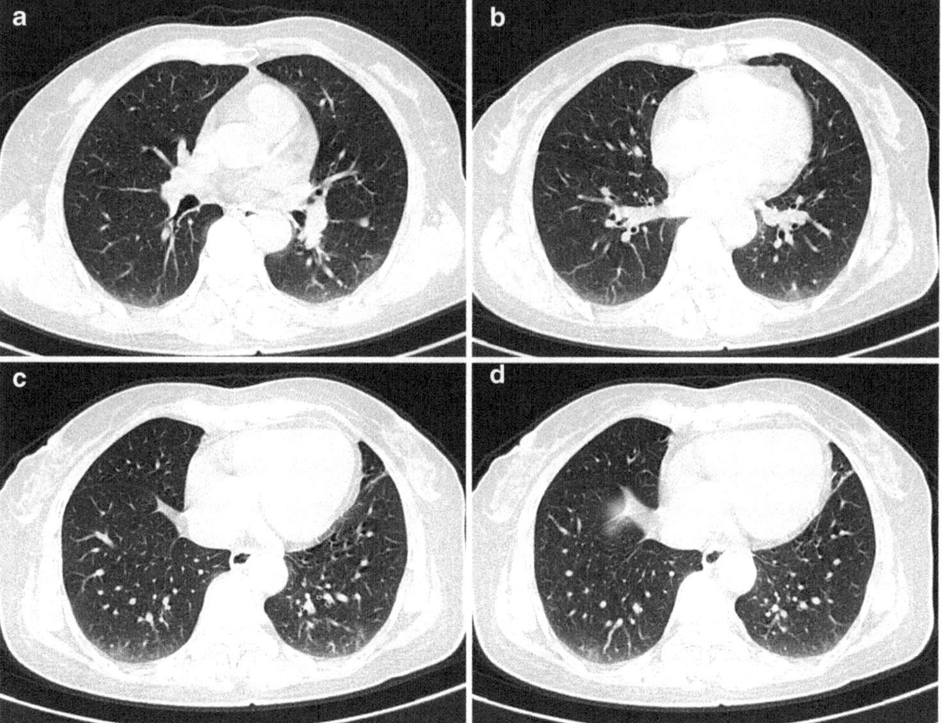

Fig. 4.85 Follow-up CT images 26 days after initial scan

Case 28

Medical History and Clinical Manifestations

A 48-year-old male was admitted in the hospital with systemic fatigue accompanied by headache and diarrhea for 8 days. Laboratory test results indicated elevated C-reactive protein (34.1 mg/L). The patient returned home from Wuhan, China before symptom onset. The SARS-CoV-2 nucleic acid test was positive during hospitalization.

Imaging Features

Initial chest CT showed patchy ground-glass shadow with unclear boundary and thickened vascular in the subpleural or around bronchovascular bundle of the lower lobe of the right lung (Fig. 4.86).

Follow-up chest CT (6 days after initial CT examination) showed that the ground-glass shadow of the lower lobe of the right lung was

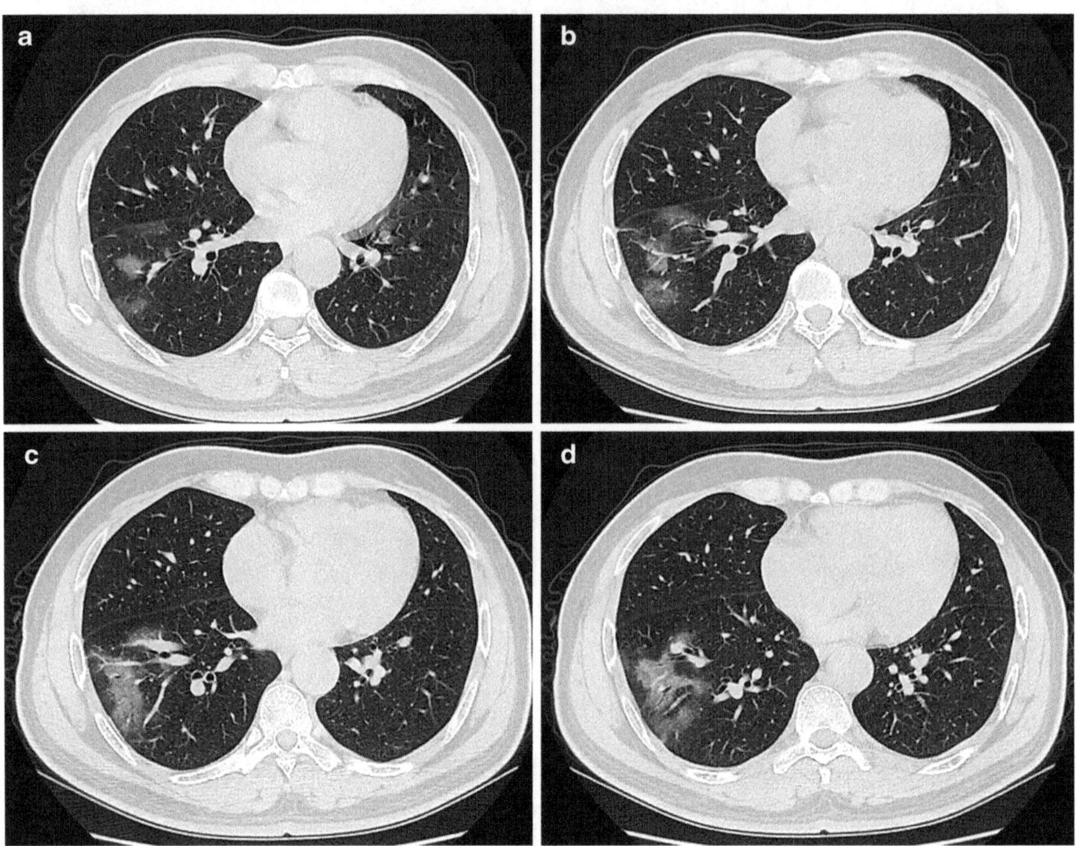

Fig. 4.86 Initial CT images

reduced, the scope was narrowed, and fibrosis was observed inside (Fig. 4.87).

After 13 days follow-up and reexamination, CT showed further absorption of the disease, remained light ground-glass shadow in the lower lobe of the right lung with unclear boundary (Fig. 4.88).

Comments: The main clinical manifestations of the patient's first visit were headache and gastrointestinal symptoms, without respiratory symptoms, but chest CT was a typical manifestation of COVID-19, showing a subpleural ground-glass shadow and a thickened vascular shadow. The ground-glass lesions were gradually absorbed, and no consolidation was observed.

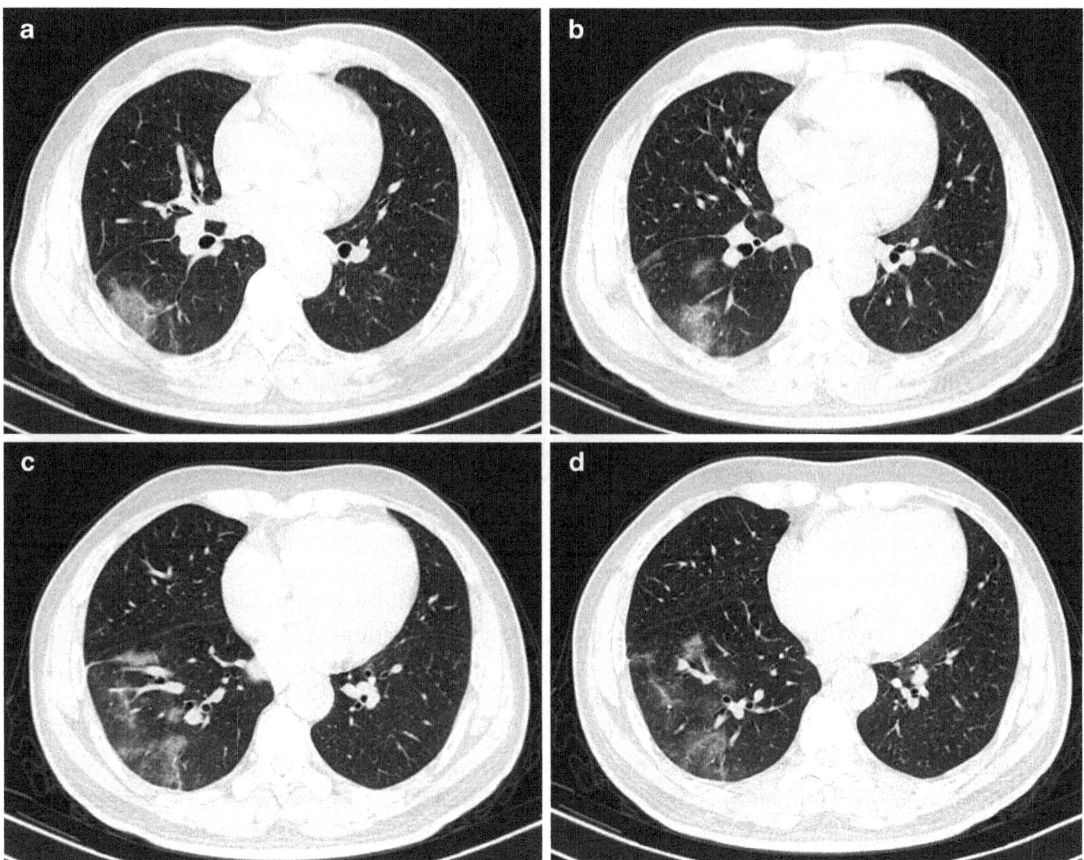

Fig. 4.87 Follow-up CT images 6 days after initial scan

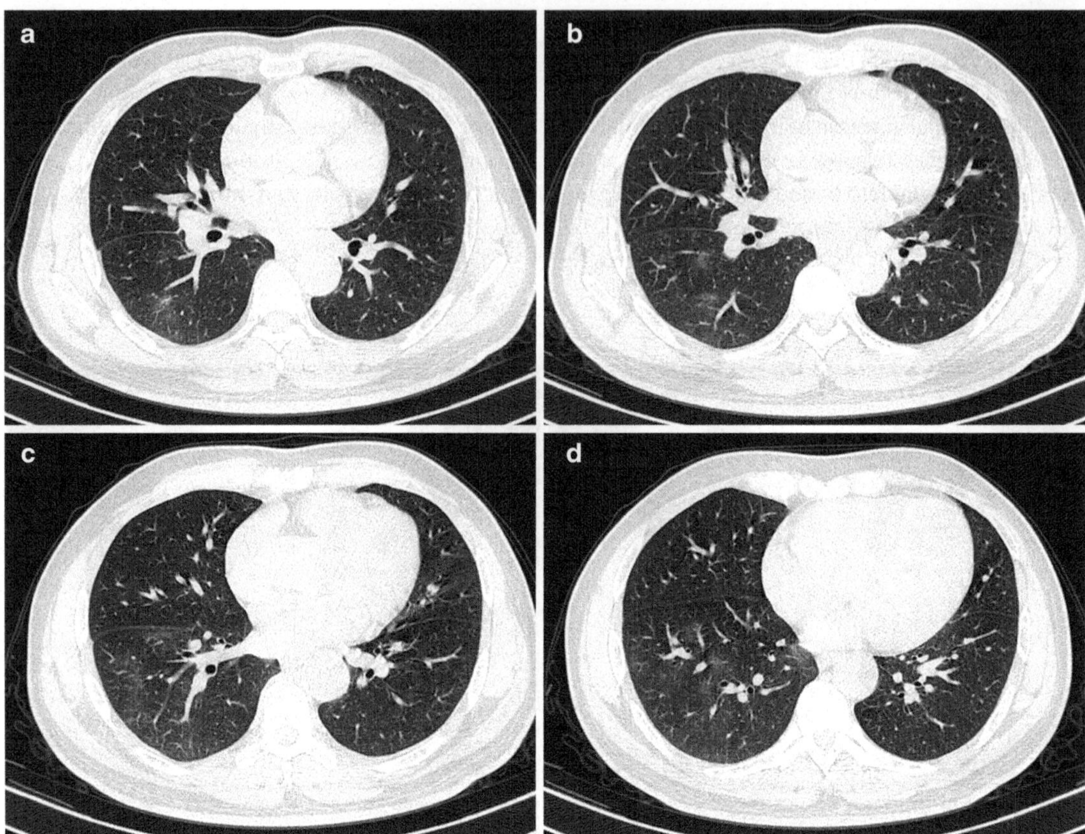

Fig. 4.88 Follow-up CT images 13 days after initial scan

Case 29

Medical History and Clinical Manifestations

A 55-year-old male was admitted in the hospital with fever for 5 days (highest body temperature: 38.6 °C). Laboratory test results indicated a normal white blood cell count of 6.9×10^9/L, 72.7% neutrophils, and 18.1% lymphocytes. There was elevated C-reactive protein (8.63 mg/L). The oxygen saturation at rest was 92.4% on the third day after admission. The patient had no confirmed COVID-19 close contact history. The SARS-CoV-2 nucleic acid test was positive on the day of admission.

Imaging Features

Initial chest CT showed a few small flaky ground-glass shadows under the pleura of both lungs, with blurred edges (Fig. 4.89).

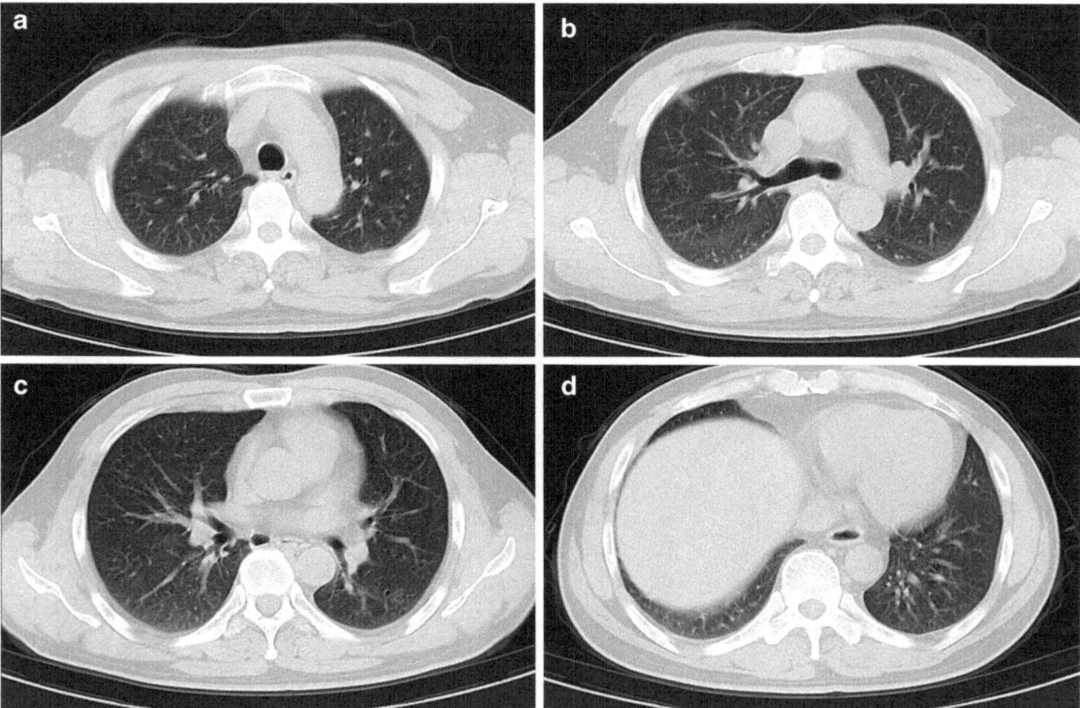

Fig. 4.89 Initial CT images

After 6 days, CT reexamination showed that the lesions developed rapidly, showing diffuse distribution of ground-glass shadows in both lungs, with crazy-paving pattern, gridded changes, thickened blood vessels, and air bronchi signs (Fig. 4.90).

On the 13th day, reexamination of chest CT showed that bilateral lungs presented ground-glass and stripy shadows under the pleura, with clear edges, and the lesions tended to be fibrotic (Fig. 4.91).

Comments: The patient was a common COVID-19 patient at the time of admission, and his condition became worse on the third day after admission, when the oxygen saturation at rest was 92.4%, meanwhile the imaging performance also changed rapidly. The patient was classified as severe case according to clinical and imaging findings.

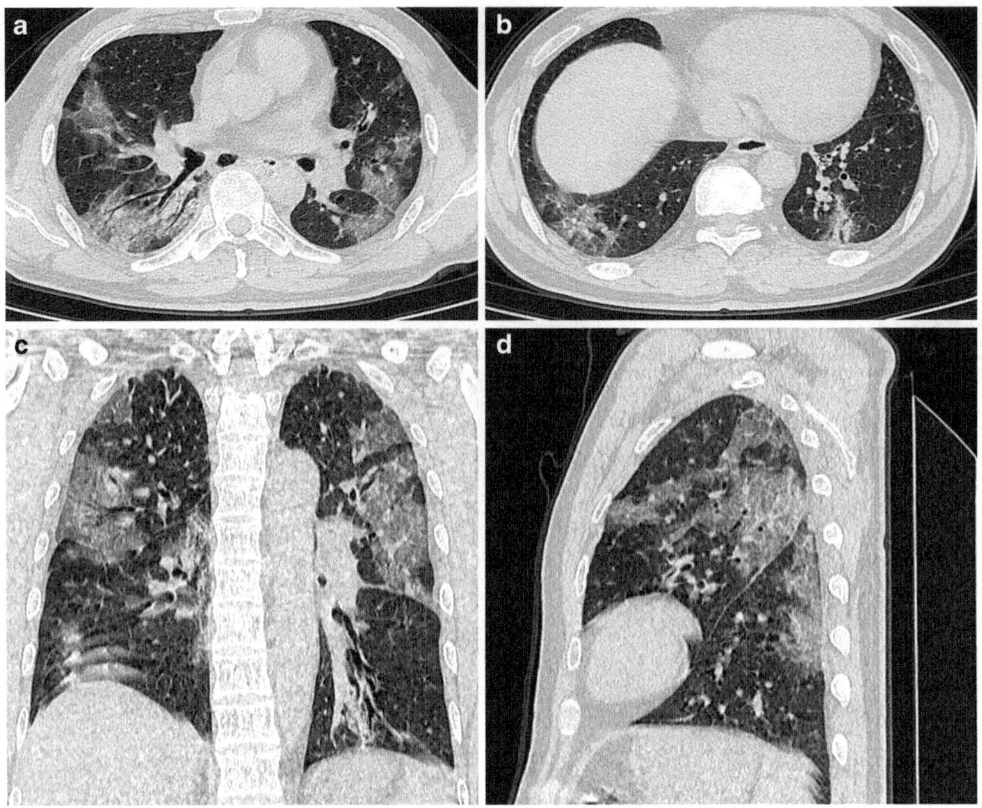

Fig. 4.90 Follow-up CT images 6 days after initial scan

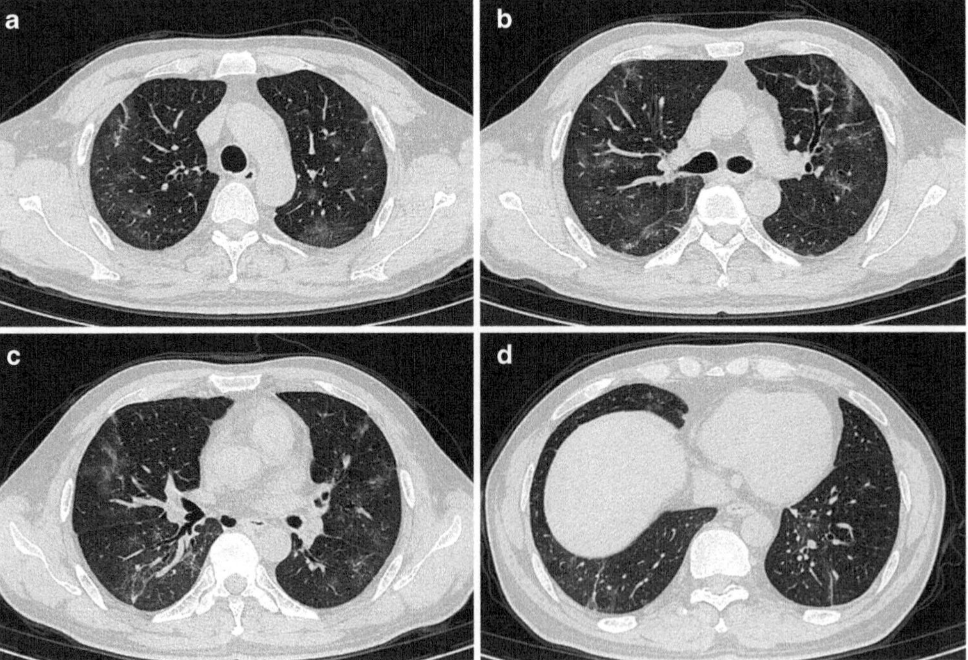

Fig. 4.91 Follow-up CT images 13 days after initial scan

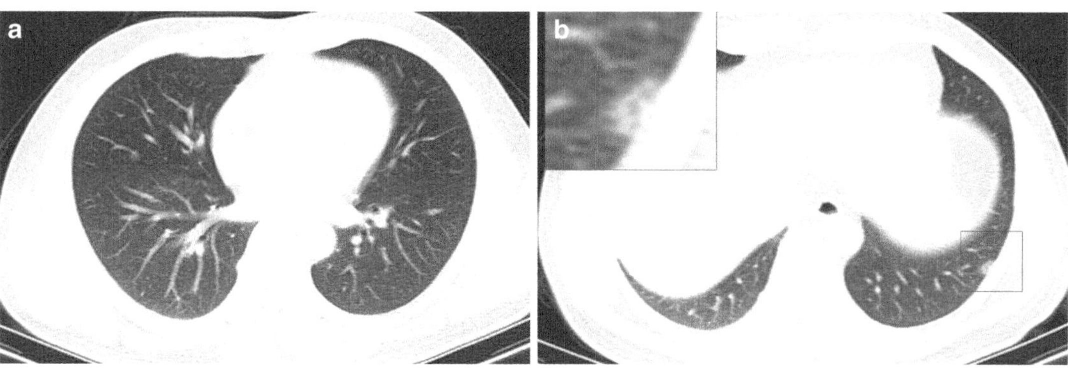

Fig. 4.92 Initial CT images

Case 30

Medical History and Clinical Manifestations

A 41-year-old male patient was hospitalized for cough, expectoration 3 days, fever (maximum temperature 38.8 °C) and fatigue 2 days. Laboratory test results indicated a normal white blood cell count of 7.5×10^9/L, 72.9% neutrophils, and 23.1% lymphocytes. The C-reactive protein was less than 0.499 mg/L. The patient lived in Wuhan, China for nearly half a year. The SARS-CoV-2 nucleic acid test was positive.

Imaging Features

Chest CT showed patchy GGOs in the subpleural areas of both lungs with blurred margins (Fig. 4.92).

Follow-up chest CT (5 days after initial CT examination) showed multiple subpleural consolidation and nodular shadows with blurred edges scattered in bilateral lung fields, The lesions in the middle lobe of the right lung showed air bronchogram (**c**: red arrow), and the subpleural shadow in the lower lobe of the left lung showed obvious progress and increased range compared with the previous slice (Fig. 4.93).

Follow-up chest CT (14 days after initial CT examination) showed multiple consolidation in both lungs, which were flaky and nodular, with subpleural distribution. Fibrous foci appeared (**c**: red arrow) (Fig. 4.94).

Comments: The imaging feature of this patient is that in the course of progression, the main manifestation is consolidation.

Case 31

Medical History and Clinical Manifestations

A 33-year-old male was admitted in the hospital with fever for 2 days (highest body temperature: 37.8 °C). Laboratory tests indicated no obvious abnormalities. The patient had contact history with people returning from Wuhan, China 2 weeks ago. The SARS-CoV-2 nucleic acid test was positive.

Imaging Features

Initial chest CT showed multiple ground-glass shadows thickened blood vessel distribution under the pleura, in both lungs (Fig. 4.95).

Follow-up chest CT (17 days after initial CT examination) showed that multiple ground-glass shadows in both lungs were significantly reduced compared with the scope of the previous lesion, with reticular and striated shadows in the lesion (Fig. 4.96).

Follow-up chest CT (23 days after initial CT examination) showed multiple light GGOs and fibrous lesions in both lungs. The lesion

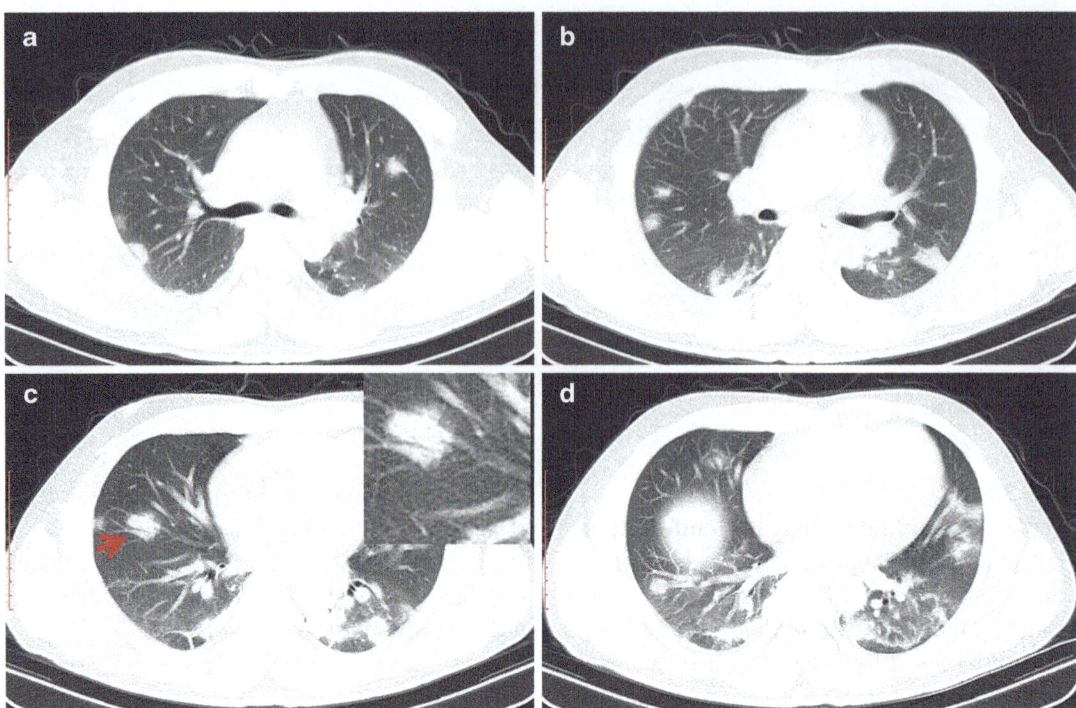

Fig. 4.93 Follow-up CT images 5 days after initial scan

scope was further narrowed and the density was reduced (Fig. 4.97).

Comments: The case shows the dynamic change of CT in a common type of patient. In the course of the development of the lesions, ground-glass shadow was the main feature without alveolar consolidation.

Case 32

Medical History and Clinical Manifestations

A 55-year-old female was admitted in the hospital with fever for 6 days, and occasional cough. Laboratory test results indicated a normal white blood cell count of 5.7×10^9/L, 76.8% neutrophils, and 18.9% lymphocytes. The patient had a history of contact with a confirmed case (the patient's sister). The SARS-CoV-2 nucleic acid test was positive.

Imaging Features

Initial CR chest radiography showed multiple patchy consolidation with blurred margins in subpleural areas of both lungs (Fig. 4.98).

Then chest CT showed scattered nodules and consolidation in the subpleural lobes of the two lungs, with air bronchi signs (**b**, **d**: red frame). A thick cord subpleural shadow was also found (**c**, **d**: black red arrow) (Fig. 4.99).

Follow-up chest CT (2 days after initial CT examination) showed decreased density of subpleural consolidation in each lobe of both lungs, and reticular changes (**a**, **b**, **d**: red frame) and air bronchi were observed in some parts. The lesions in the upper lobe were more larger and the lesions in the lower lobe were smaller than before (Fig. 4.100).

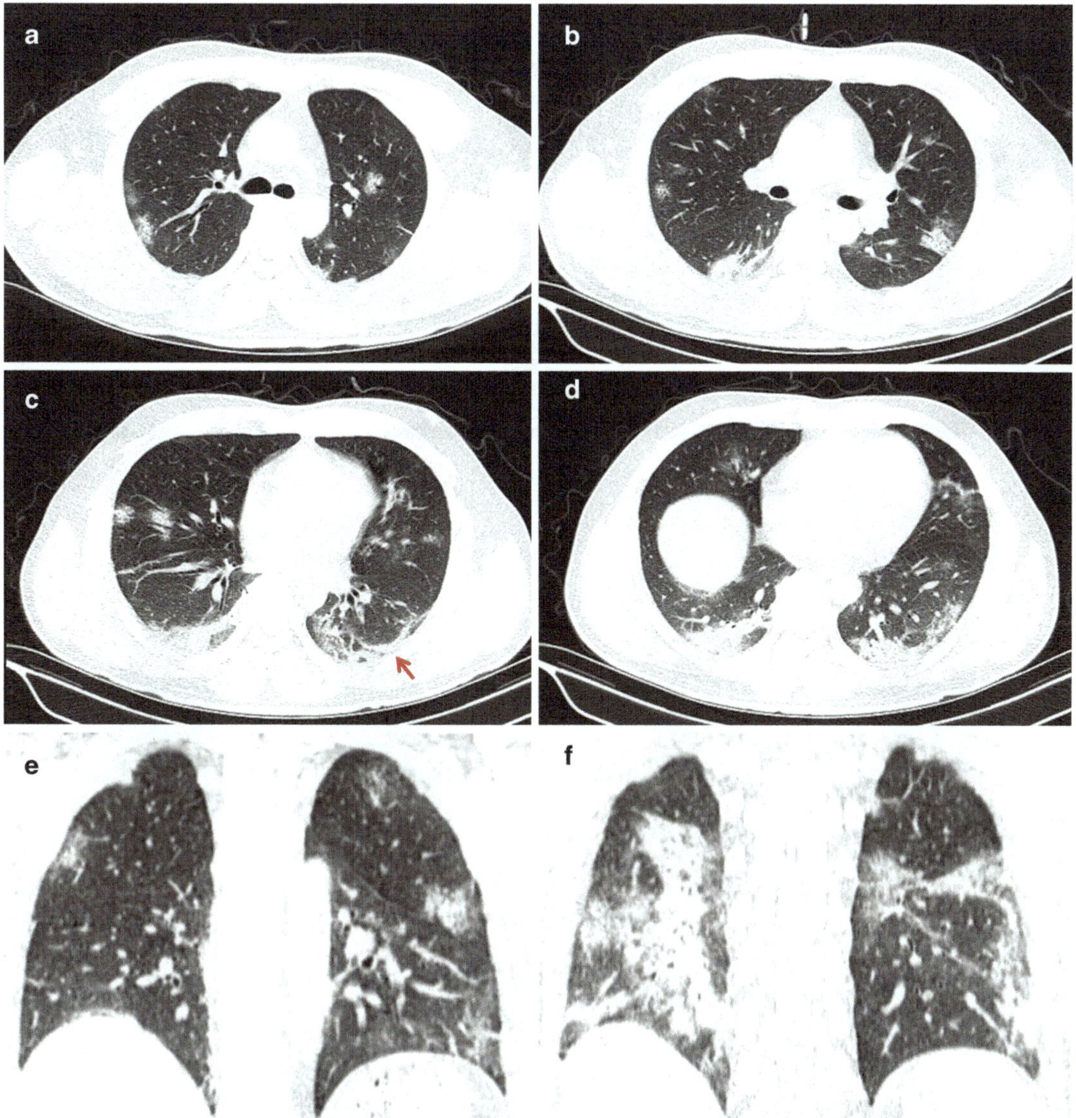

Fig. 4.94 Follow-up axial chest CT (**a–d**) and reconstructed coronal (**e**, **f**) images 14 days after initial scan

Follow-up chest CT (5 days after initial CT examination) showed that the subpleural consolidation in the two lungs was further attenuated, and the scope was narrowed. The subpleural shadows of both lungs become fiber like curves (**c**, **d**: red arrows) (Fig. 4.101).

Follow-up chest CT (35 days after initial CT examination) showed the lesions of bilateral lungs had been completely absorbed (Fig. 4.102).

Comments: In the course of the improvement of the case, the image showed a subpleural fibroid curve, which was finally completely absorbed. It can be inferred that the fibroid curve under pleura is not fibrosis, but alveolar collapse.

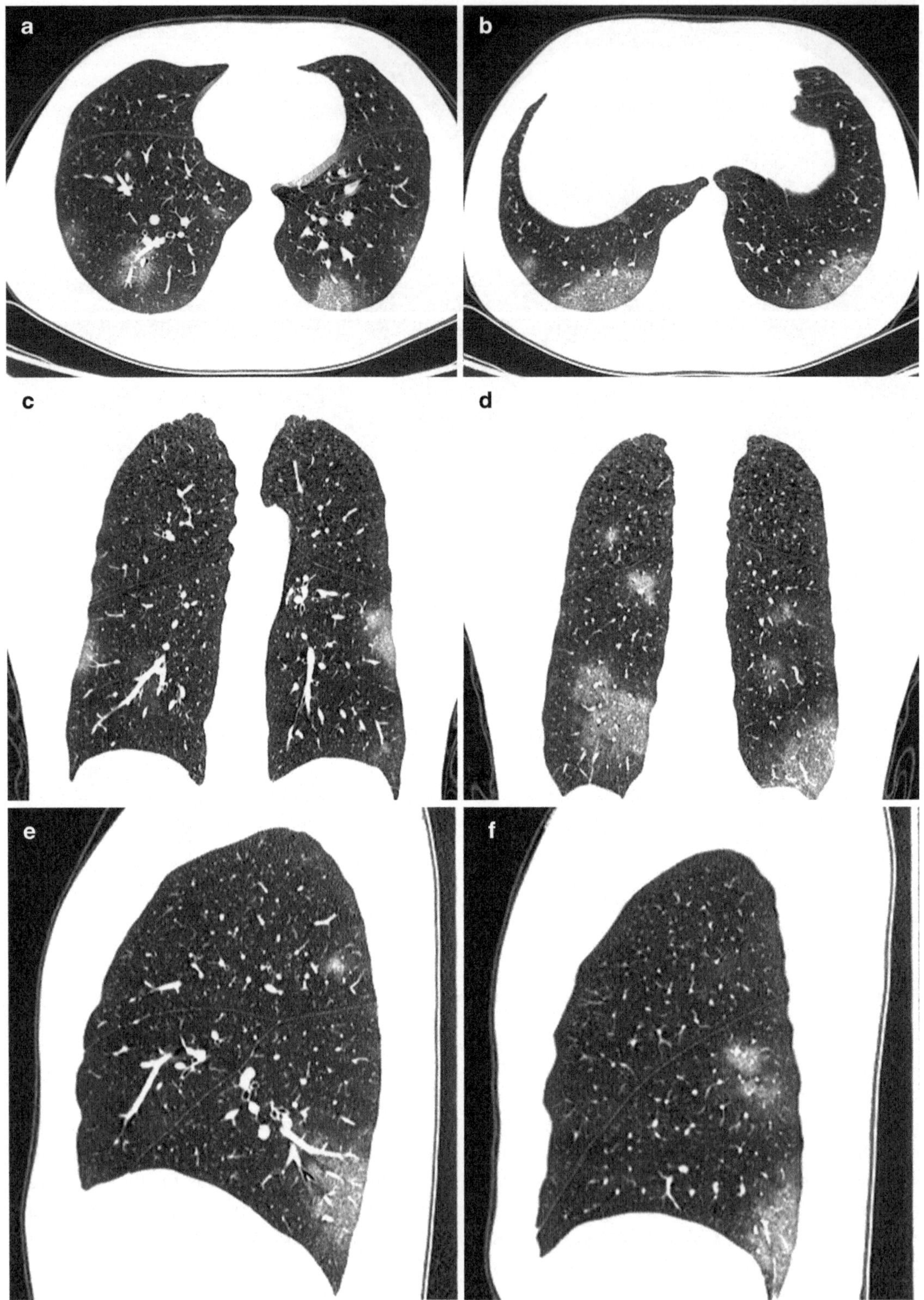

Fig. 4.95 Follow-up axial chest CT (**a**, **b**), reconstructed coronal (**c**, **d**) and sagittal (**e**, **f**) images 3 days after initial scan

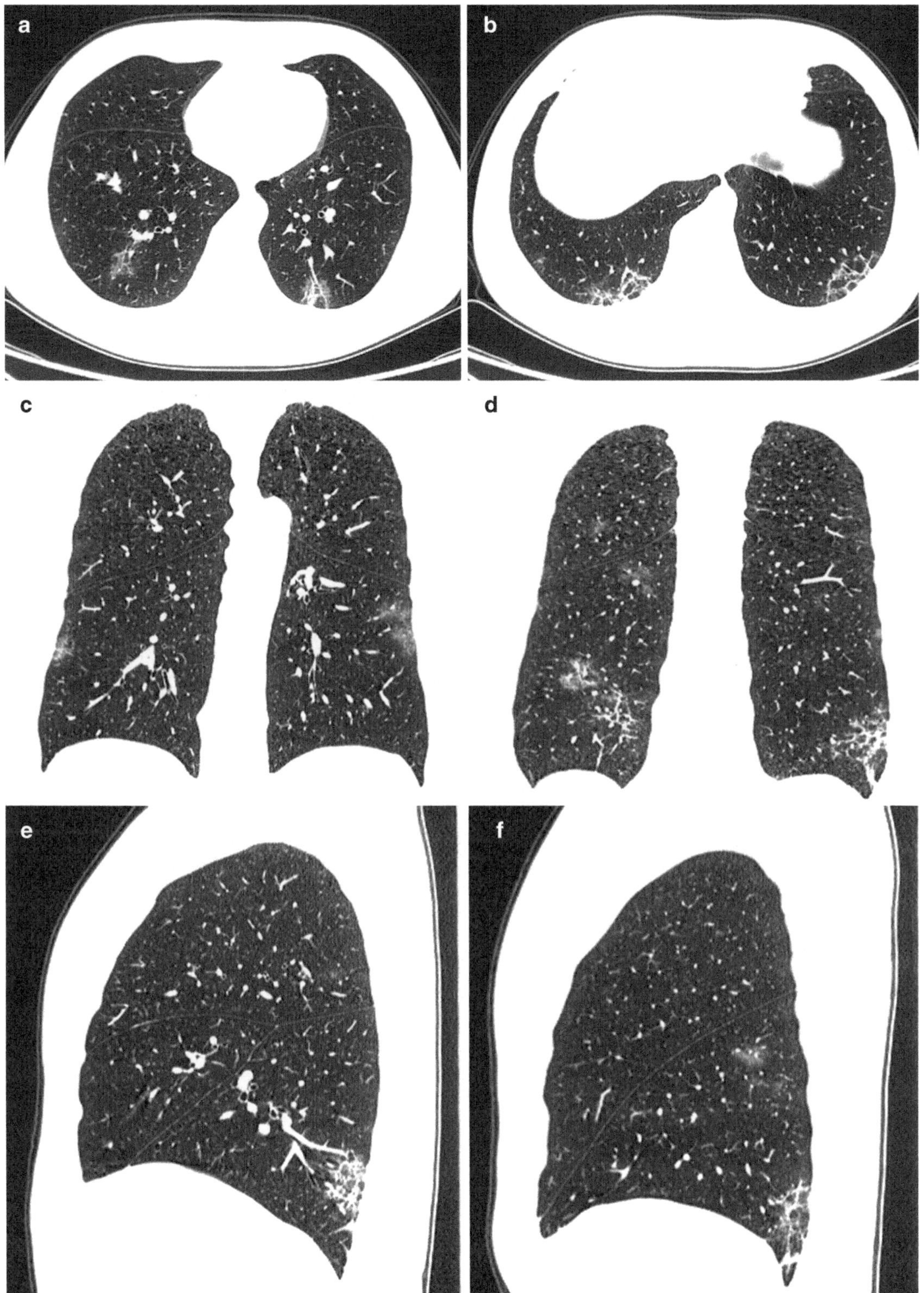

Fig. 4.96 Follow-up axial chest CT (**a**, **b**), reconstructed coronal (**c**, **d**) and sagittal (**e**, **f**) images 17 days after initial scan

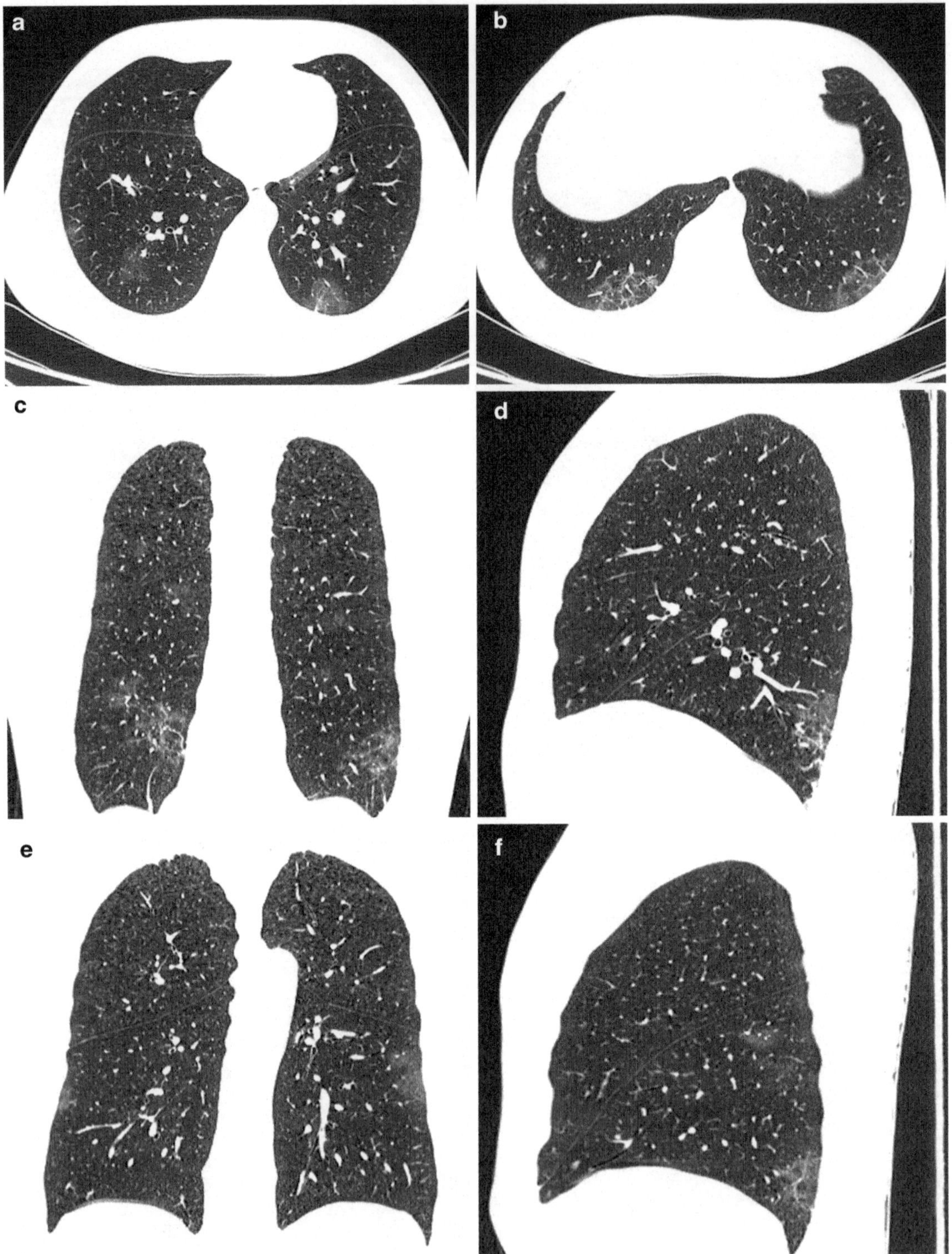

Fig. 4.97 Follow-up axial chest CT (**a**, **b**), reconstructed coronal (**c**, **d**) and sagittal (**e**, **f**) images 23 days after initial scan

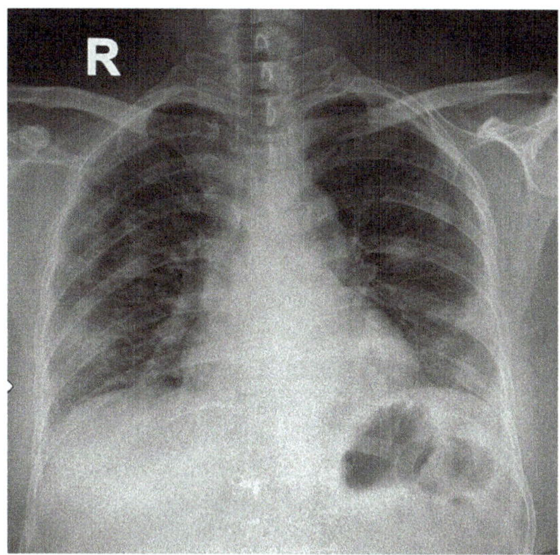

Fig. 4.98 Initial chest radiography image

Case 33

Medical History and Clinical Manifestations

A 64-year-old female was admitted in the hospital for low fever (highest body temperature: 37.8 °C) 5 days, dry cough and paroxysms 2 days. Laboratory test results indicated white blood cell count of 3.5×10^9/L, 66.1% neutrophils, and 26.5% lymphocytes. The patient has no definite epidemiological history. On the day of admission, the SARS-CoV-2 nucleic acid test was positive.

Imaging Features

Initial chest CT showed multiple subpleural consolidation and ground-glass shadows in bilateral lungs, with crazy-paving pattern (**b**: red frame), and fibrous lesions (**c**: red arrows) in the lower lobes of both lungs (Fig. 4.103).

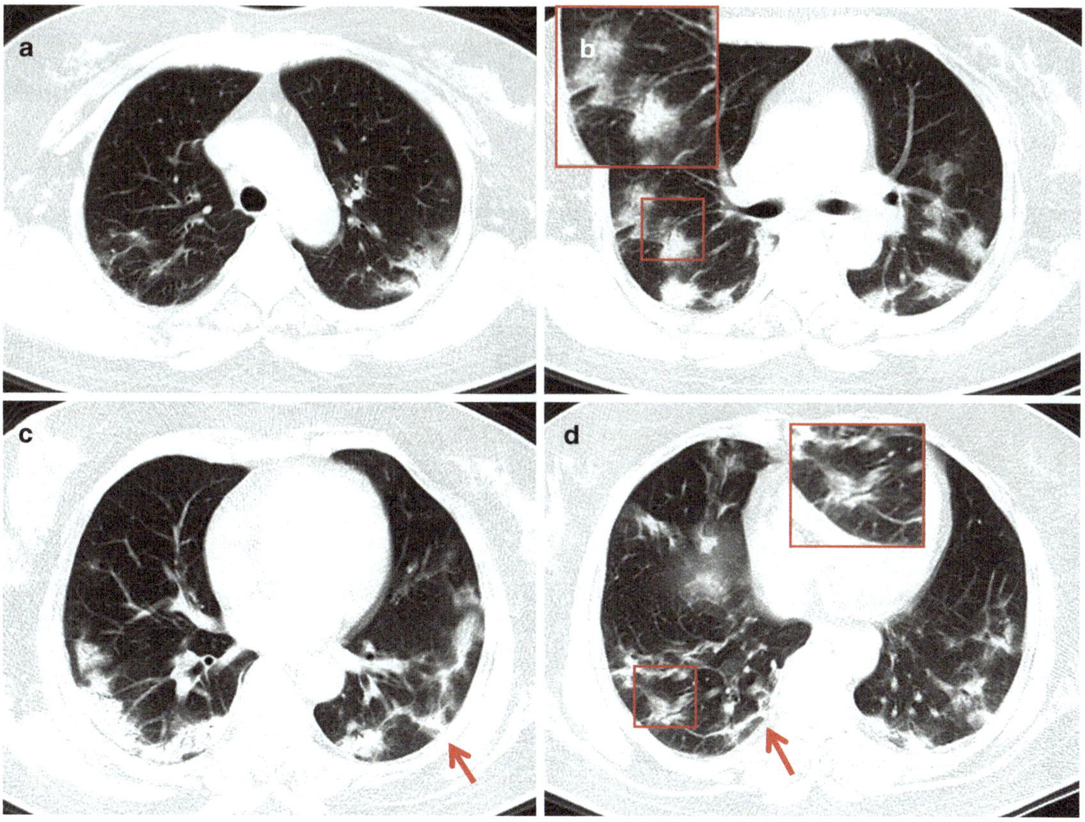

Fig. 4.99 Initial CT images

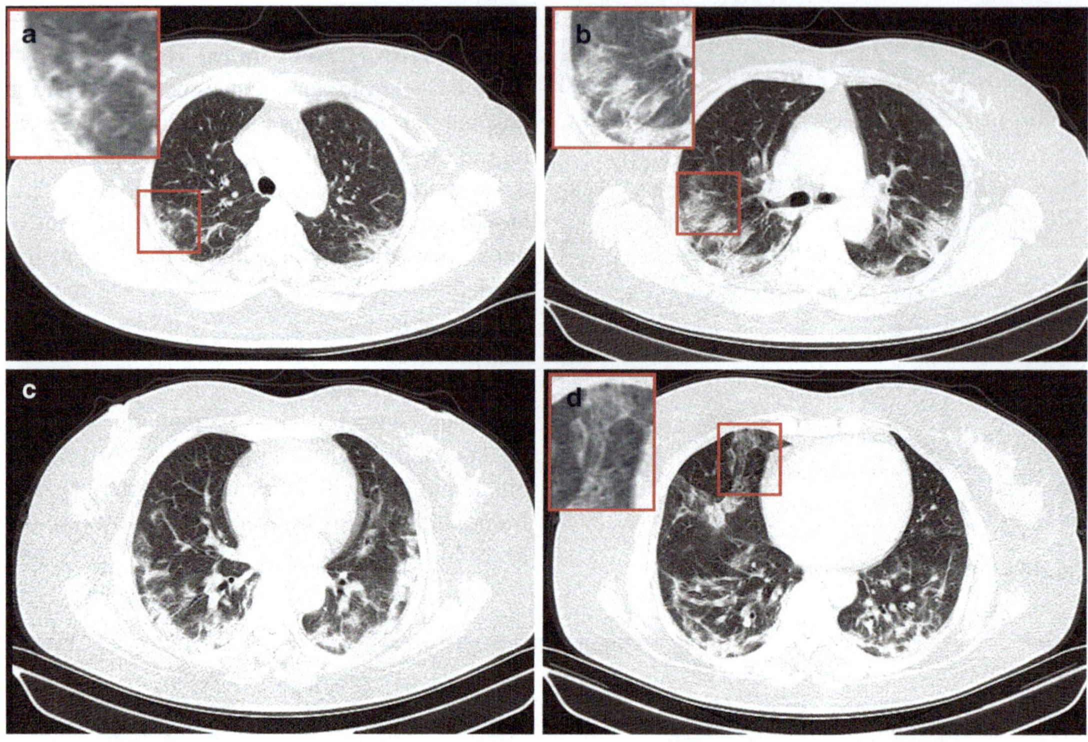

Fig. 4.100 Follow-up CT images 2 days after initial scan

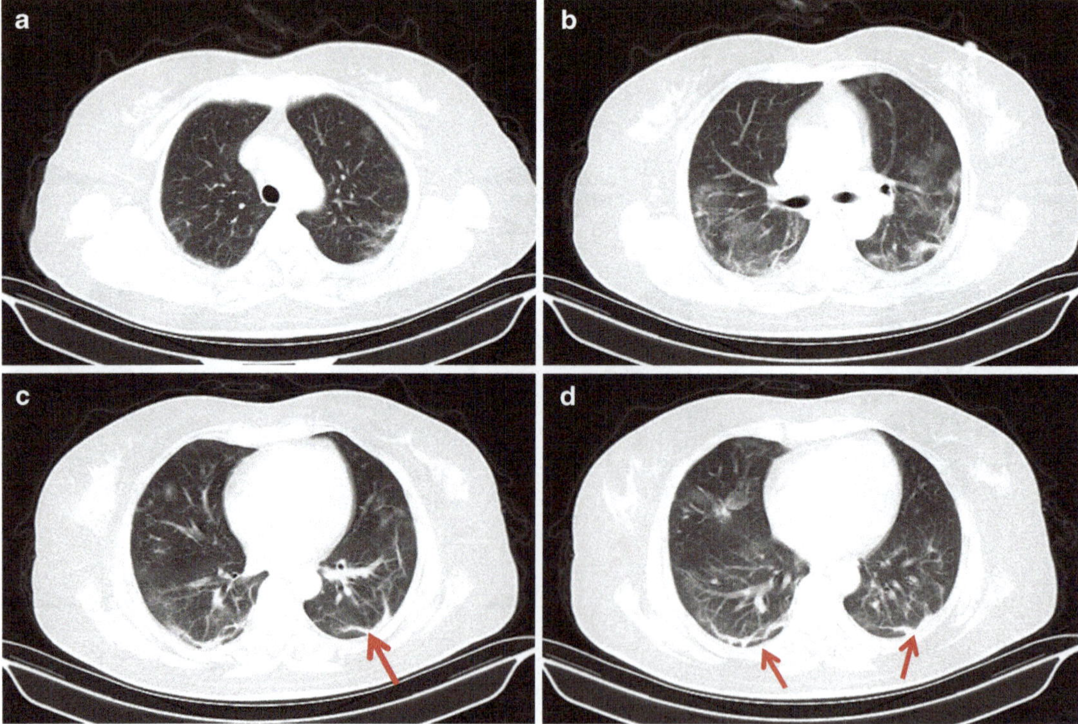

Fig. 4.101 Follow-up CT images 5 days after initial scan

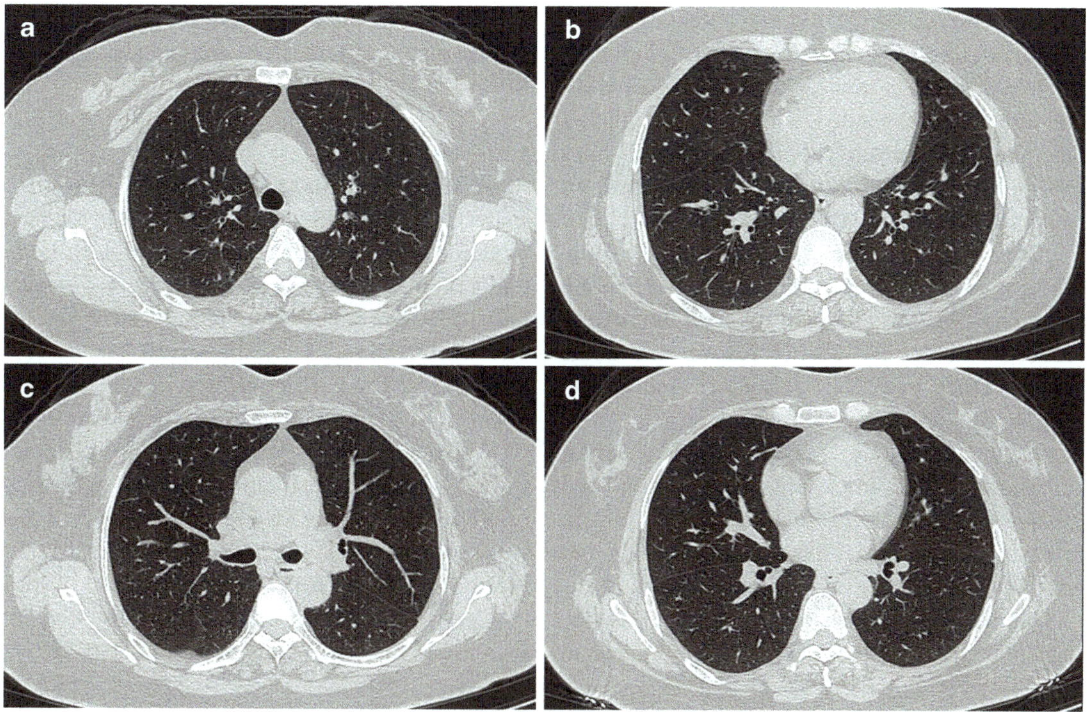

Fig. 4.102 Follow-up CT images 35 days after initial scan

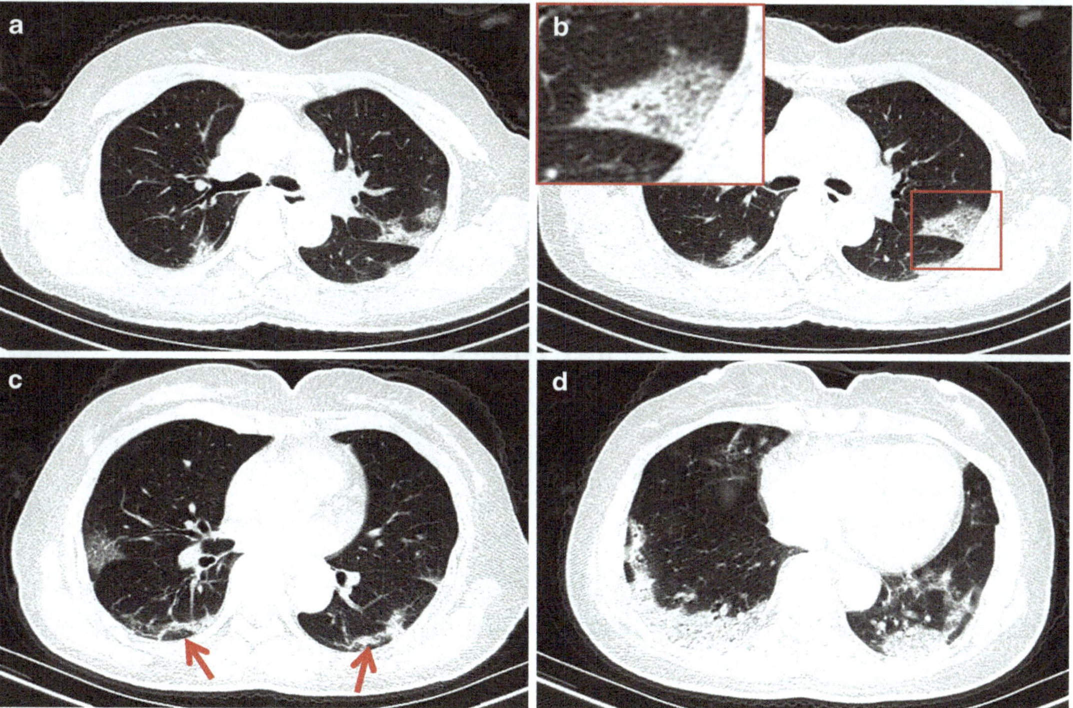

Fig. 4.103 Initial CT image

Follow-up chest CT (3 days after initial CT examination) showed that the scope of subpleural consolidation and ground-glass shadows of bilateral lungs were expanded, with crazy-paving pattern, and the shadow of subpleural fibrous lesions changed into lamellar consolidation shadows (red frame) (Fig. 4.104).

After 6 days follow-up and reexamination, CT showed the scope of subpleural consolidation and ground-glass shadows of bilateral lungs were reduced and density was increased, and some lesions turned to fibrotic lesions (**c**: red arrow) (Fig. 4.105).

On the 15th day, reexamination of chest CT showed that subpleural consolidation and ground-glass shadows remarkable absorbed in bilateral lungs, remaining fibrosis (**b–d**: red arrows) (Fig. 4.106).

Comments: The case presented typical imaging features, such as the density shadow of ground glass in the subpleural of both lungs, with crazy-paving pattern, fibrosis and gradual absorption in the lesion.

Case 34

Medical History and Clinical Manifestations

A 33-year-old female was admitted in the hospital for fever with chills 4 days (highest body temperature: 38.7 °C). Laboratory test results indicated a normal white blood cell count of 4.6×10^9/L, 34.3% lymphocytes, and 60.7% neutrophils. The C-reactive protein was less than 0.499 mg/L. Exposure history: The patient lived in Wuhan, China for years, returning to hometown 5 days prior to symptom onset. On the day of admission, the SARS-CoV-2 nucleic acid test was positive.

Imaging Features

Chest radiography showed patchy density increase in the lower lung areas (Fig. 4.107).

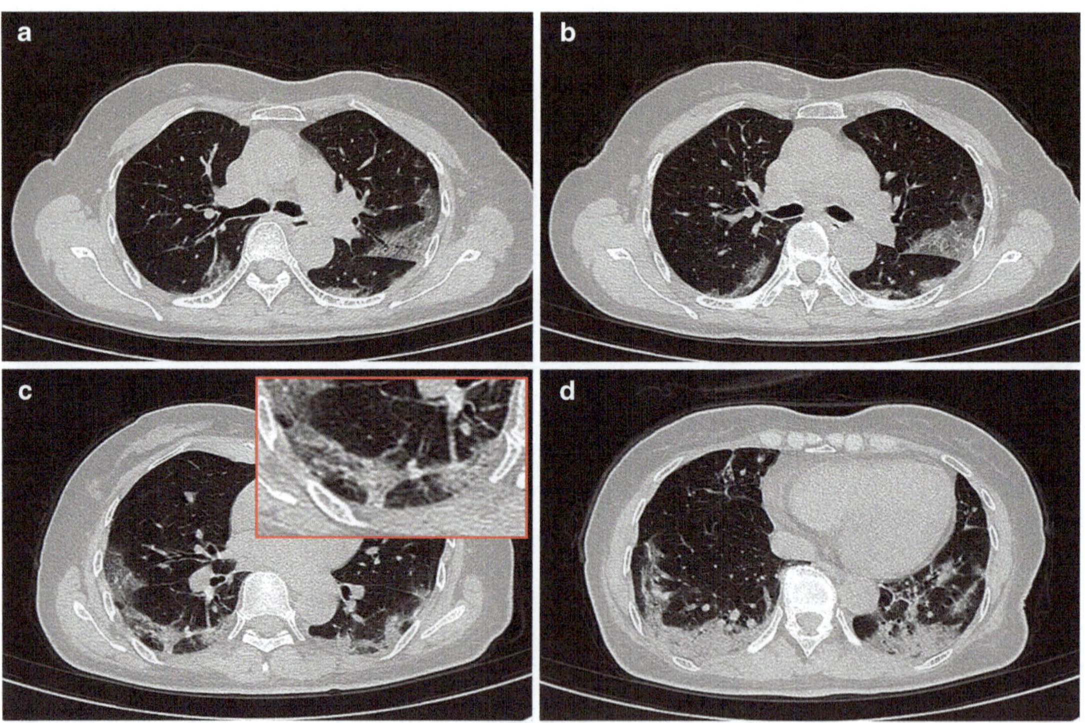

Fig. 4.104 Follow-up CT images 3 days after initial scan

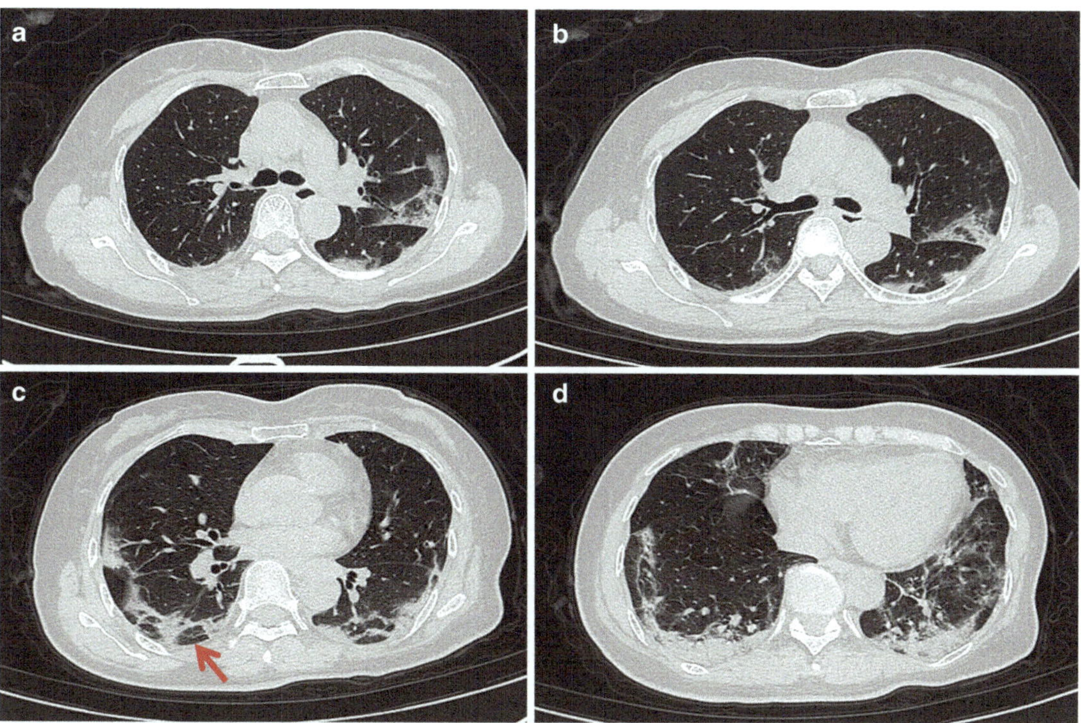

Fig. 4.105 Follow-up CT images 6 days after initial scan

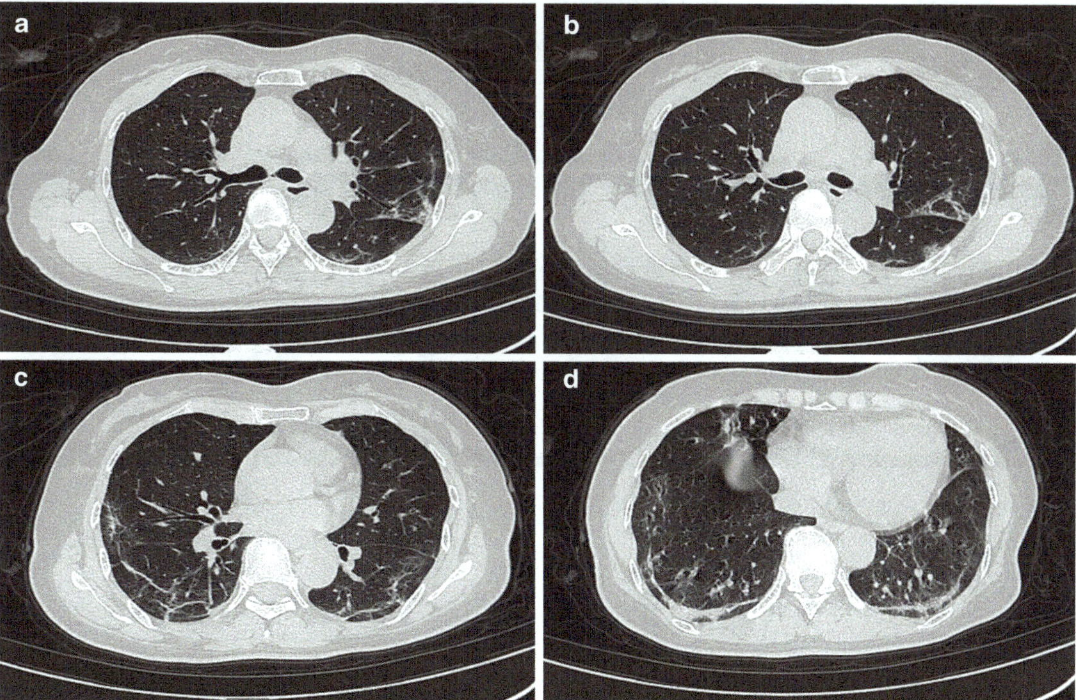

Fig. 4.106 Follow-up CT images 15 days after initial scan

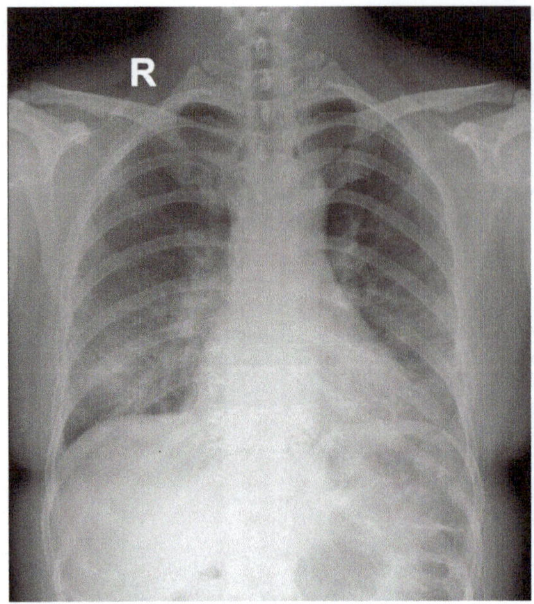

Fig. 4.107 Initial chest radiography image

Chest CT showed scattered nodules and patchy consolidation in bilateral lungs, with crazy-paving signs and microvascular thickening (**c**, **e**, **f**: red frame). The pleura is slightly thickened on both sides (**b**: white arrows) (Fig. 4.108).

Follow-up chest CT (3 days after initial CT examination) showed that the consolidations in bilateral lungs were resolved, nodules were reduced, thickened interlobular septa were obvious in the lesion, and fibrous lesions were increasing (Fig. 4.109).

After 8 days follow-up, CT showed that the lesions of consolidation in bilateral lungs were significantly resolved and presented as GGOs. The nodules were significantly absorbed and the density was reduced, and subpleural fibrous lesions were increased (Fig. 4.110).

On the tenth day, chest CT showed the lesions in bilateral lungs resolved completely (Fig. 4.111).

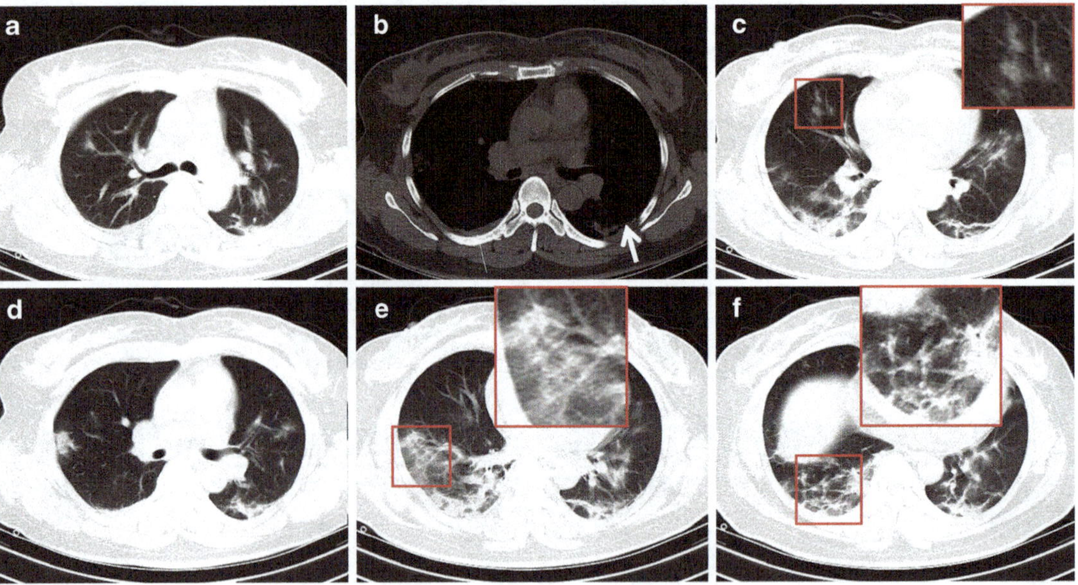

Fig. 4.108 Initial CT image

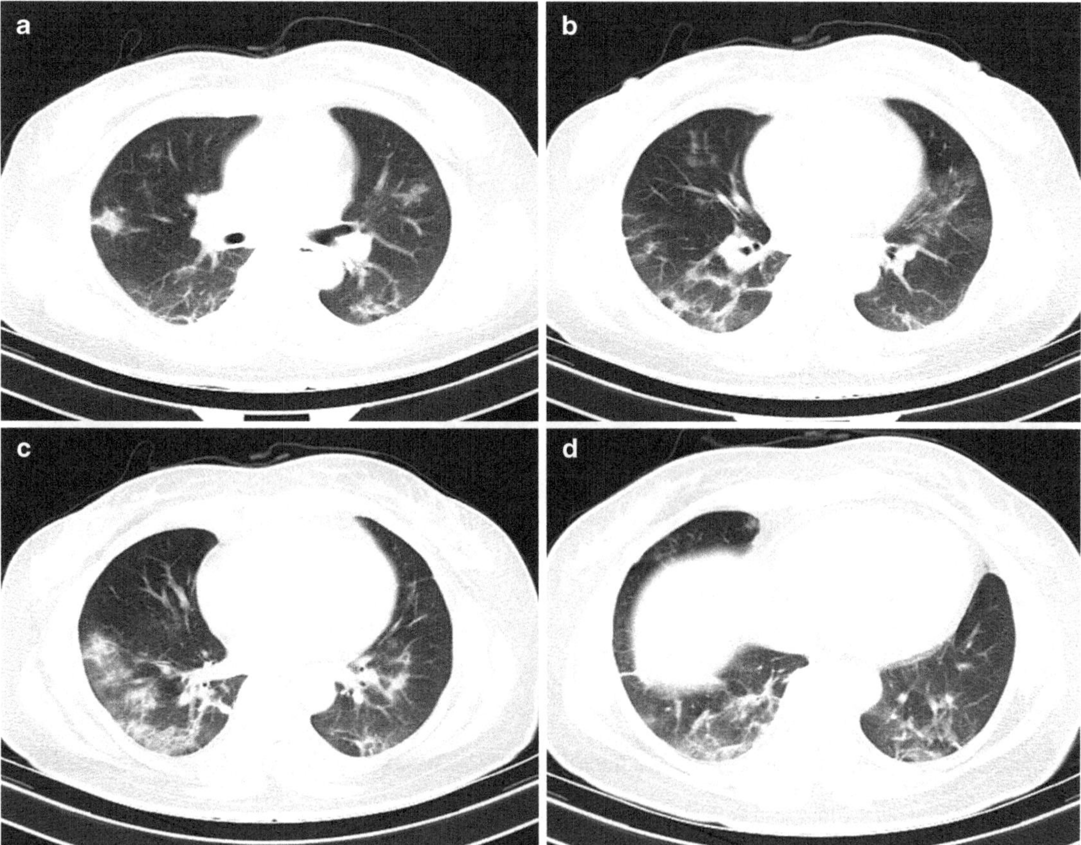

Fig. 4.109 Follow-up CT images 3 days after initial scan

Comments: The chest radiograph of this patient showed the lesions of consolidation of the lower lung field and lobular pneumonia in the early stage. The chest CT showed a tendency of fibrosis which was completely absorbed finally.

Case 35
Medical History and Clinical Manifestations

A 36-year-old female was admitted in the hospital with diarrhea lasted for 3 days and fever for 2 days (highest body temperature: 38.5 °C). The patient suffered from cough and low fever 5 days ago, but the initial pharynx swab SARS-CoV-2 nucleic acid test was negative. Laboratory test results indicated a normal white blood cell count of 4.9×10^9/L, 32.0% lymphocytes, and 57.3% neutrophil percentage. Exposure history: She had a close contacting history with confirmed COVID-19 patient. The SARS-CoV-2 nucleic acid test was positive on the day of admission.

Imaging Features

Initial chest CT showed a small patchy subpleural consolidation (**a**: red arrow) in dorsal segment of the right lower lobe (Fig. 4.112).

Follow-up chest CT (5 days after initial CT examination) showed the lesion progressed. The lesion of subpleural consolidation significantly increased with blurred edges and air bronchial signs (**a**, **b**: red frame), (**c**: red arrow). The lesion extends to the posterior segment of the right upper lobe of the lung (Fig. 4.113).

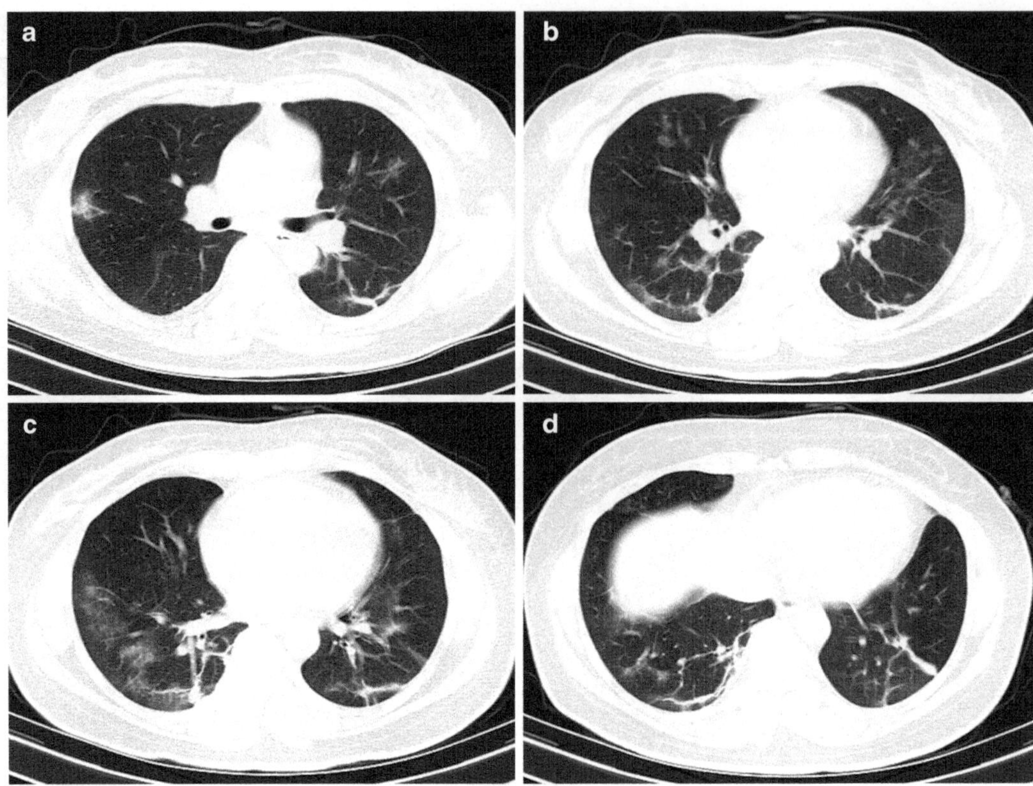

Fig. 4.110 Follow-up CT images 8 days after initial scan

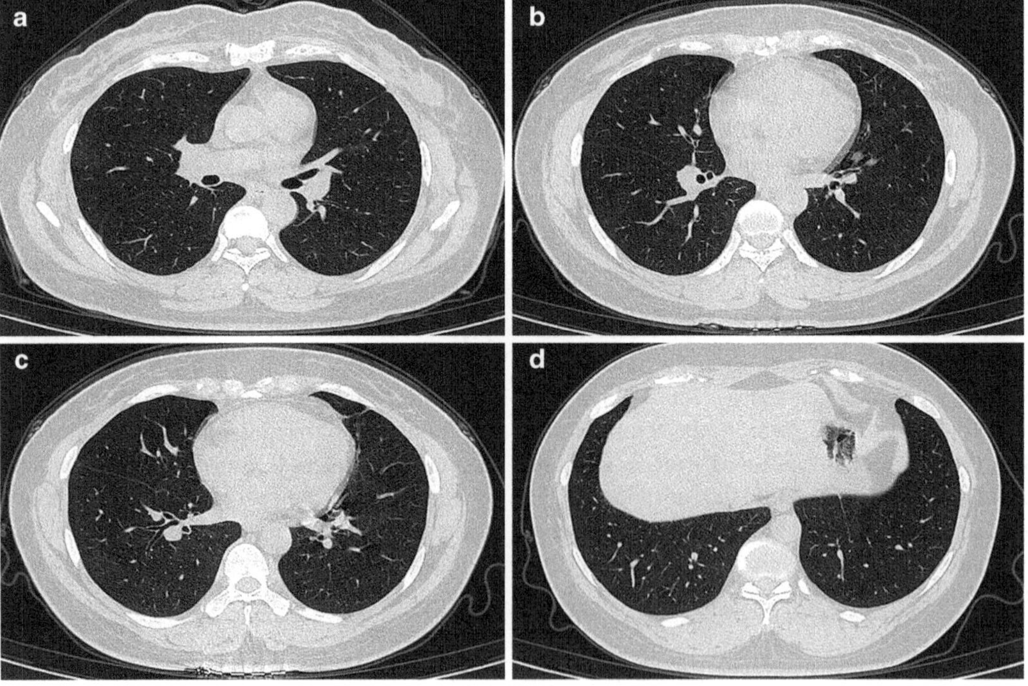

Fig. 4.111 Follow-up CT images 10 days after initial scan

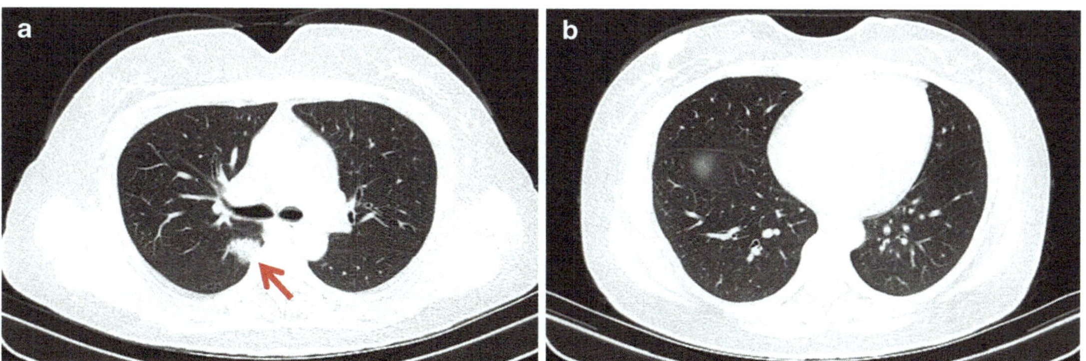

Fig. 4.112 Initial CT image

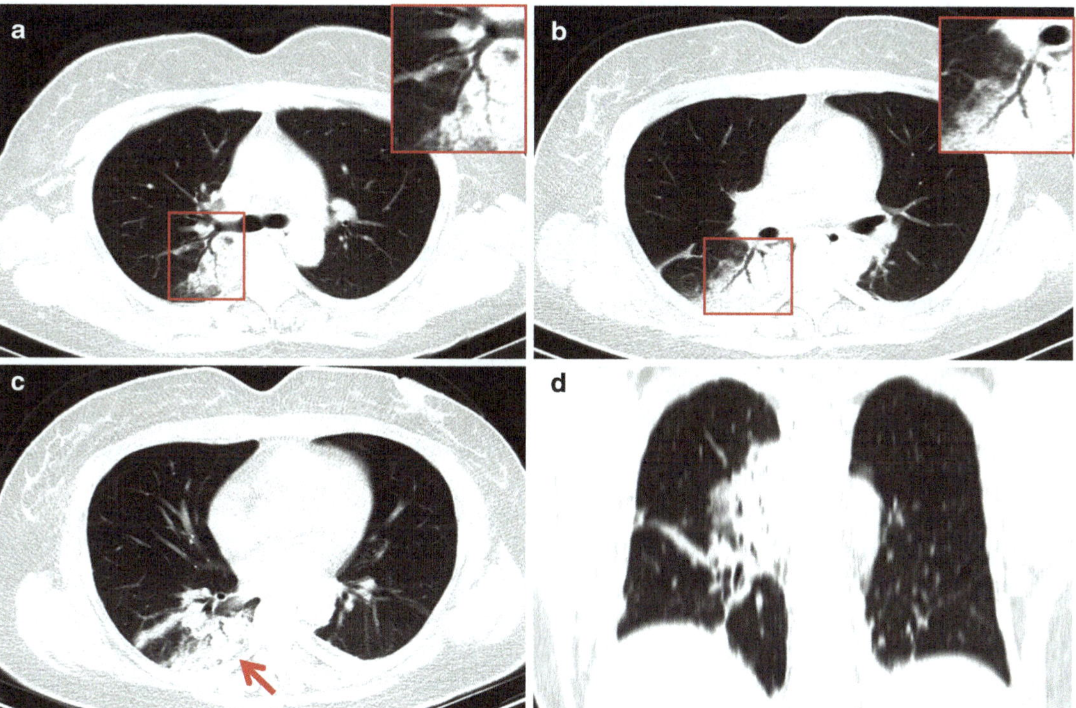

Fig. 4.113 Follow-up CT images 5 days after initial scan

After 12 days follow-up and reexamination, CT showed small patches and fibrous lesions in the upper and lower lobes of the right lung, the lesions reduced. Fibrosis lesions showed up in the lower lobe of both lungs (black arrow) (Fig. 4.114).

Comments: The CT features of this case were small solid lesion in the early stage. The lesion was found to involve the upper and lower lobes of the right lung during the progress. It is suggested that the upper part of the right pulmonary oblique fissure is not well developed.

Case 36

Medical History and Clinical Manifestations

A 25-year-old female was admitted in the hospital with dry cough for 2 days and fever for 1 day (highest body temperature: 37.2 °C). Laboratory test

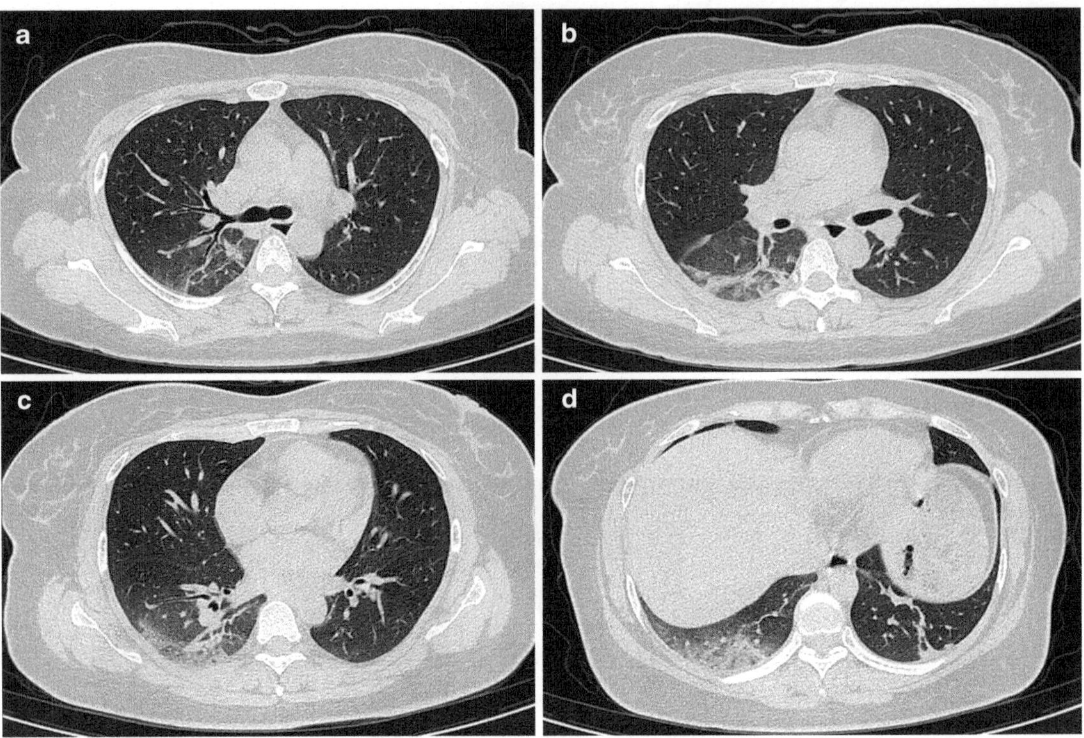

Fig. 4.114 Follow-up CT images 12 days after initial scan

results indicated decreased blood leukocyte count and lymphocyte count. Exposure history: She had a close contacting history with confirmed COVID-19 patient (her aunt). The SARS-CoV-2 nucleic acid test was positive 2 days after admission.

Imaging Features

Initial chest CT showed multiple patchy GGOs in bilateral lungs. The lesions were mainly distributed along the subpleura, with microvascular thickening and reticular pattern (Fig. 4.115).

Follow-up chest CT (2 days after initial CT examination) showed multiple nodular and large ground-glass shadows in both lungs. Compared with the previous images, some new lesions appeared and the scope of lesions expanded, and consolidation appeared (Fig. 4.116).

Follow-up chest CT (12 days after Initial CT examination) showed that the scope and density of multiple lesions in bilateral lungs were smaller and decreased than those in the previous images (Fig. 4.117).

Follow-up chest CT (15 days after Initial CT examination) showed multiple patchy ground-glass shadows in bilateral lungs, which were further decreased in size and density (Fig. 4.118).

Comments: This was an ordinary COVID-19 patient. Her CT showed a typical subpleural distribution of ground-glass shadow, with reticulated paving stone sign. And the lesions were slightly enlarged with a small amount of consolidation in a short time, and the lesions obviously absorbed after 15 days therapy.

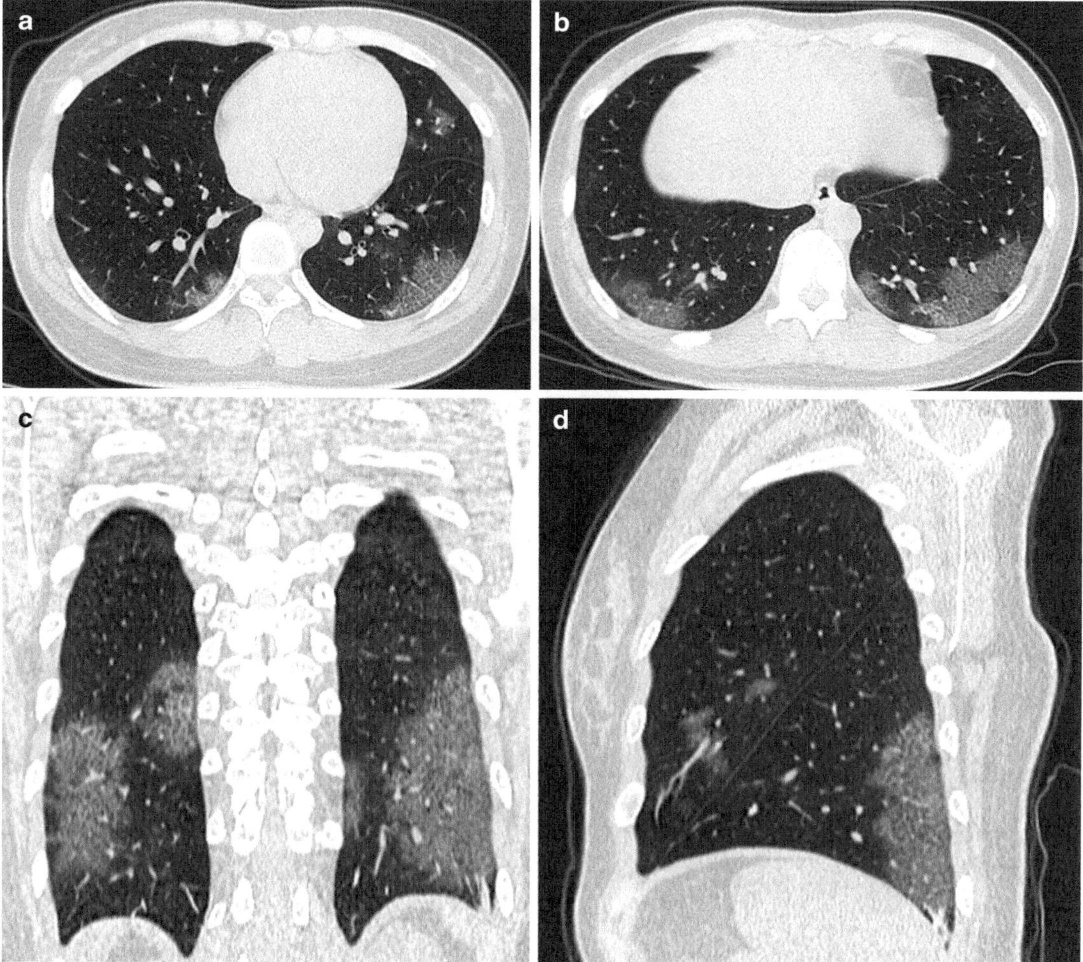

Fig. 4.115 Initial axial chest CT (**a**, **b**), reconstructed coronal (**c**) and sagittal (**d**) images of the patient

Case 37

Medical History and Clinical Manifestations

A 33-year-old female was admitted in the hospital for 3 days with cough. Laboratory test results indicated decreased white blood cell count of 2.7×10^9/mL, normal lymphocytes percentage 24.8%, and neutrophils percentage of 63.9%. Exposure history: She had been on a business trip to Jingzhou, Hubei province, China 7 days before her illness. The SARS-CoV-2 nucleic acid test was positive on the day of admission.

Imaging Features

Chest radiography showed no obvious abnormal signs (Fig. 4.119).

Chest CT showed a ground-glass nodule (**b**: red frame) in the lower lobe of the left lung, and the edge of lesion was slightly blurred (Fig. 4.120).

Follow-up chest CT (4 days after initial CT examination) showed multiple ground-glass nodules under the pleura of the lower lobe of both lungs, mainly in the lower lobe of the left lung, the

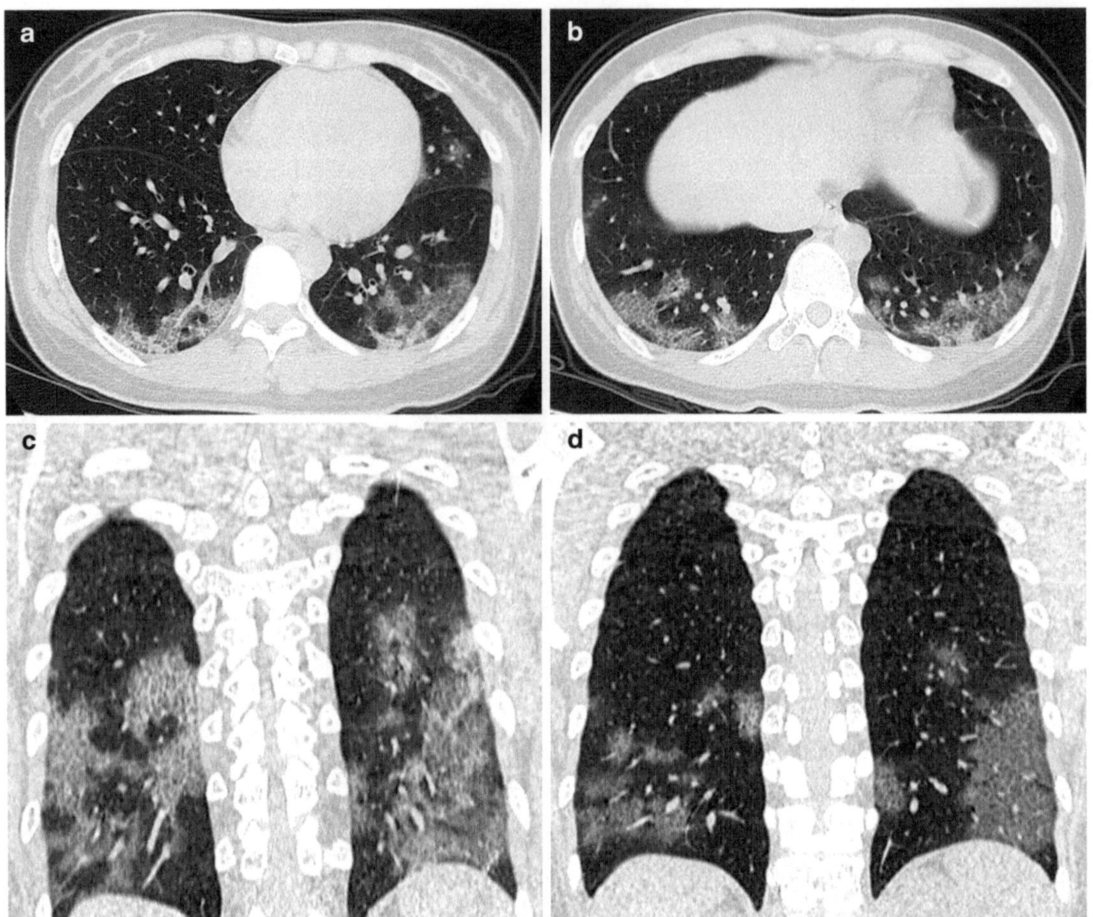

Fig. 4.116 Follow-up axial chest CT (**a**, **b**) and reconstructed coronal (**c**, **d**) images 2 days after initial scan

edge was slightly blurred, and there was a small grid shadow (**b**: red frame) in it (Fig. 4.121).

Follow-up chest CT (13 days after initial CT examination) showed multiple subpleural lesions in the lower lobe of both lungs, with clear edge, obvious absorption, and partial fibrosis (**a**: red arrow) (Fig. 4.122).

Comments: This was a mild COVID-19 patients. The lesions in CT obviously increased and enlarged 4 days after admission, showing a typical ground-glass nodule shadow with reticulated paving stone sign. He was getting better quickly.

Case 38

Medical History and Clinical Manifestations

A 39-year-old male was admitted in the hospital for 4 days with fever (highest body temperature: 38.2 °C), cough, and muscle soreness. Laboratory test results indicated a normal white blood cell count of 6.3×10^9/L, 65.2% neutrophils, and 26.2% lymphocytes. Exposure history: He had a close contacting history with his wife's brother who returned home from Wuhan, China. The patient's wife and brother have been diagnosed with COVID-19. The SARS-CoV-2 nucleic acid test was positive 3 days after admission.

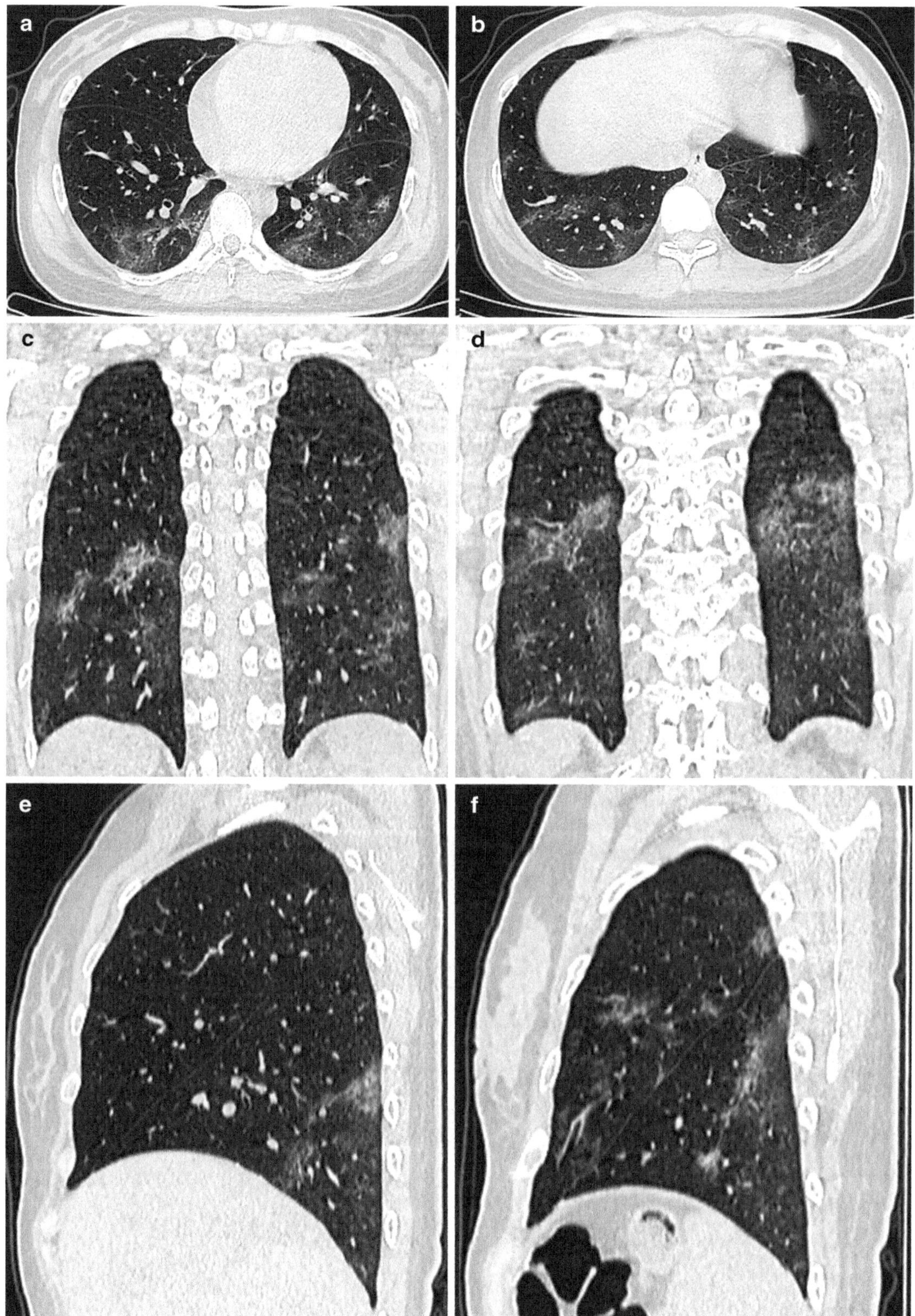

Fig. 4.117 Follow-up axial chest CT (**a**, **b**), reconstructed coronal (**c**, **d**) and sagittal (**e**, **f**) images 12 days after initial scan

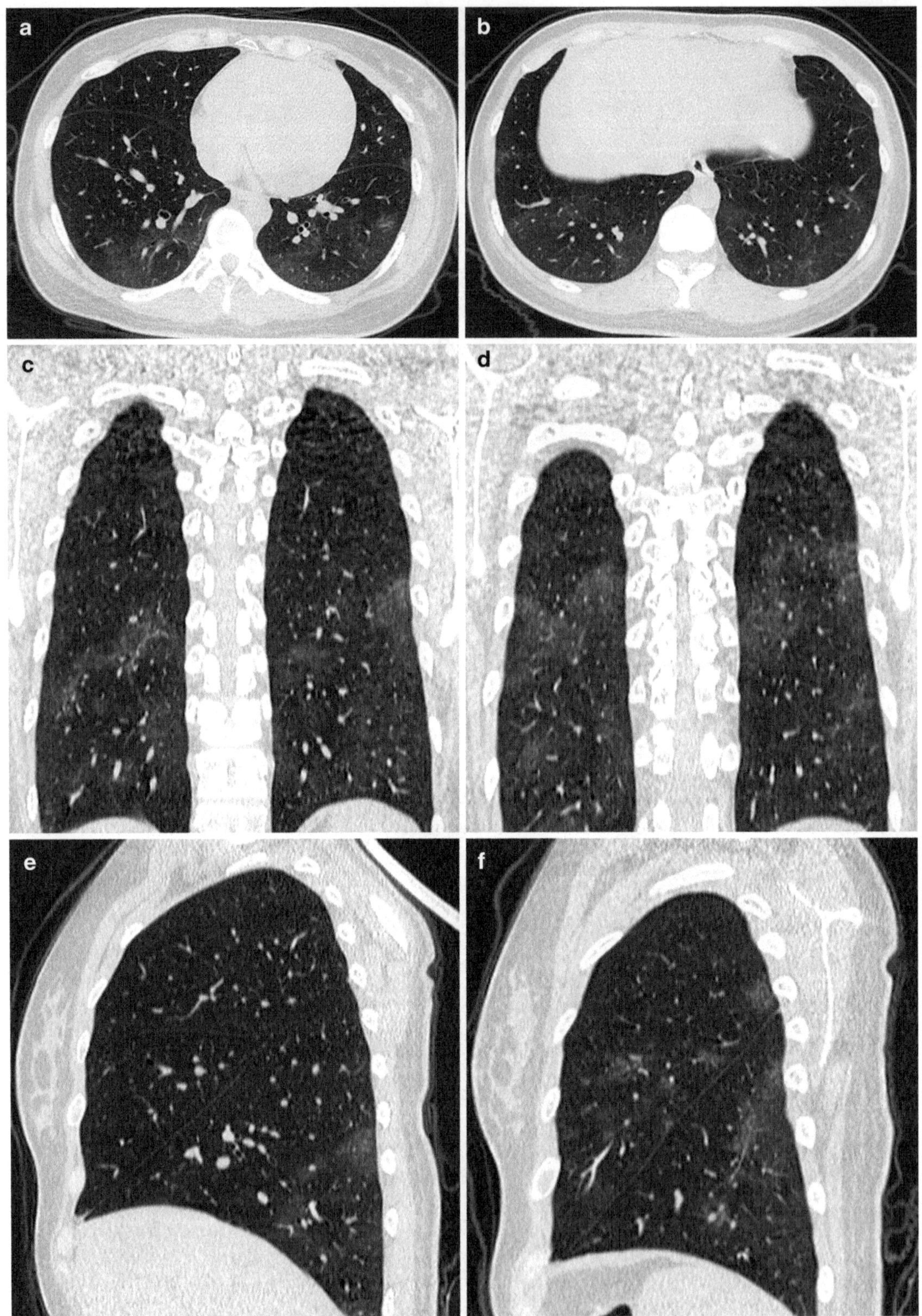

Fig. 4.118 Follow-up axial chest CT (**a**, **b**), reconstructed coronal (**c**, **d**) and sagittal (**e**, **f**) images 15 days after initial scan

Imaging Features

Initial chest CT showed multiple nodular and patchy ground-glass opacities in the subpleural area of the right middle lobe, lower lobe, and the upper lobe of left lung (Fig. 4.123).

Follow-up chest CT (2 days after initial CT examination) showed multiple patchy ground-glass opacities in the subpleural area progressed. Crazy-paving pattern was seen in the focus of the right lower lung, with partial consolidation (Fig. 4.124).

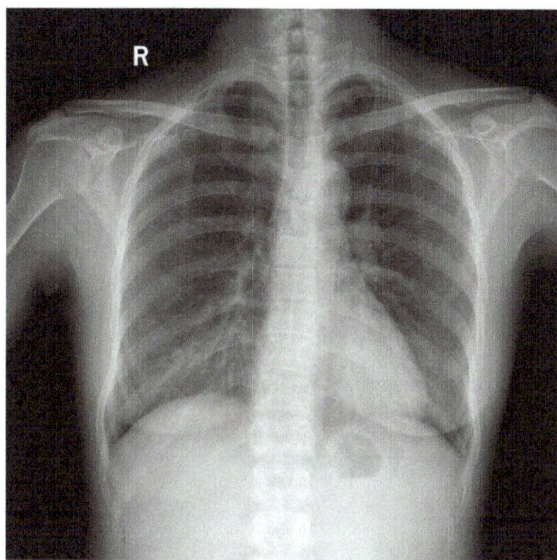

Fig. 4.119 Initial chest radiography image

Follow-up chest CT (10 days after initial CT examination) showed that the lesions in both lungs were absorbed and reduced, and the density was lower than previous images (Fig. 4.125).

Comments: This is a common COVID-19 patient. The CT findings of the chest were typical, and the lesions absorbed quickly after 10 days of treatment.

Case 39

Medical History and Clinical Manifestations

A 51-year-old male was admitted in the hospital for 3 days with fever (highest body temperature: 38.4 °C). Laboratory test results indicated a normal white blood cell count of 6.5×10^9/L, 29.2% lymphocytes, and decreased neutrophils of 51.6%. C-reactive protein 7.4 mg/L was normal. Exposure history: The patient lived in Xiangyang, Hubei province, China for a long time. He drove home via through Wuhan, China and contacted friends in Wuhan, who had confirmed COVID-19 after then. The patient had a history of hypertension and was undergoing antihypertensive therapy.

Imaging Features

Chest radiography showed a small patchy density increase in the middle field of the right lung (Fig. 4.126).

Chest CT showed a semisolid nodule with blurred edge in the middle lobe of the right lung (Fig. 4.127).

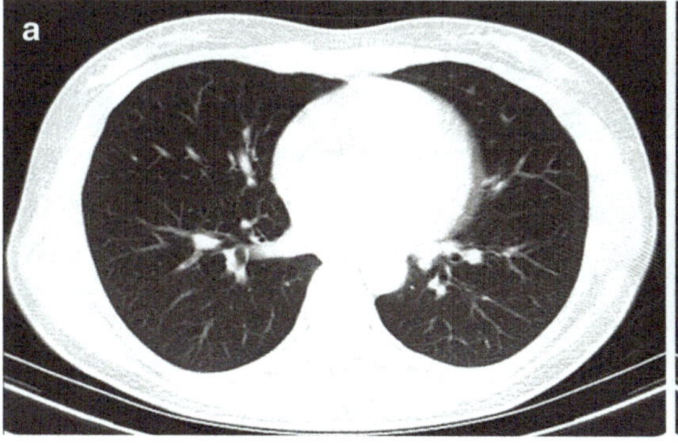

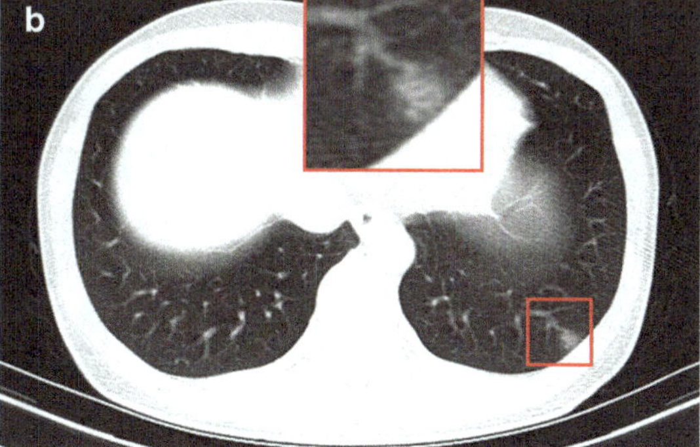

Fig. 4.120 Initial CT image

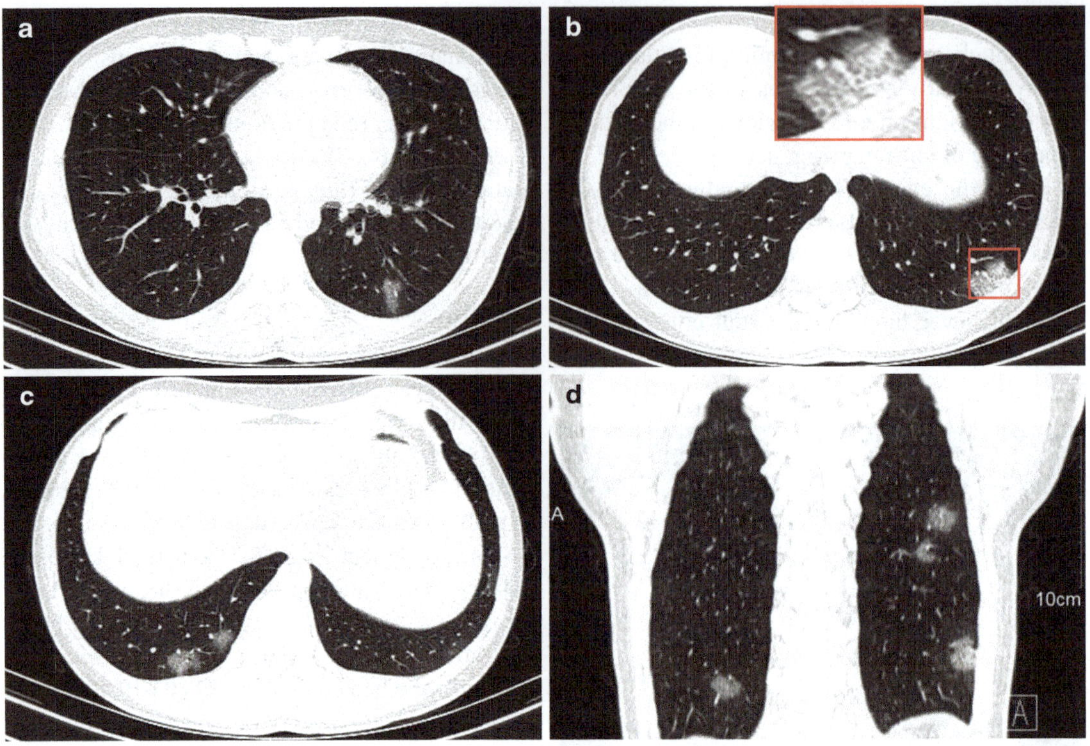

Fig. 4.121 Follow-up axial chest CT (**a–c**) and reconstructed coronal (**d**) images 4 days after initial scan

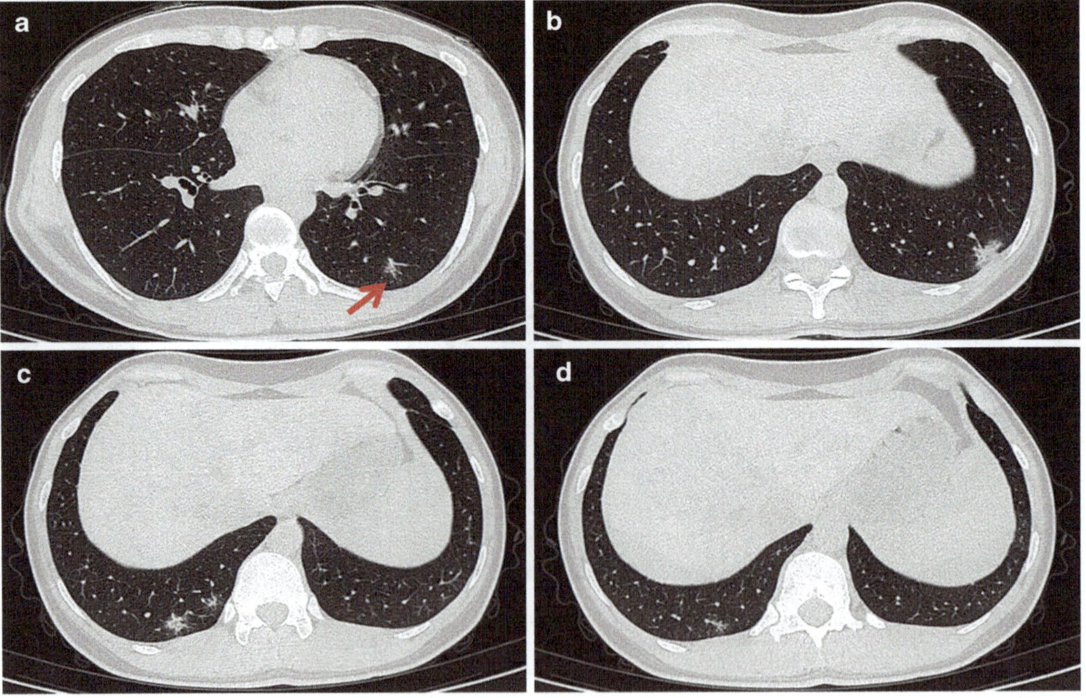

Fig. 4.122 Follow-up CT images 13 days after initial scan

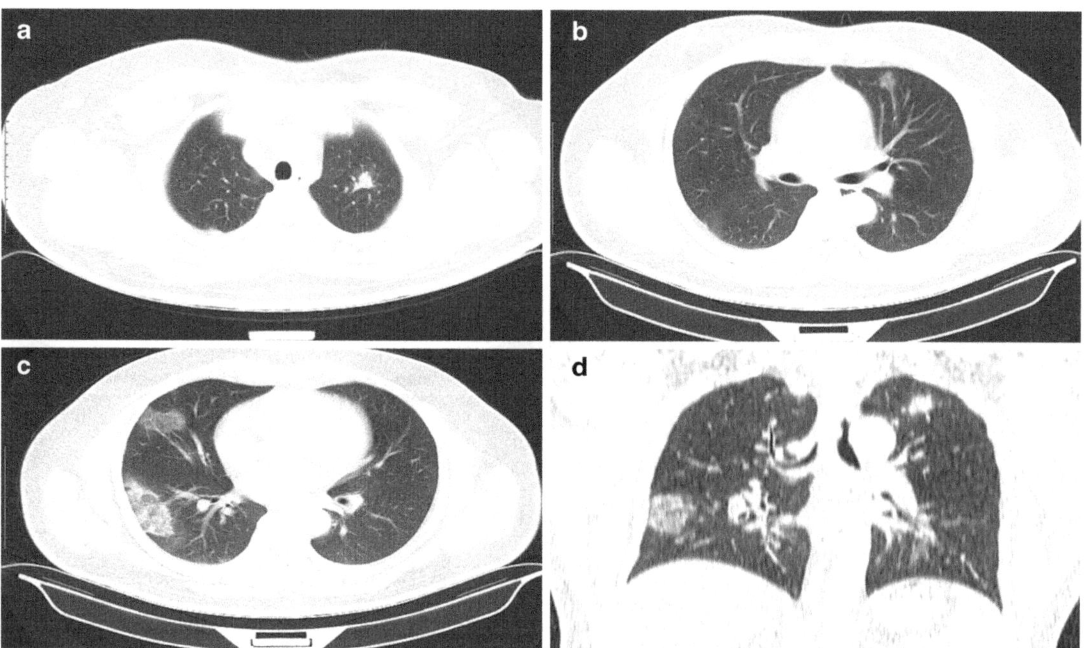

Fig. 4.123 Initial axial chest CT (**a–c**) and reconstructed coronal (**d**) images of the patient

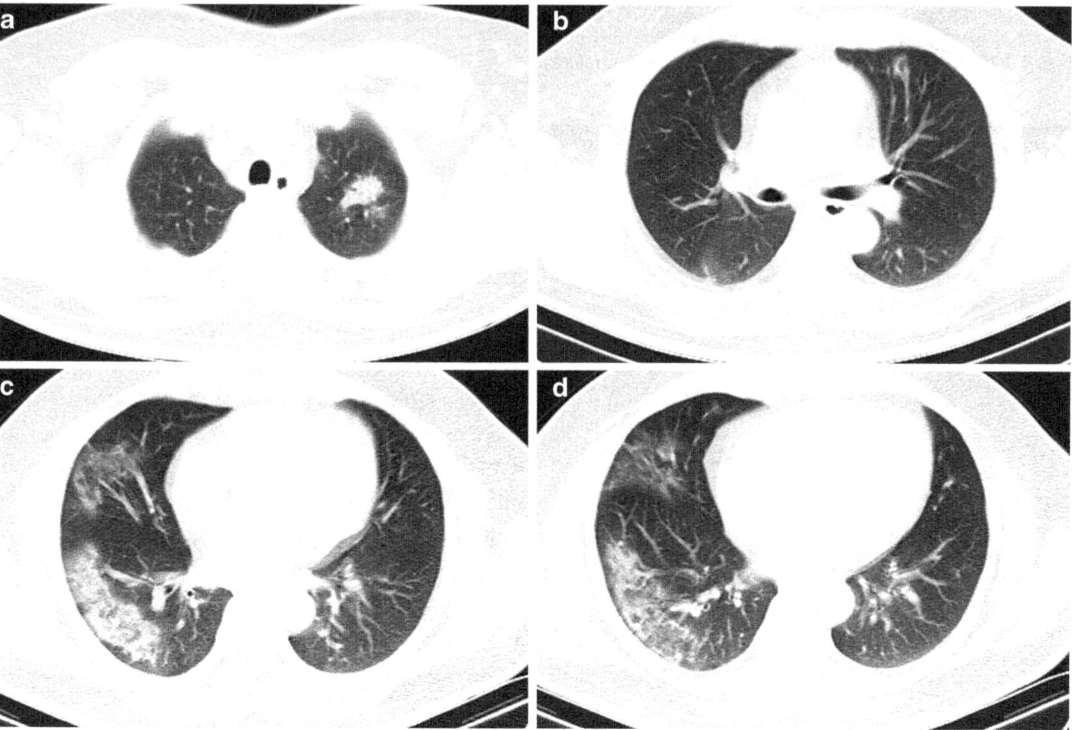

Fig. 4.124 Follow-up CT images 2 days after initial scan

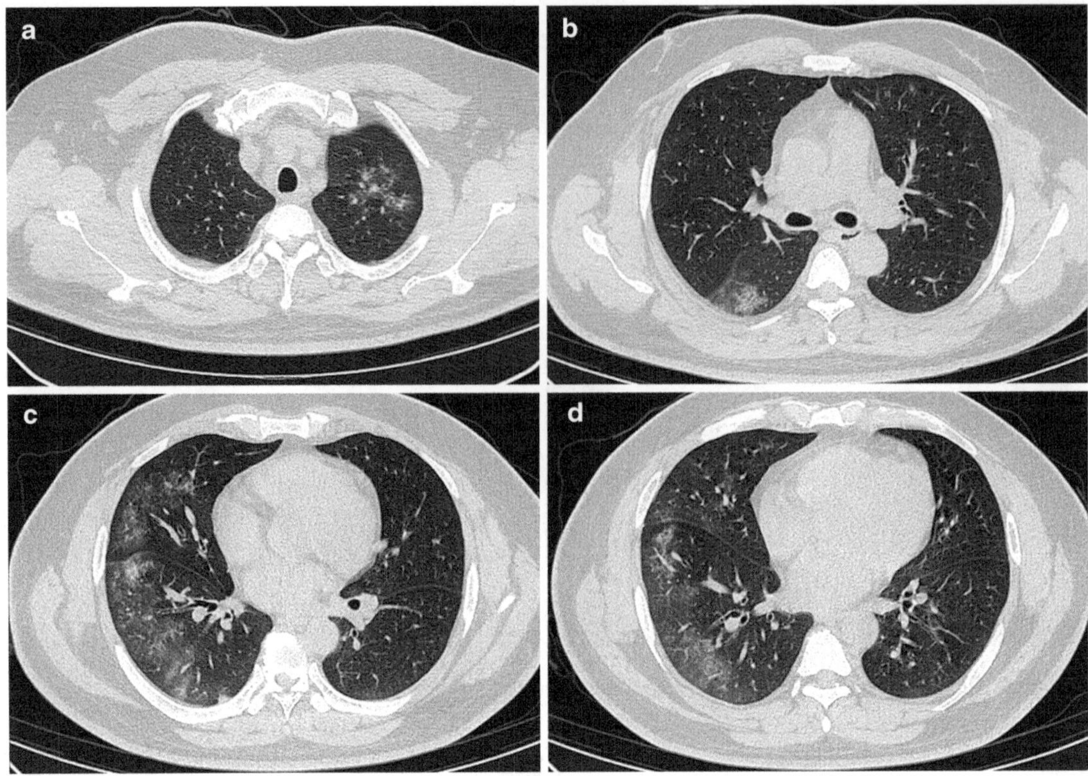

Fig. 4.125 Follow-up CT images 10 days after initial scan

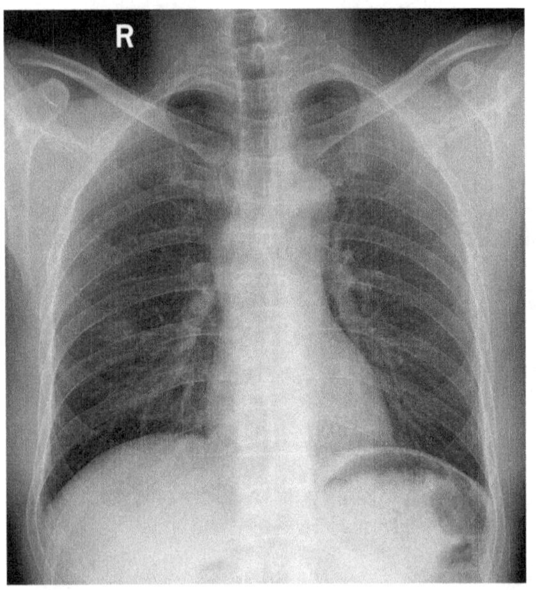

Fig. 4.126 Initial chest radiography image

Follow-up chest CT (4 days after initial CT examination) showed uneven patchy solid shadow with "halo sign" along bronchovascular bundles in the middle lobe of the right lung (Fig. 4.128).

After 15 days follow-up and reexamination, CT showed that the lesion was absorbed and tended to disappear compared with the previous images (Fig. 4.129).

Comments: This was a mild case of COVID-19. CT showed solitary solid nodules, which progressed in a short time, but soon improved.

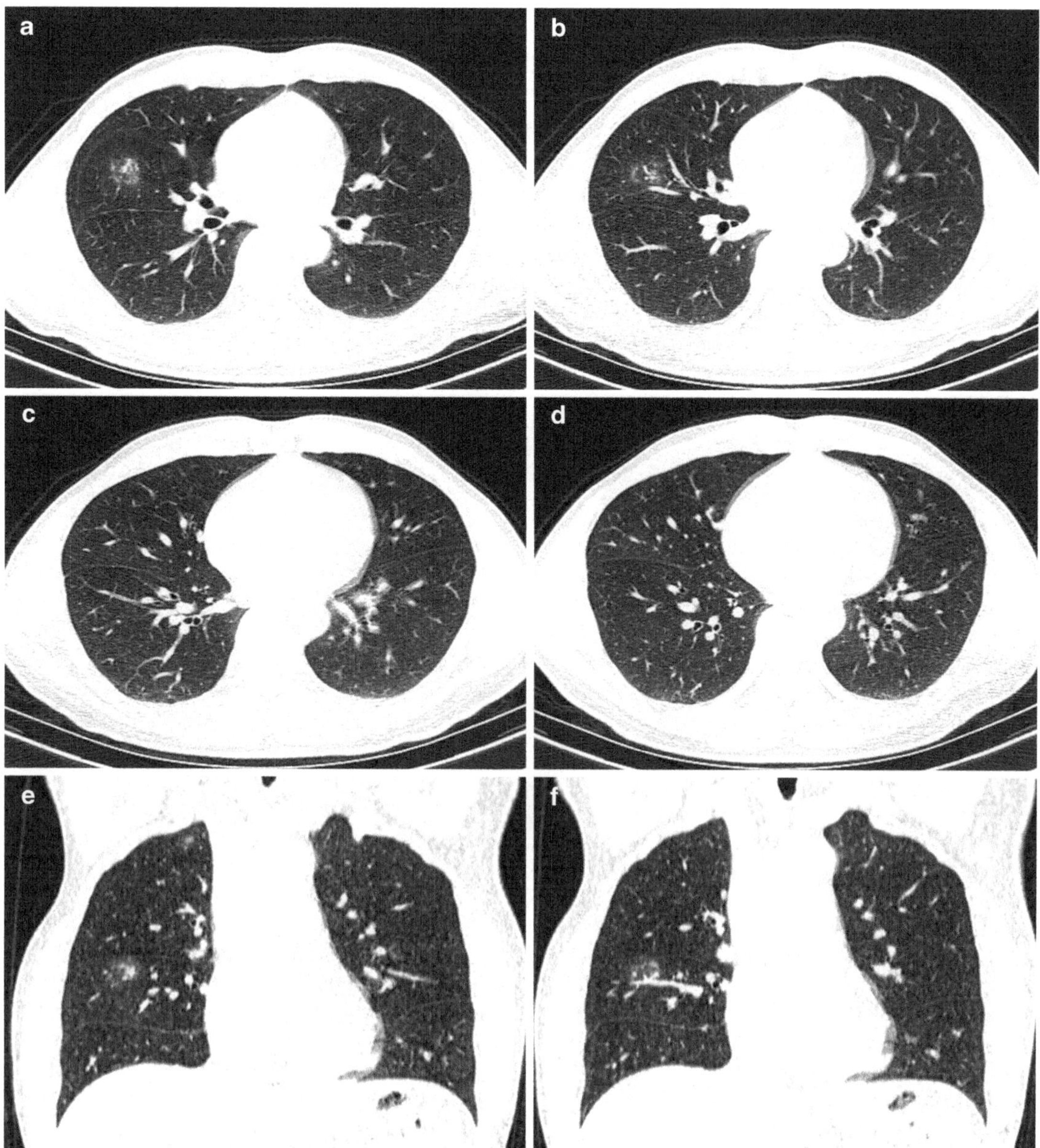

Fig. 4.127 Initial axial chest CT (**a–d**) and reconstructed coronal (**e**, **f**) images of the patient

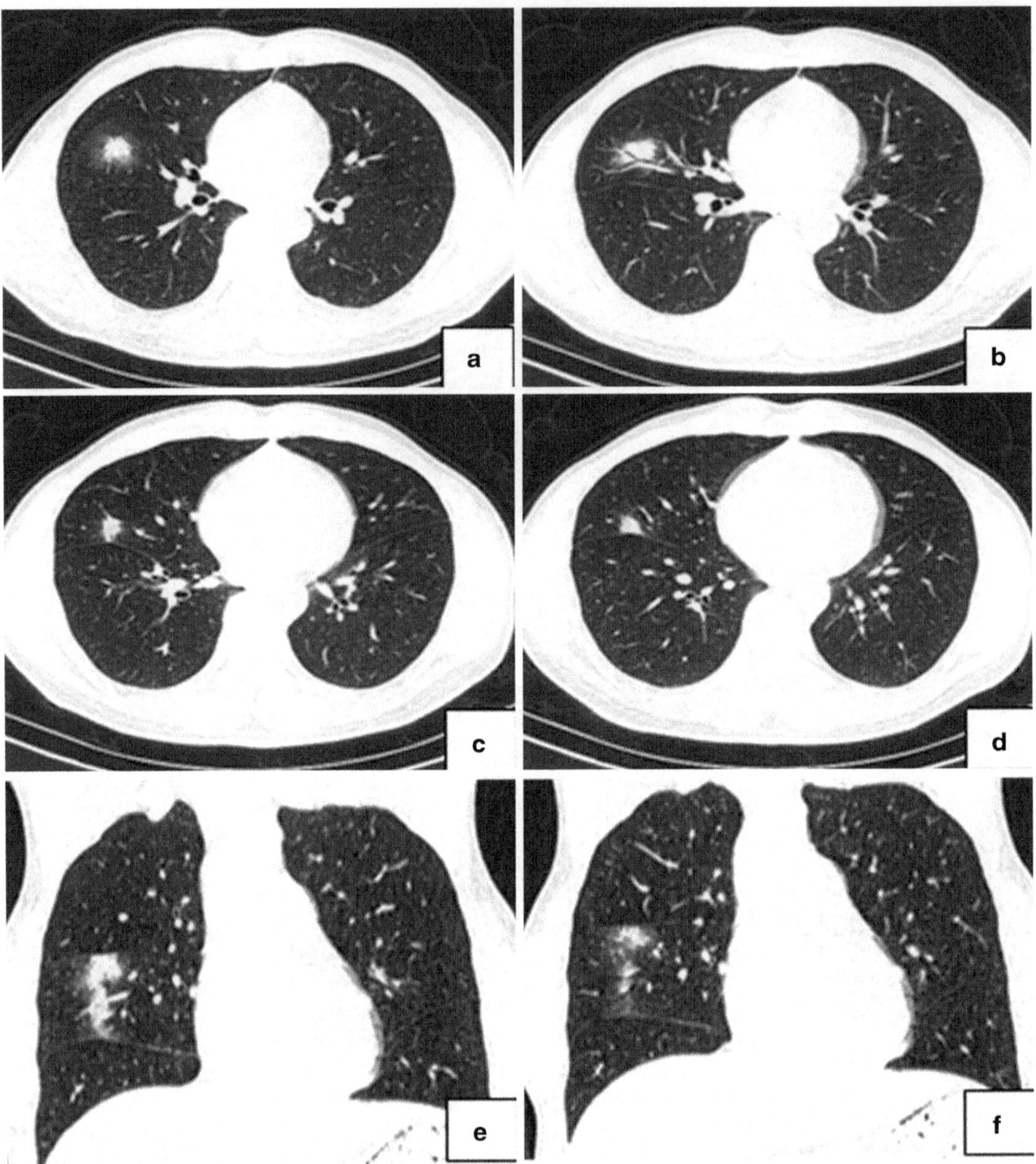

Fig. 4.128 Follow-up axial chest CT (**a–d**) and reconstructed coronal (**e, f**) images 4 days after initial scan

4.3 Severe Typical Case and Its Outcome

Case 40

Medical History and Clinical Manifestations

A 41-year-old female was admitted in the hospital for 10 days with dry cough and 3 days with fever (highest body temperature: 38.7 °C) and fatigue. Laboratory test results indicated the neutrophil percentage increased, and the lymphocyte count and percentage was decreased, the eosinophil count and percentage decreased, and the erythrocyte sedimentation rate, C-reactive protein, and IL-6 increased. The resting oxygen

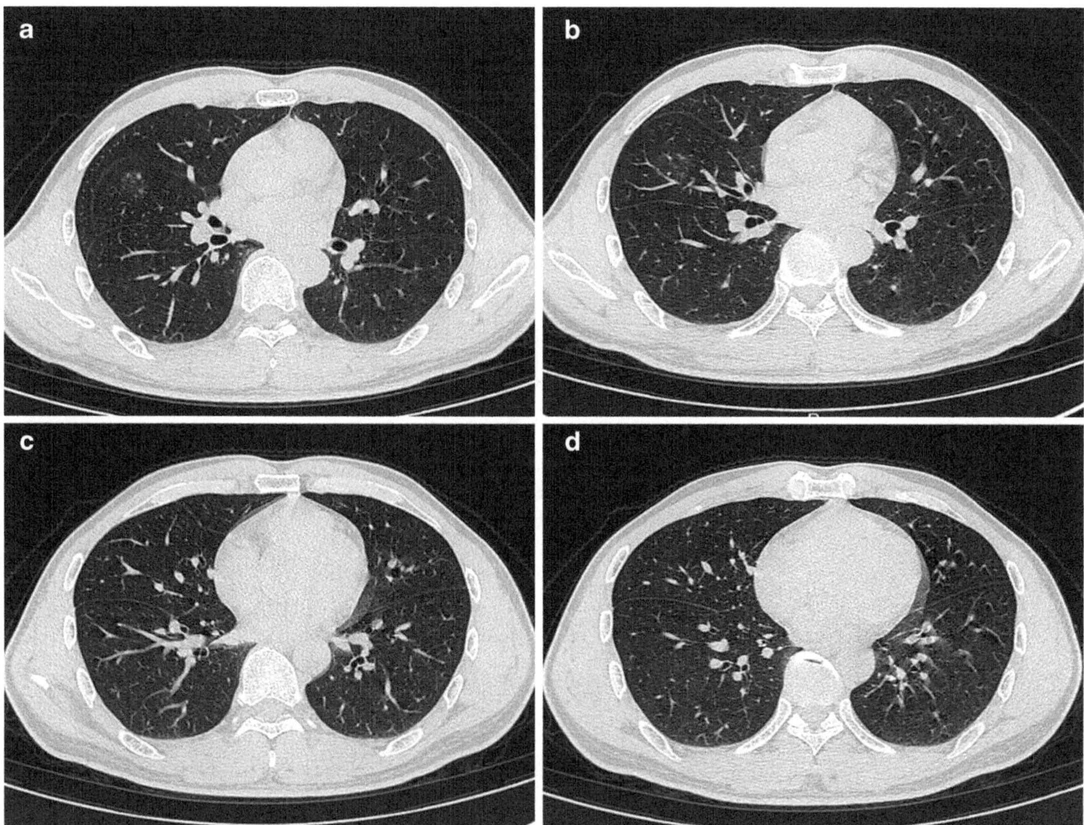

Fig. 4.129 Follow-up CT images 15 days after initial scan

saturation of this patient was 91%. Exposure history: There was no obvious close contacting with COVID-19 patient. The SARS-CoV-2 nucleic acid test was positive on the day of admission. He had a history of type 2 diabetes.

Imaging Features

Initial chest CT showed multiple nodular and large ground-glass shadows in both lungs, and the lesion boundary was clear. Thickened vascular shadow, air bronchial sign, and nodular antihalo sign could be seen in the lesions (Fig. 4.130).

Follow-up chest CT (9 days after initial CT examination) showed the lesions in both lungs were absorbed and reduced, but the density increased and became solid (Fig. 4.131).

Follow-up chest CT (18 days after initial CT examination) showed that the lesions in both lungs were significantly absorbed, and reduced in density (Fig. 4.132).

Comments: Middle-aged male patients with an underlying medical condition of diabetes and decreased lymphocyte count and percentage, increased erythrocyte sedimentation rate, increased C-reactive protein and IL-6, and decreased oxygen saturation suggested that the condition was severe. After 18 days effective therapy, the patient improved rapidly and the pulmonary lesions were also reduced.

Case 41

Medical History and Clinical Manifestations

A 33-year-old female was admitted in the hospital for 7 days with fever (highest body temperature: 40.2 °C), occasionally cough and runny nose. Laboratory test results indicated a normal white blood cell count of 4.33×10^9/L, 74.1% neutrophils, and decreased lymphocytes of 19.1%. There were elevated blood levels for erythrocyte sedimentation rate (21 mm/h), C

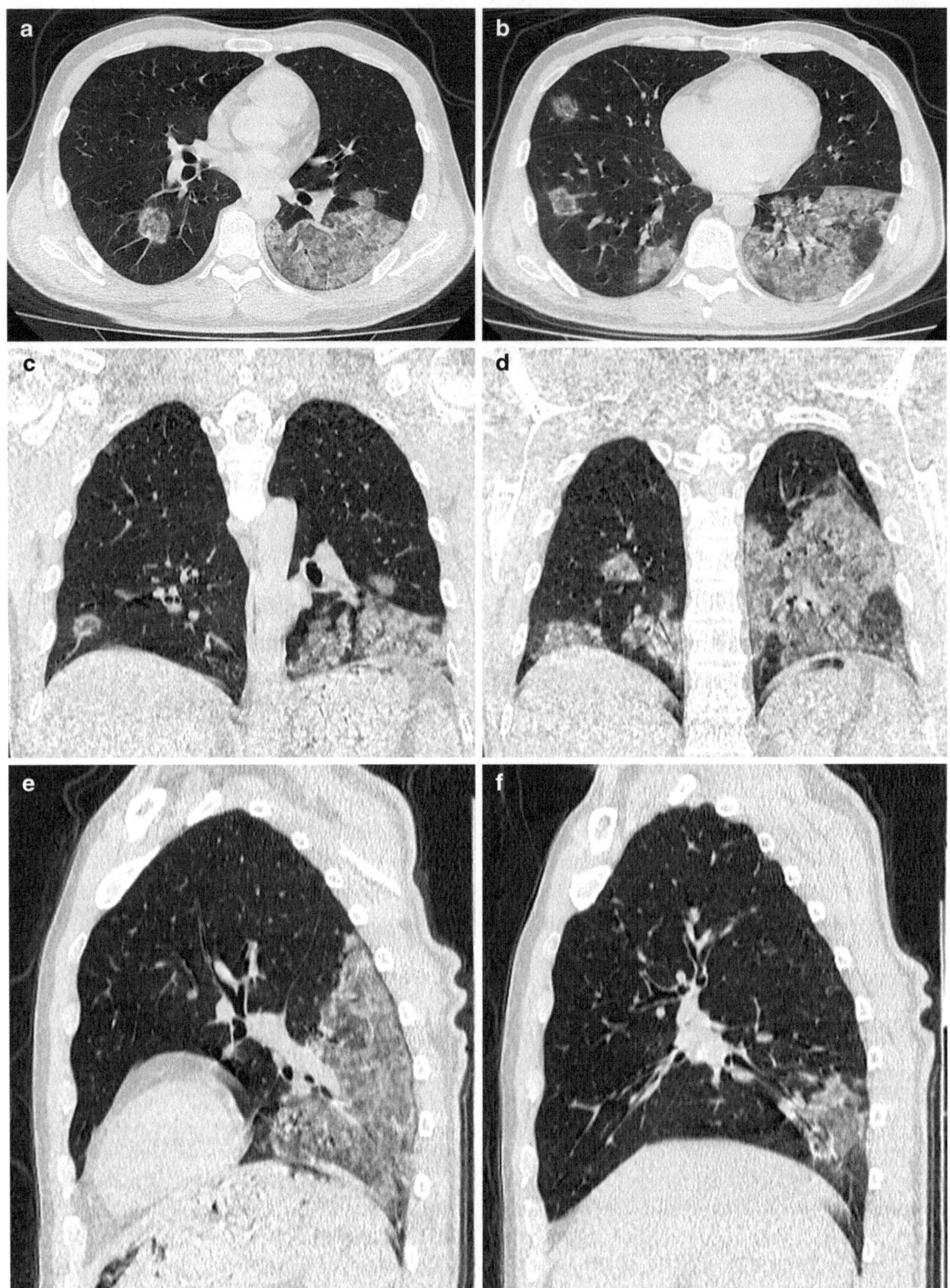

Fig. 4.130 Initial axial chest CT (**a**, **b**), reconstructed coronal (**c**, **d**) and sagittal (**e**, **f**) images of the patient

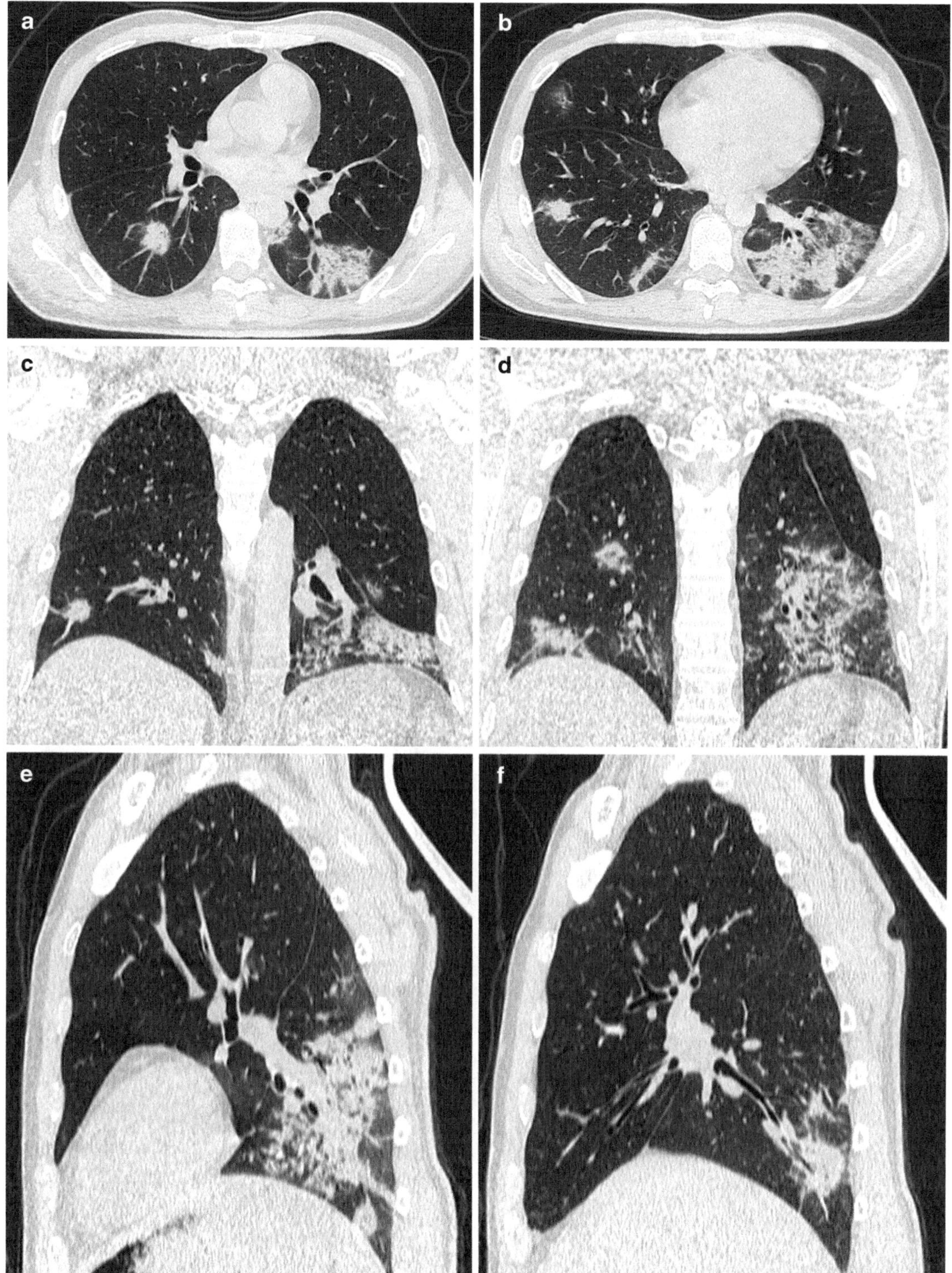

Fig. 4.131 Follow-up axial chest CT (**a**, **b**), reconstructed coronal (**c**, **d**) and sagittal (**e**, **f**) images 9 days after initial scan

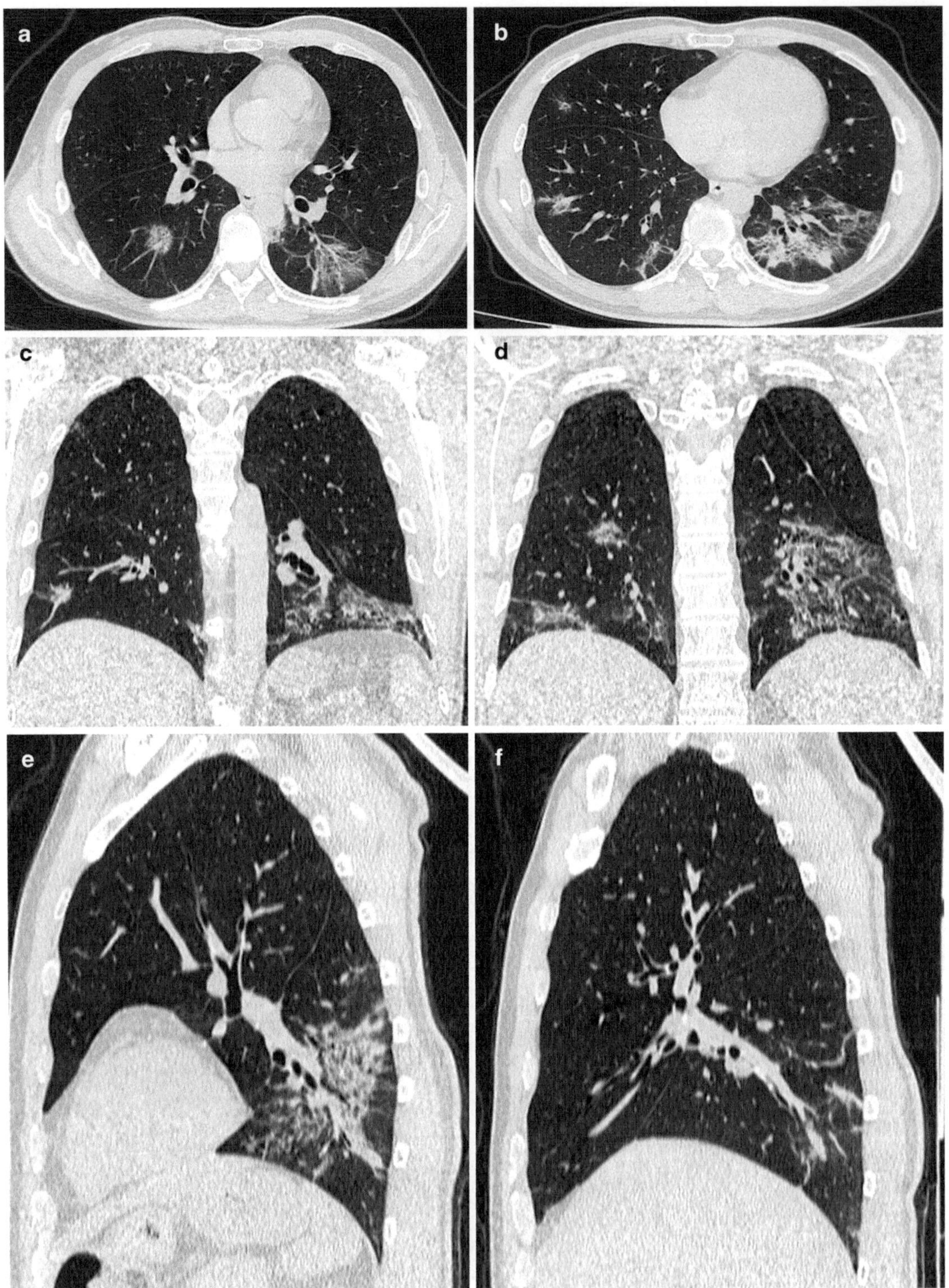

Fig. 4.132 Follow-up axial chest CT (**a**, **b**), reconstructed coronal (**c**, **d**) and sagittal (**e**, **f**) images 18 days after initial scan

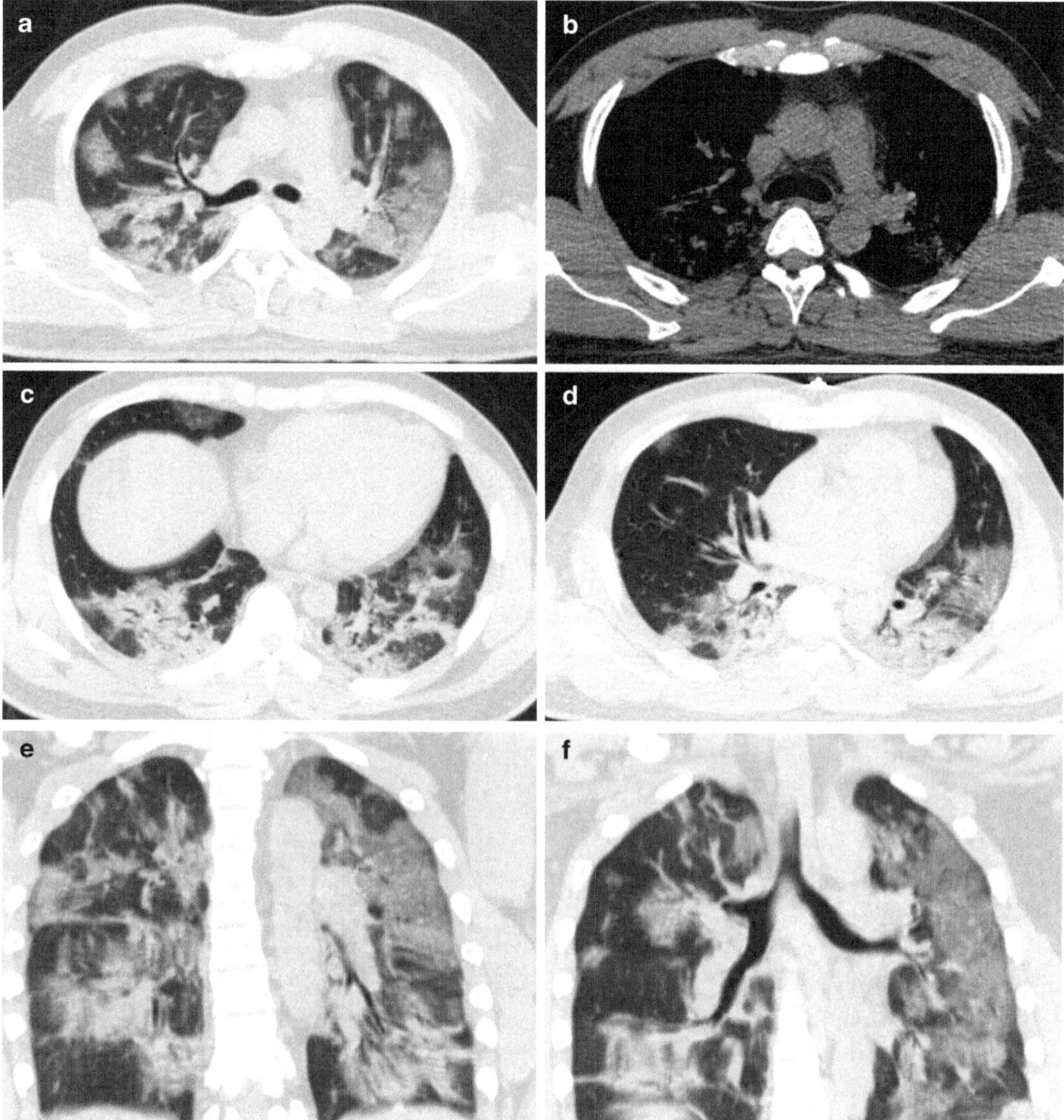

Fig. 4.133 Initial axial chest CT (**a–d**) and reconstructed coronal (**e**, **f**) images of the patient

reactive protein/(35.14 mg/L), and procalcitonin (0.112 ng/mL). The arterial oxygen partial pressure (PaO_2)/inhaled oxygen concentration (FiO_2) was 165.8 mmHg. Exposure history: The patient worked in Wuhan, China and more than 20 people suffered from fever in the workplace. The SARS-CoV-2 nucleic acid test was positive on the day of admission.

Imaging Features

Initial chest CT showed multiple patchy and large ground-glass opacities and consolidation in both lungs. The lesions were more obvious in the subpleural area of both lungs, with "grid-like changes" (black arrow) and "air bronchial sign," also fibrosis can be seen around the focus (Fig. 4.133).

Follow-up chest CT (10 days after initial CT examination) showed the ground-glass shadows and consolidation of bilateral lungs were significantly absorbed, and the lesions were relatively scattered; multiple fibrous cord foci (**c–e**: white arrows) appeared in both lungs (Fig. 4.134).

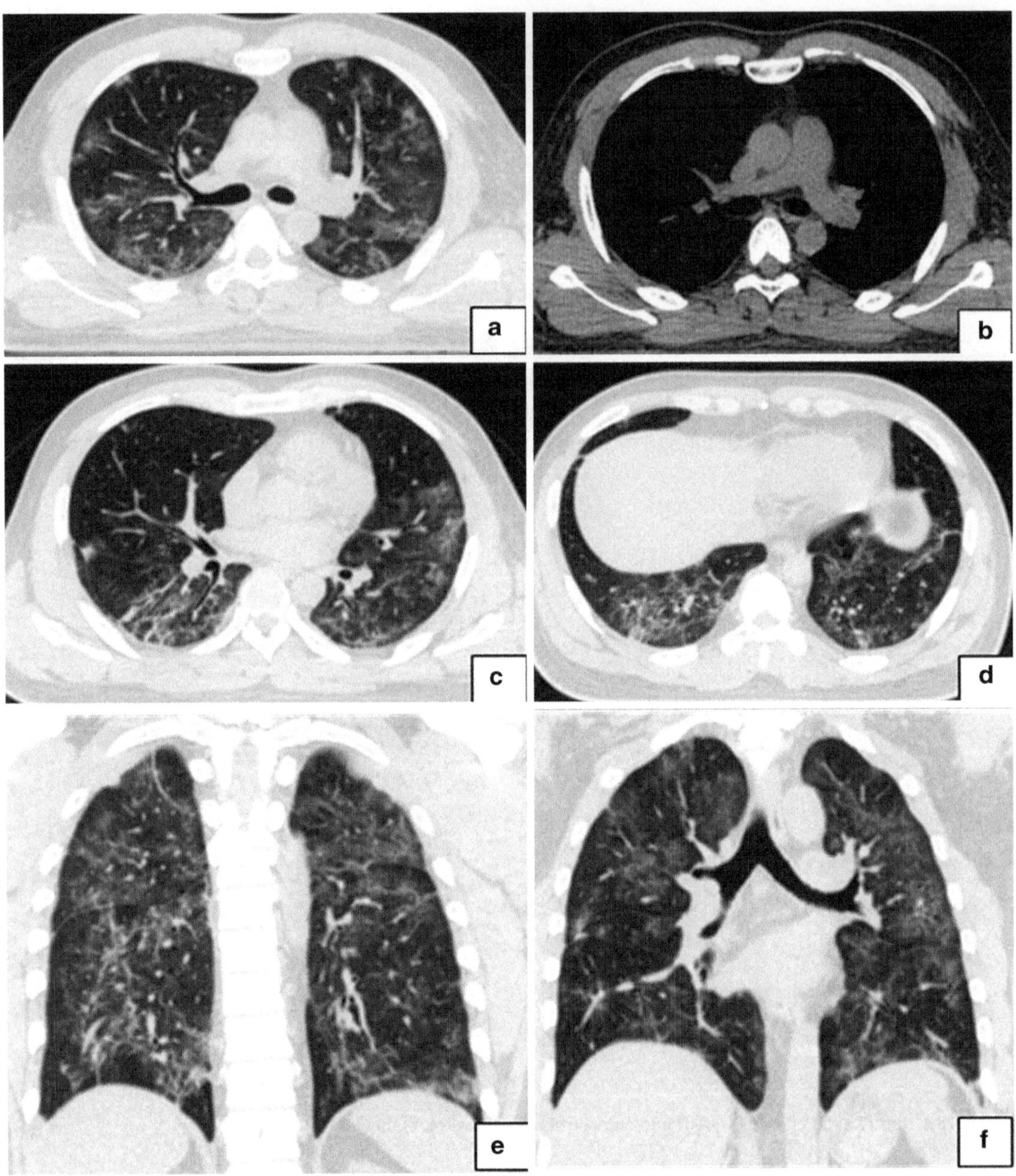

Fig. 4.134 Follow-up axial chest CT (**a–d**) and reconstructed coronal (**e**, **f**) images 10 days after initial scan

Follow-up chest CT (23 days after Initial CT examination) showed the inflammatory lesions in both lungs were further absorbed, remaining a small amount of patchy GGOs (Fig. 4.135).

Comments: The patient was a clinically severe patient with typical imaging findings for the first CT images. This case showed the dynamic changes of chest CT from admission to recovery and discharge. However, after two consecutive negative the SARS-CoV-2 nucleic acid test, patchy ground-glass shadow was still in both lungs, suggesting that the patient might still need to isolation.

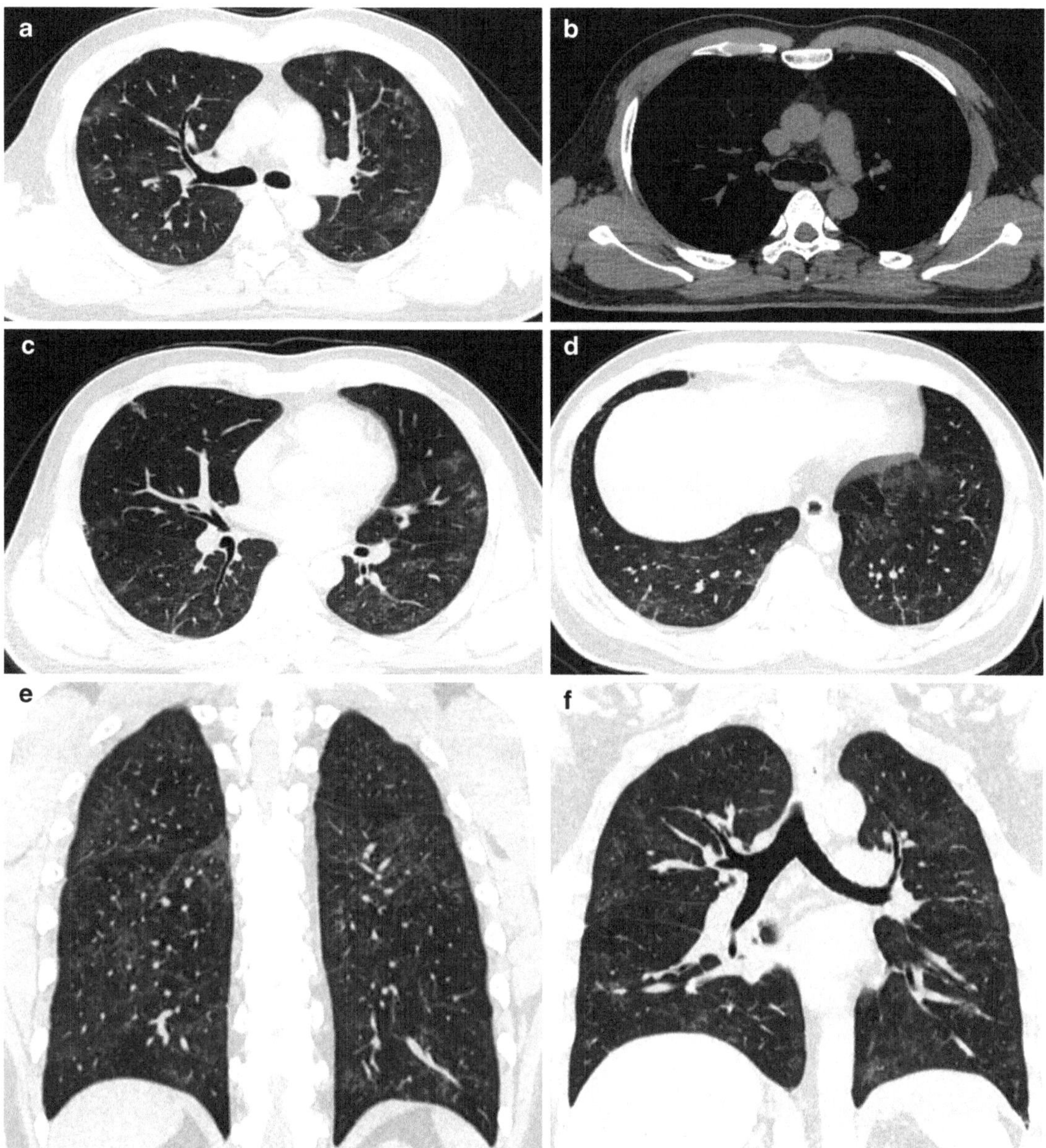

Fig. 4.135 Follow-up axial chest CT (**a–d**) and reconstructed coronal (**e**, **f**) images 23 days after initial scan

Imaging Features of COVID-19 in Elder People

5

Xiaopei Xu, Zhujing Shen, Hui Mao, Bin Lin, and Minming Zhang

It has been generally reported that elderly individuals, especially those with underlying disease, are most vulnerable to SARS-CoV-2 infection. After being infected with SARS-CoV-2, elderly patients, typically aged over 65, are more prone to severe symptoms and conditions, requiring care at the intensive care unit (ICU) [1, 2]. The elderly COVID-19 patients usually have poor outcomes with higher mortality than other age groups. A recent report from studying 339 elderly COVID-19 patients found that more than 70% of the enrolled patients were in severe or critical conditions, while 42.8% developed complication with bacterial infection. Acute respiratory distress syndrome (ARDS) was reported in 21.0% of these patients. The mortality rate was 19.2% [3]. Another retrospective study on 113 deceased patients found that more than 83% of them were aged 60 or older [4]. This may be related to the weakened immune system and respiratory function of the elderly. Accordingly, the CT imaging manifestation of elderly patients appears severer and more progressive than that of young and middle-aged patients. The inflammation is mostly subpleural and often involving bilateral lungs, mainly presenting as ground-glass opacities (GGO) and consolidations in pulmonary CT. As the disease is rapidly progressive, diffuse bilateral lesions could develop in 4–7 days [5].

In addition, there are a higher proportion of the elderly COVID-19 patients who have underlying chronic diseases, such as diabetes, hypertension, cardiovascular disease, cerebrovascular disease, and chronic obstructive pulmonary disease. Existing lung diseases or disorders may lead to atypical imaging manifestation in the early stage. Thus, comparing the images from prior exams or using dynamic or multiple time point scans to interrogate abnormalities should be strongly considered. Because coexistence of basic diseases complicates the symptoms and conditions, multiple diseases affect each other; the difficulty of treatment is greatly increased. Therefore, in the process of clinical diagnosis and treatment, a comprehensive evaluation of elderly patients should be conducted in order to identify high-risk elderly patients who may develop severe/critical conditions. Timely interventions should be taken to improve the prognosis.

X. Xu · B. Lin (✉) · M. Zhang
Department of Radiology, the Second Affiliated Hospital, Zhejiang University School of Medicine, Hangzhou, China
e-mail: xiaopeix@zju.edu.cn; zjdxlinbin@zju.edu.cn; zhangminming@zju.edu.cn

Z. Shen · H. Mao
Department of Radiology and Imaging Sciences, Emory University School of Medicine, Atlanta, GA, USA
e-mail: shenzhujing@zju.edu.cn; hmao@emory.edu

M. Zhang, B. Lin (eds.), *Diagnostic Imaging of Novel Coronavirus Pneumonia*,
https://doi.org/10.1007/978-981-15-5992-1_5

Case 1

Medical History and Clinical Manifestations

A 79-year-old female was admitted in the hospital for 6 h with low fever (highest body temperature: 37.5 °C). Laboratory examination indicated a normal white blood cell count of 4.43 × 10^9/L, 62.4% neutrophil, and 26.9% lymphocyte. There were elevated blood levels for erythrocyte sedimentation rate (41 mm/h) and C-reactive protein (10.54 mg/L). The patient lived in Wuhan, China for a long time. She had been to a hospital in Wuhan, China and traveled to Guilin, Guangxi Province, China in days prior to symptom onset. The SARS-CoV-2 nucleic acid was positive. The patient developed respiratory failure 17 days after onset and was given invasive ventilation.

Imaging Features

Initial chest CT showed patchy ground glass opacities in bilateral lungs, the "reticular pattern" (**a**. red arrow) in the left lung, dilated of blood vessels (**c**. red arrow), and ground-glass opacities with "halo sign" in the right upper lobe (Fig. 5.1).

Follow-up chest CT (17 days after initial CT examination) showed multiple lamellar ground-glass opacities on both lungs, showing air bronchogram (red arrow) and enlarged consolidation lesion (Fig. 5.2).

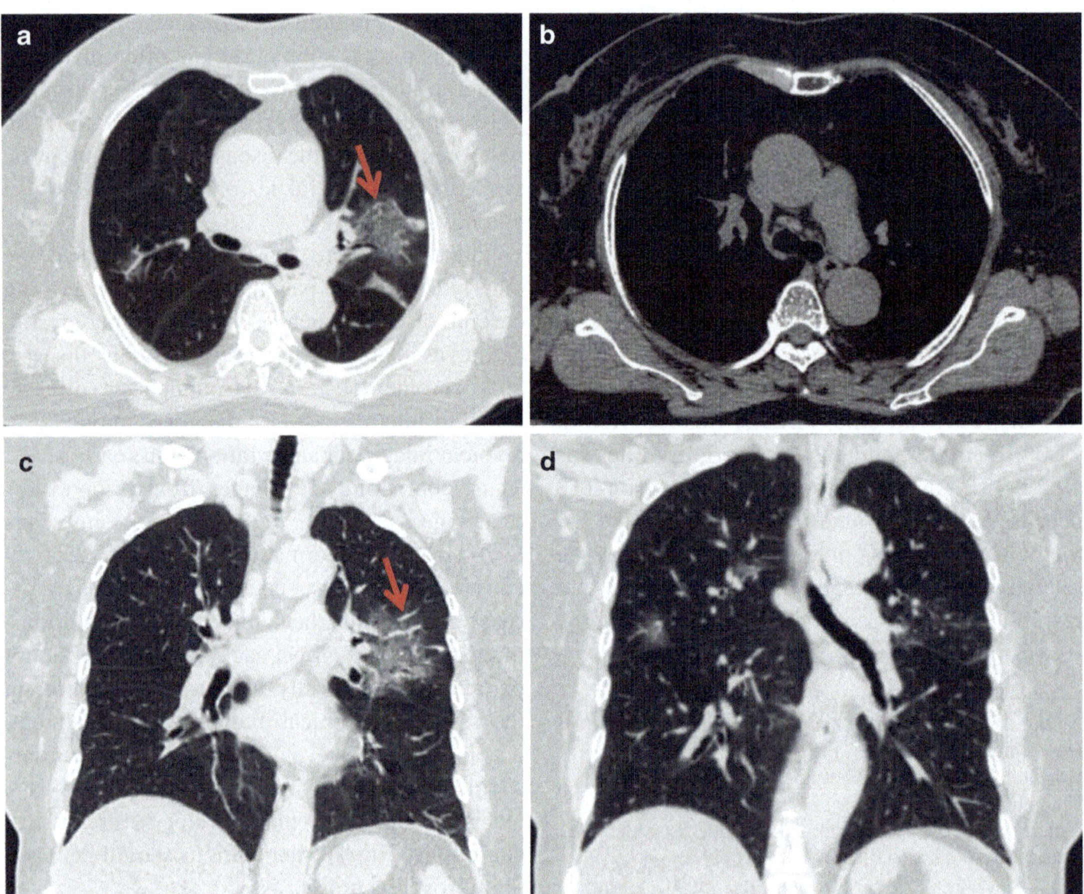

Fig. 5.1 Initial axial chest CT (**a**, **b**), reconstructed coronal (**c**, **d**) images of the patient

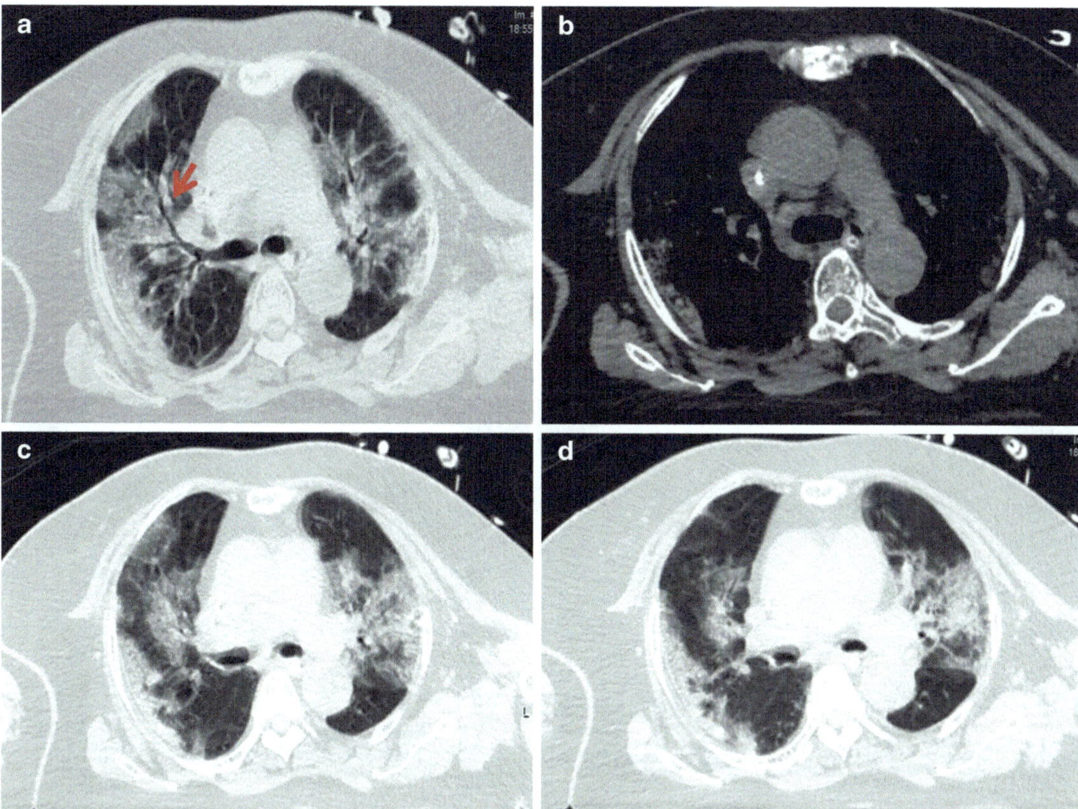

Fig. 5.2 Follow-up CT images 17 days after initial scan

Follow-up chest CT (35 days after initial CT examination) showed that the multiple ground-glass opacities of both lungs were resolved, the solid component of the lesion increased slightly, the fibrosis lesions increased significantly, and small amount of pleural effusion on the right side of the chest appeared (Fig. 5.3).

Comments: In the elderly female patients, ground-glass opacity was the main CT image at the onset of the disease, with a little consolidation. With the aggravation of the disease, the CT image showed diversity, consolidation increased, and the disease was extensive, involving multiple lung lobes. During treatment, the patient was found to be simultaneously infected with gram-negative bacilli. The course of the disease was prolonged, CT showed more consolidation, fibrosis, and a small amount of pleural effusion on the right side of the chest.

Case 2

Medical History and Clinical Manifestations

A 71-year-old female was admitted in the hospital with fever (highest body temperature: 37.5 °C) for 4 days after cold exposure, chills, and shortness of breath after activity. Laboratory test results showed low white blood cell count of 3.53×10^9/L, high neutrophil percentage of 86.5%, and low lymphocyte percentage of 8%. There were elevated blood levels for erythrocyte sedimentation rate (21 mm/h) and C-reactive protein (22.54 mg/L). The patient lived in Wuhan,

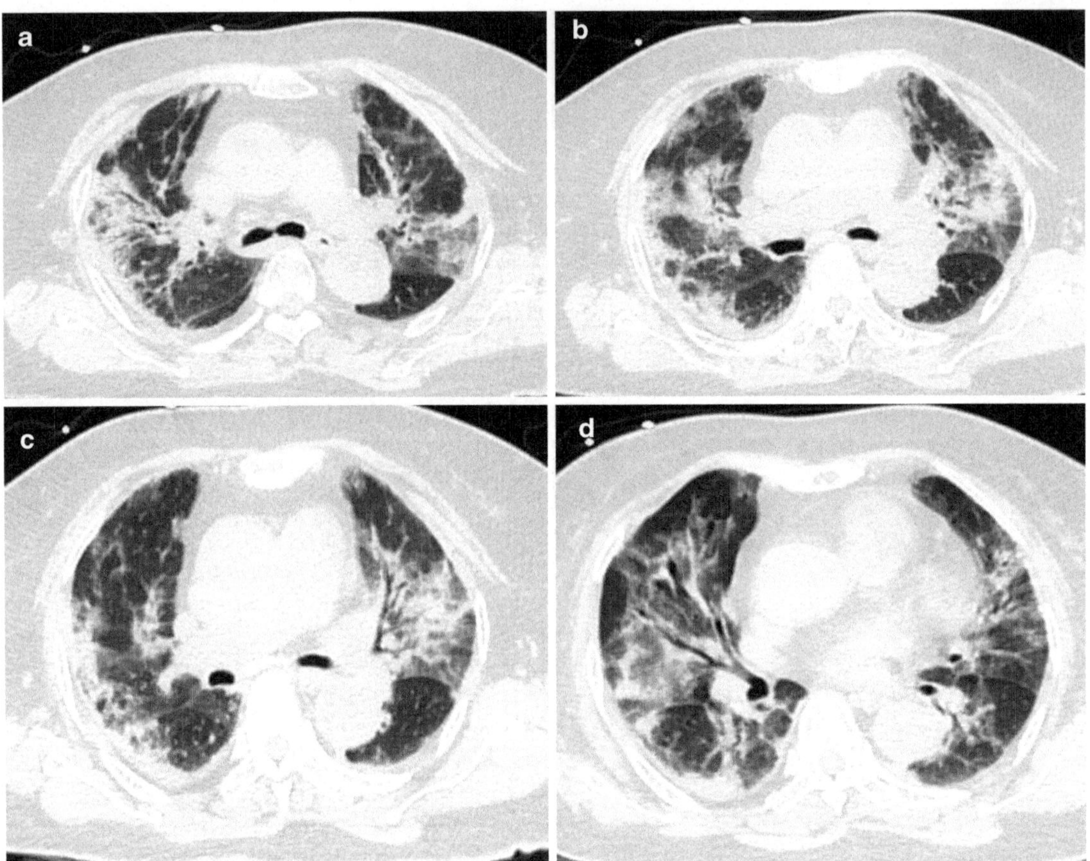

Fig. 5.3 Follow-up CT image 35 days after initial scan

China for a long time and went to Guilin, China in the days prior to symptom onset. The SARS-CoV-2 nucleic acid test was positive.

Imaging Features

Initial chest CT shows multiple flaky and curved ground-glass opacities under the pleura and along the bronchial vascular bundles, "reticular pattern" (**b**. red arrow) can be seen in the left lower lobe subpleural area, and scattered fibrous cord foci (**a**. red arrow) can be seen in the left lung base. Reconstructed coronal images showed that there were mainly ground-glass-like changes, and a few fibrous lesions (**d**, **e**, **f**. red arrow) were seen in the right apex and left lower lobe (Fig. 5.4).

After 10 days of treatment, the SARS-CoV-2 nucleic acid test was still positive, while follow-up chest CT showed that the multiple inflammatory lesions were obviously absorbed, became lighter, and the distribution was more scattered than before (Fig. 5.5).

After 25 days of treatment, the SARS-CoV-2 nucleic acid test was negative for two times. Follow-up chest CT (25 days after initial CT

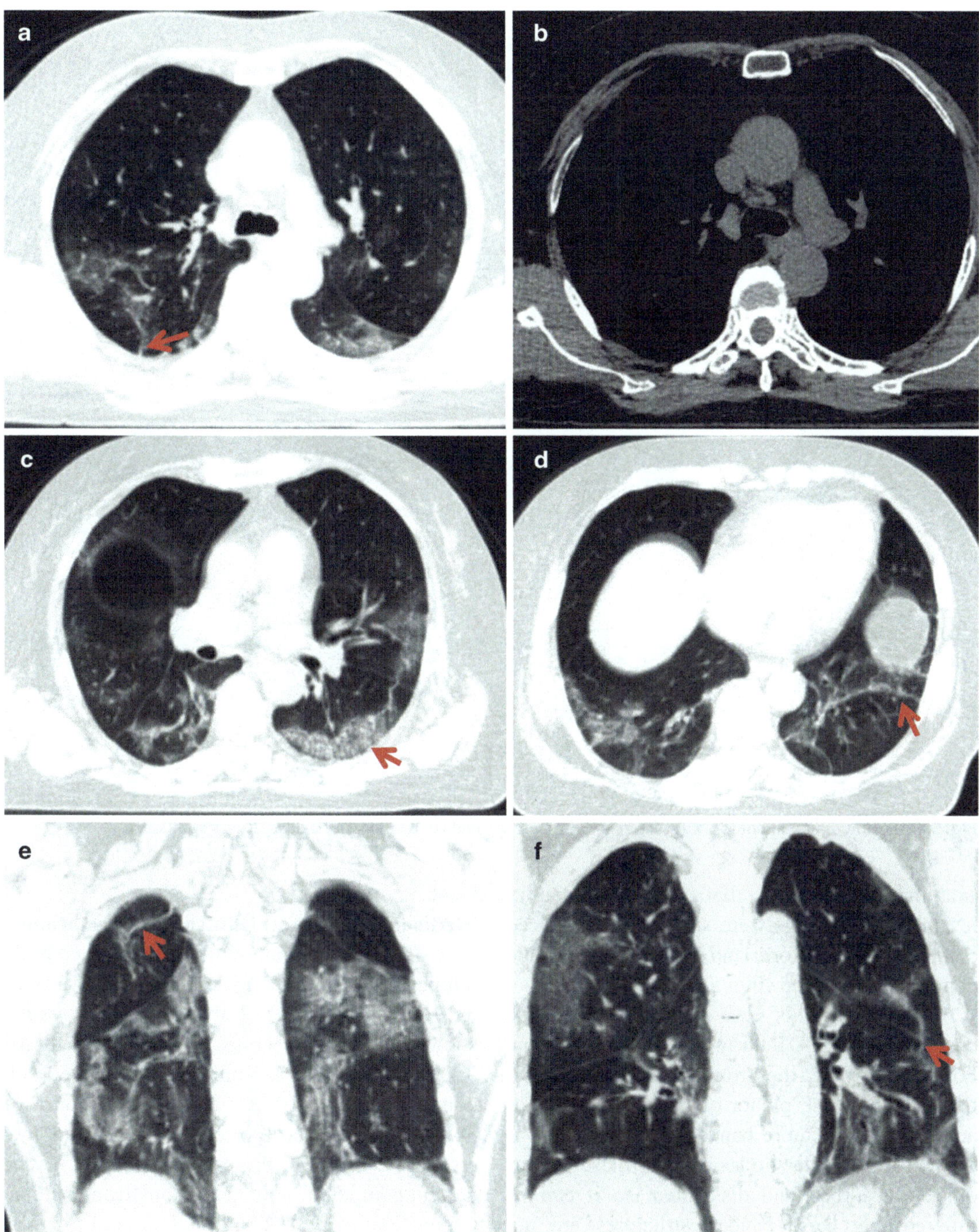

Fig. 5.4 Initial axial chest CT (**a**–**d**), reconstructed coronal (**e**, **f**) images of the patient

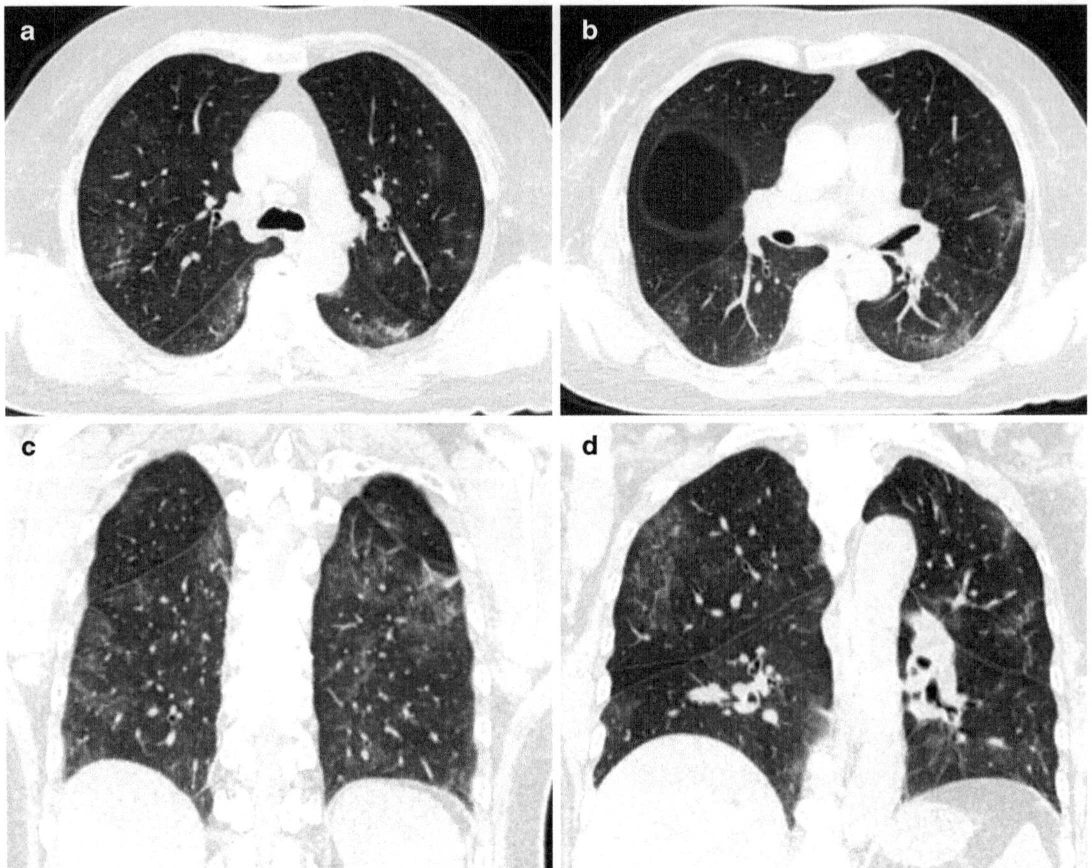

Fig. 5.5 Follow-up axial chest CT (**a**, **b**), reconstructed coronal (**c**, **d**) images 10 days after initial scan

examination) showed that the inflammatory lesions of both lungs were significantly reduced compared with before, and most of them were completely absorbed (Fig. 5.6).

Comments: This case shows the dynamic changes of chest CT during the transformation. For the first time, the ground-glass shadow distributed under the pleura of the two lungs was accompanied by more banded structures. It was thought to be a fibrotic lesion. But these lesions quickly absorbed and dissipated, so it can be inferred that these banded structures are not fibrosis but atelectasis.

Case 3

Medical History and Clinical Manifestations

A 72-year-old male with fever (highest body temperature: 38.4 °C) and chills was admitted in the hospital. Laboratory test results showed a normal white blood cell count of 8.15×10^9/L, 73.6% neutrophil, red blood cell count of 3.90×10^{12}/L, and platelet count of 345×10^9/L. There were elevated blood levels for C-reactive protein (56.2 mg/L). The patient contacted with the persons from Wuhan, China. The SARS-CoV-2 nucleic acid test was positive.

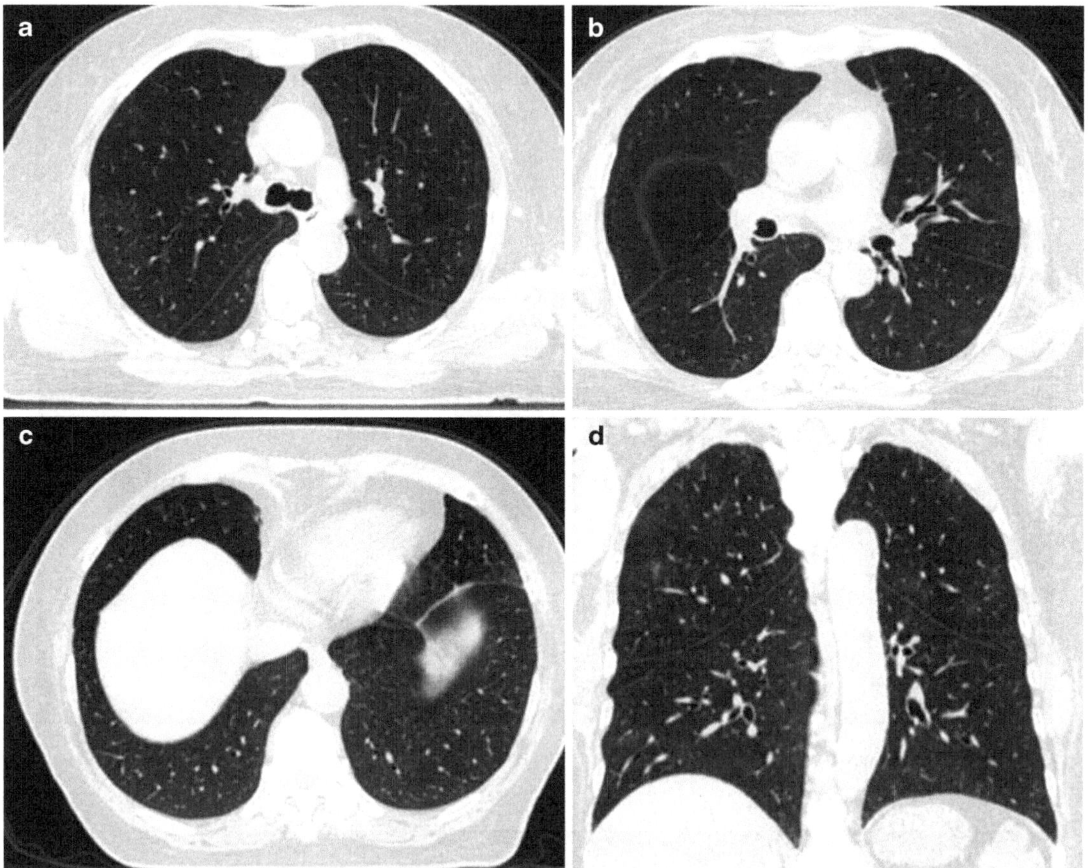

Fig. 5.6 Follow-up axial chest CT (**a**, **b**, **c**), reconstructed coronal (**d**) images 25 days after initial scan

Imaging Features

Initial chest CT showed subpleural consolidation in the lower lobe of both lungs with air bronchograms. Some bronchial tubes are twisted, and fibrosis is seen (Fig. 5.7).

Follow-up chest CT (19 days after initial CT examination) showed that the consolidation lesions were diminished, replacing ground-glass opacities with fibrosis (Fig. 5.8).

Comments: This case is an elderly male patient, presenting with clinical common type. After the treatment, it improved smoothly. The changes of CT manifestations include consolidation absorption and fibrosis.

Case 4

Medical History and Clinical Manifestations

A 67-year-old female was admitted in the hospital with fever for 2 days (highest body temperature: 38.0 °C). Laboratory test results showed low white blood cell count of 3.7×10^9/L, normal lymphocyte percentage of 21.2%, and neutrophil percentage of 68.9%. The patient's son lives in Wuhan, China and recently returned to his hometown, Ruian, Zhejiang Province, China. Both the patient and her son's SARS-CoV-2 nucleic acid tests are positive.

Imaging Features

Initial chest radiograph showed increased texture of both lungs with exudation of the right lower lobe (Fig. 5.9).

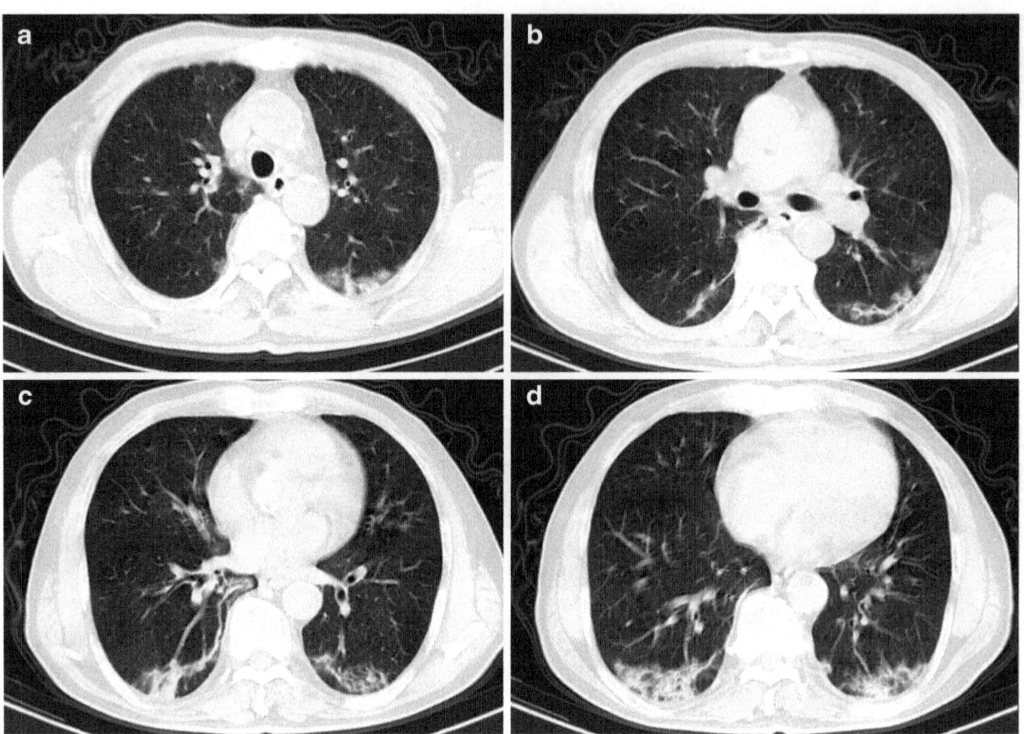

Fig. 5.7 Initial CT image of the patient

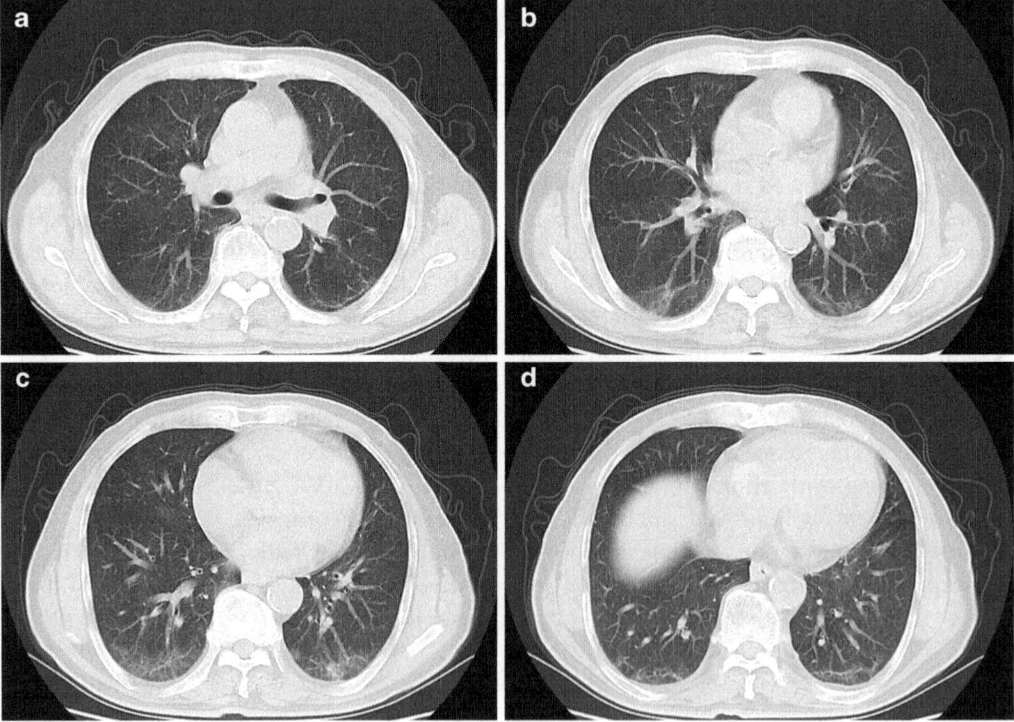

Fig. 5.8 Follow-up CT images 19 days after initial scan

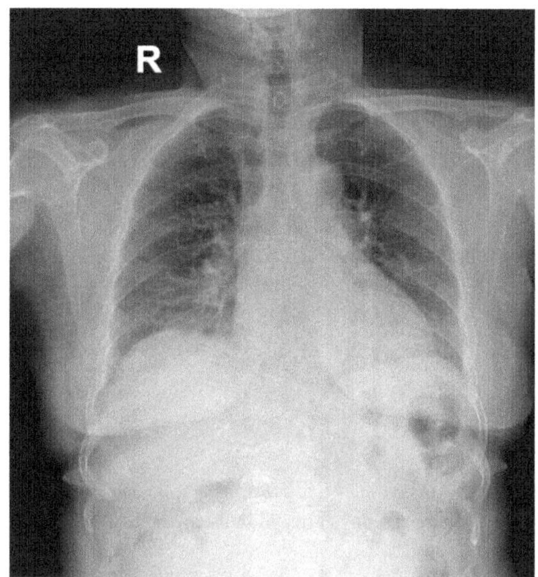

Fig. 5.9 Initial chest radiograph of the patient

Chest CT showed nodules and patchy ground-glass opacities of both lungs. Some lesions of the lower lobe of both lungs showed "reticular pattern" (Fig. 5.10).

Follow-up chest CT (5 days after initial CT examination) showed that the ground-glass opacities progressed. The "reticular pattern" and "crazy paving" became much more markedly (Fig. 5.11).

Follow-up chest CT (9 days after initial CT examination) showed that some patchy ground-glass opacity was more solid (red arrow), and some lesions became lighter (Fig. 5.12).

Follow-up chest CT (18 days after initial CT examination) showed the lesions further absorbed than the lesions in the previous images (red arrow) (Fig. 5.13).

Comments: Chest radiograph of this patient after onset showed increased texture of both

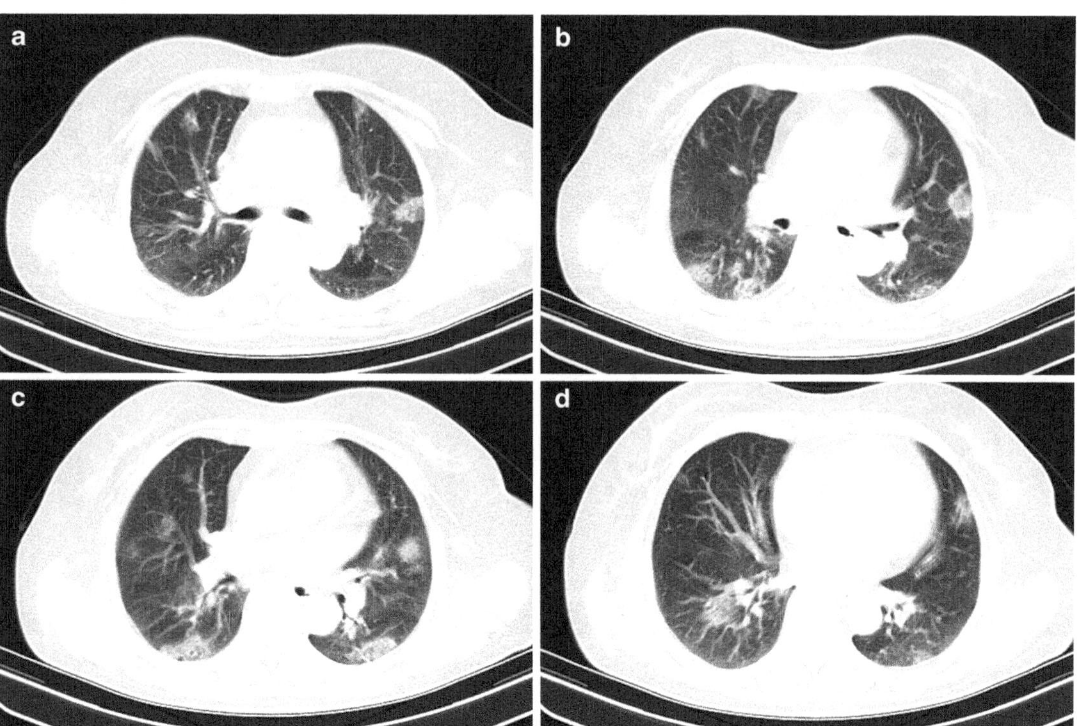

Fig. 5.10 Initial CT images of the patient

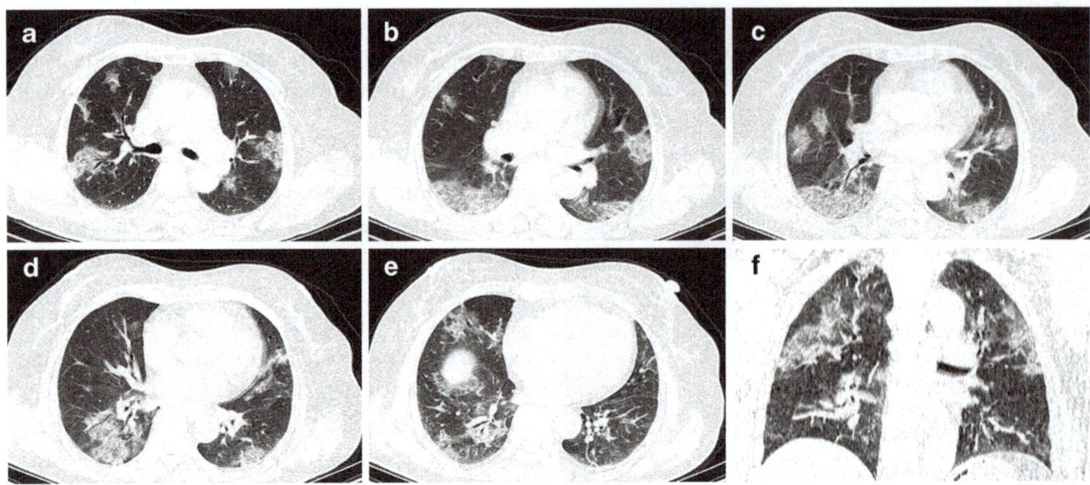

Fig. 5.11 Follow-up axial chest CT (**a**–**e**), reconstructed coronal (**f**) images 5 days after initial scan

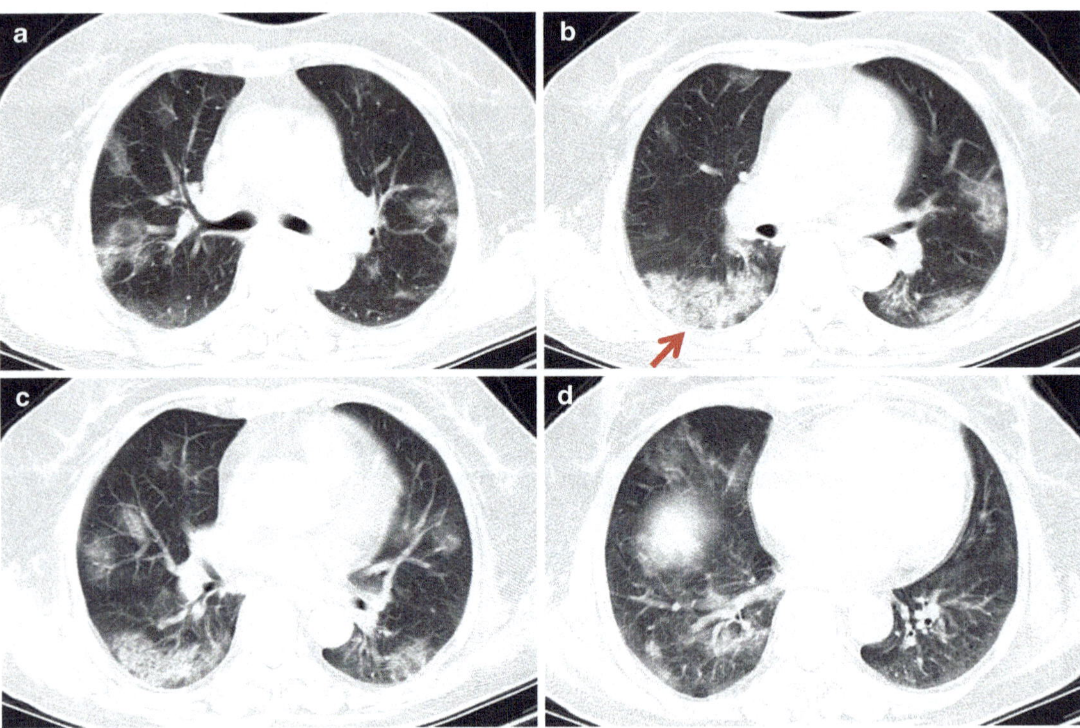

Fig. 5.12 Follow-up CT images 9 days after initial scan

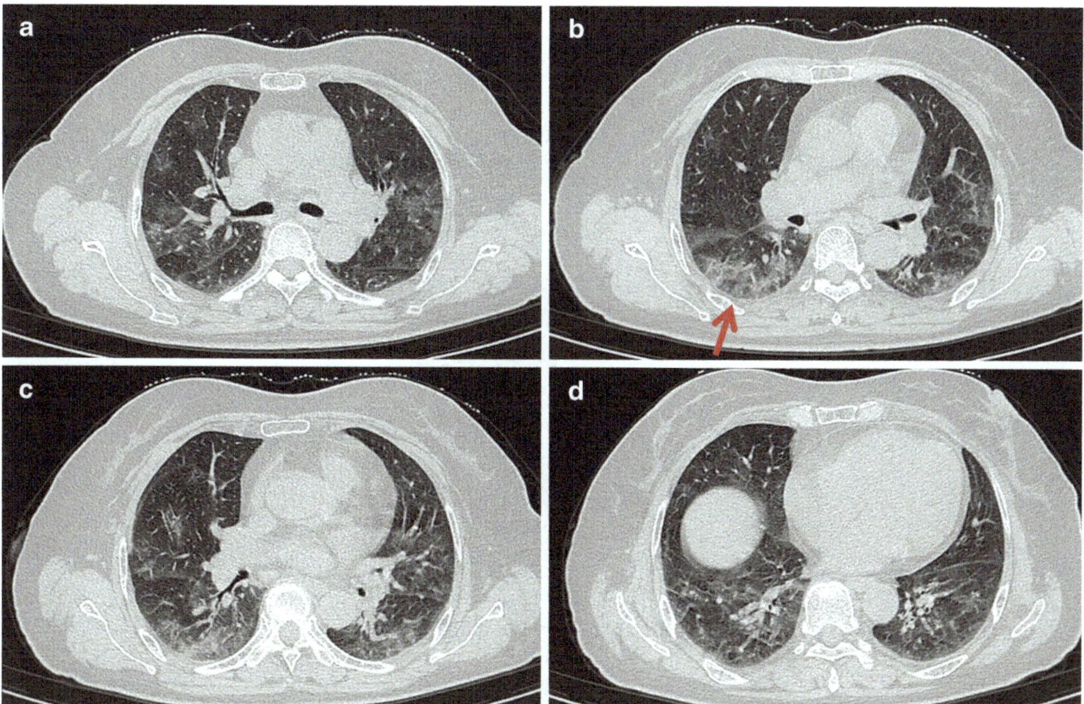

Fig. 5.13 Follow-up CT images 18 days after initial scan

lungs with exudation of the right lower lobe, suggesting changes in bronchopneumonia and these features lack specificity. The initial CT appearance is typical, the lesion is distributed under the pleura, and the sheet-like consolidation is accompanied by reticular pattern.

Case 5

Medical History and Clinical Manifestations

A 68-year-old female was admitted in the hospital with fever for 4 days (highest body temperature: 38.6 °C) accompanied by chills. Laboratory test results showed low white blood cell count of 3.9×10^9/L, C-reactive protein (<0.499 mg/L), normal lymphocyte percentage of 23.1%, and neutrophil percentage of 66.7%. Patient's son returned to Ruian, Zhejiang Province, from Wuhan, China and had a close contact with him. The SARS-CoV-2 nucleic acid test was positive.

Imaging Features

Initial radiograph showed increased texture of bilateral lungs (Fig. 5.14).

Chest CT showed scattered ground-glass opacity nodules of the two lungs, some lesions with "halo signs" (red arrows) (Fig. 5.15).

Follow-up chest CT (9 days after initial CT examination) showed multiple new lesions in both lungs, showing reticular pattern, air bronchogram, and crazy paving (Fig. 5.16).

Follow-up CT examination of 15 days after initial CT examination showed that most of the ground-glass opacities and consolidation lesions were absorbed, the density of the lesions decreased, while some fibrotic changes appeared under the pleura (Fig. 5.17).

Comments: Chest film is not sensitive to early coronary pneumonia. The initial CT of this patient showed multiple nodule lesions with "halo

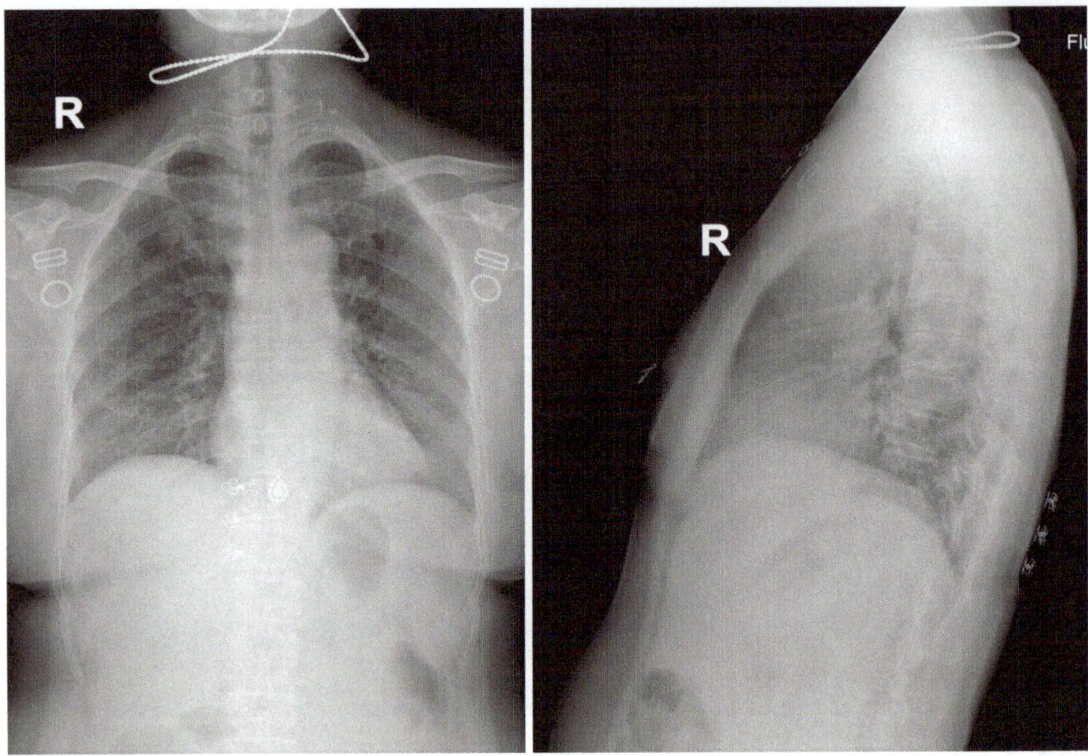

Fig. 5.14 Initial chest radiograph

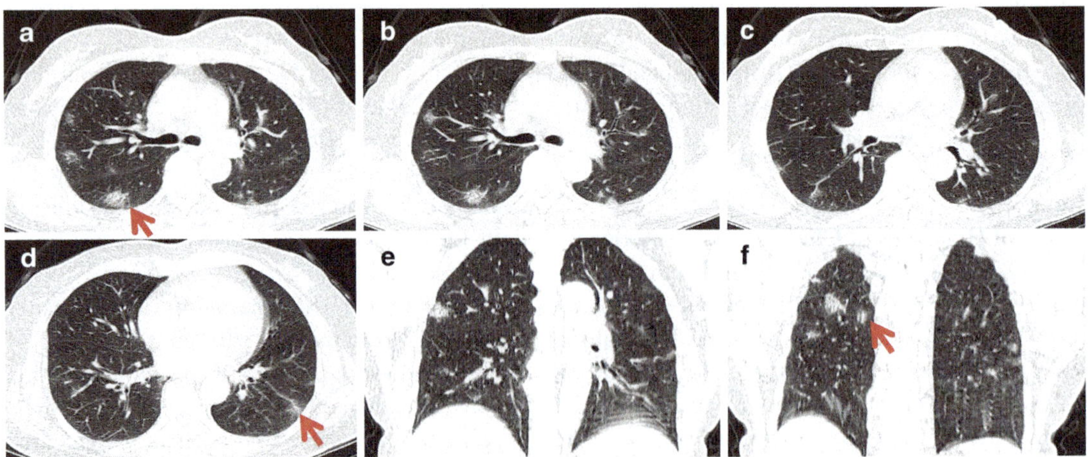

Fig. 5.15 Axial chest CT (**a–e**), reconstructed coronal (**f**) images of the patient

sign." The "halo sign" seen on CT was common in fungal infection, but not in viral pneumonia.

Case 6
Medical History and Clinical Manifestations

A 66-year-old male was admitted in the hospital with fever (highest body temperature: 37.4 °C), cough, and sputum for 3 days. Laboratory test results indicated normal white blood cell count: 5.0×10^9/L, 33.9% lymphocyte, and 52.3% neutrophil. The patient has been in contact with diagnosed COVID-19 patient. The SARS-CoV-2 nucleic acid test was positive.

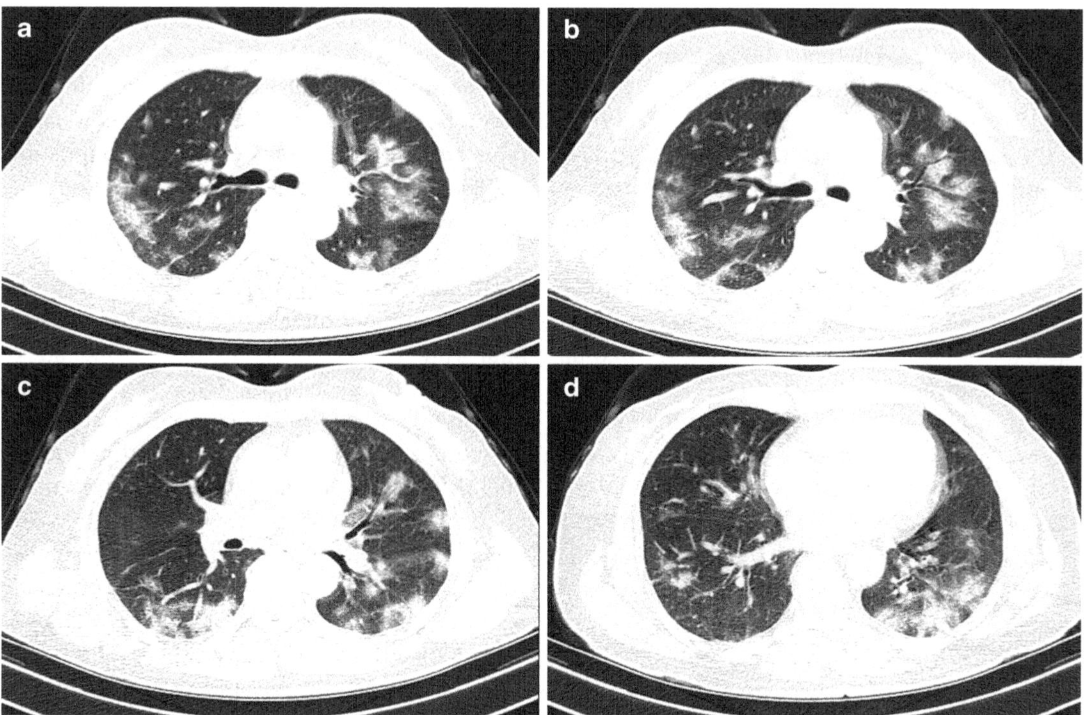

Fig. 5.16 Follow-up CT images 9 days after initial scan

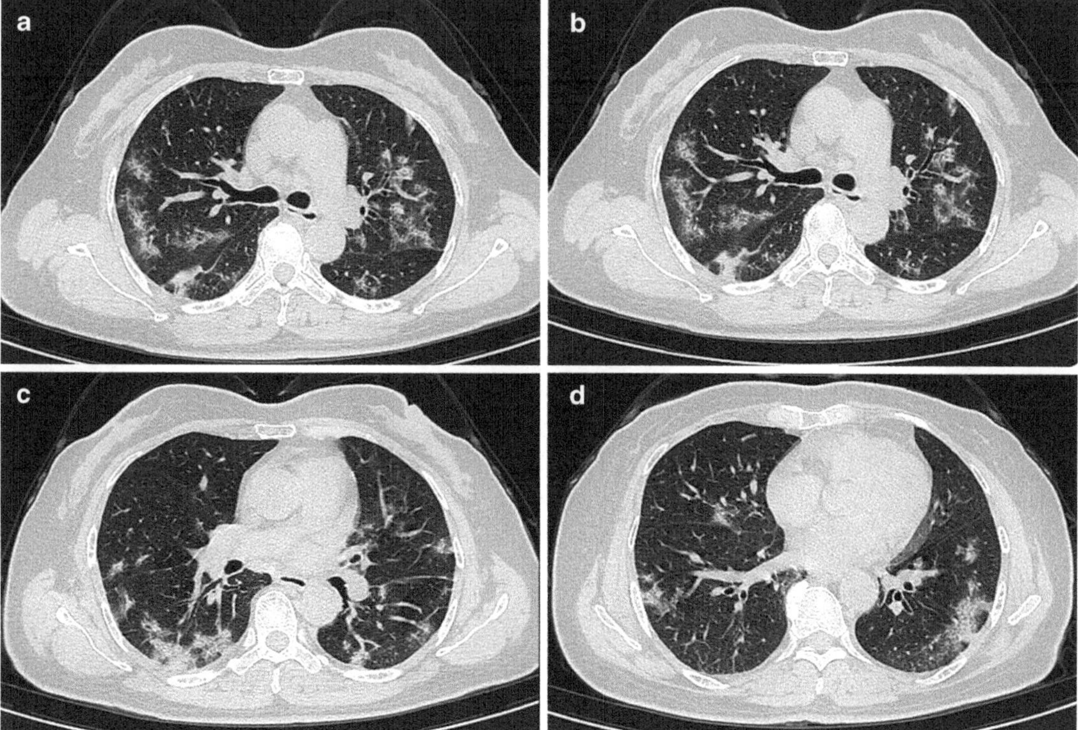

Fig. 5.17 Follow-up CT images 15 days after initial scan

Imaging Features

Initial chest radiograph showed small patch density increases in right lung (red arrow) (Fig. 5.18).

CT scan of the chest shows that there is a slightly higher ground-glass density shadow under the pleura of the posterior segment of the right upper lobe (Fig. 5.19).

Follow-up chest CT (6 days after initial CT examination) showed the lesion became consolidated and enlarged, and a new lesion showed up in the left lower lobe (Fig. 5.20).

Eleven days after the first CT examination, the follow-up chest CT showed that the focus was obviously absorbed and the density of the focus became low (Fig. 5.21).

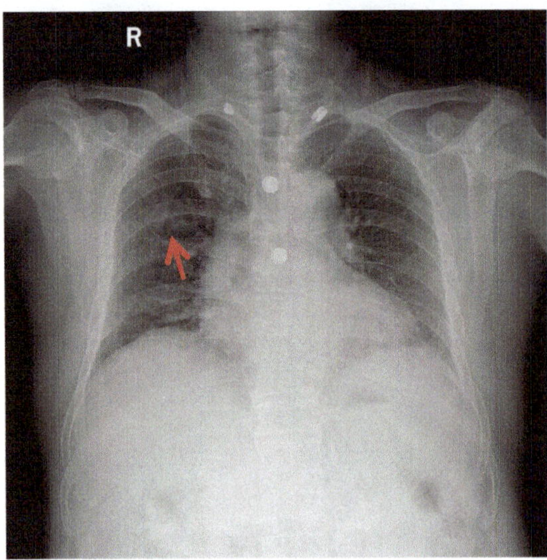

Fig. 5.18 Initial chest radiograph

Comments: The chest radiograph of this case shows that the heart shadow is enlarged to aortic type, and the exudative focus of the lung is difficult to identify and easy to miss diagnosis.

Case 7

Medical History and Clinical Manifestations

A 70-year-old male was admitted in the hospital with cough, a small amount of white sticky sputum, accompanied by fever (highest body temperature: 38.7 °C) for 1 week. Laboratory test results showed low white blood cell count of 3.0×10^9/L, normal lymphocyte percentage of 31.6%, neutrophil percentage of 58.3%, and C-reactive protein of 37.5 mg/L. Patient's spouse was diagnosed with COVID-19 and the couple was in close contact a week ago. The SARS-CoV-2 nucleic acid test was positive. In the non-oxygenated state, the patient's oxygen saturation continued to be below 93%, and the clinical typing was severe.

Imaging Features

Chest CT showed multiple ground-glass opacities with reticular pattern (red arrow) under the pleura of both lungs, with the right lower lobe as the focus, and thickened small blood vessel opacities were seen in some lesions (Fig. 5.22).

Follow-up chest CT (5 days after initial CT examination) showed the multiple reticular lesions obviously progressed than the previous images (Fig. 5.23).

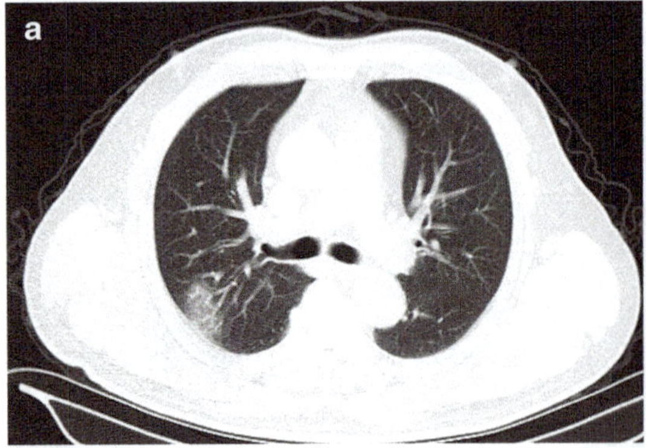

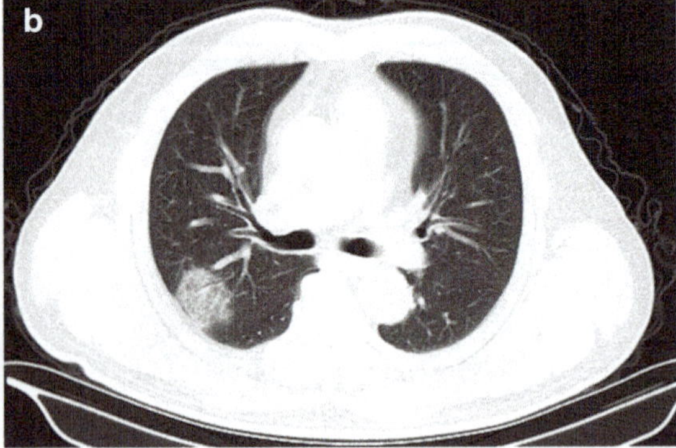

Fig. 5.19 Initial CT image

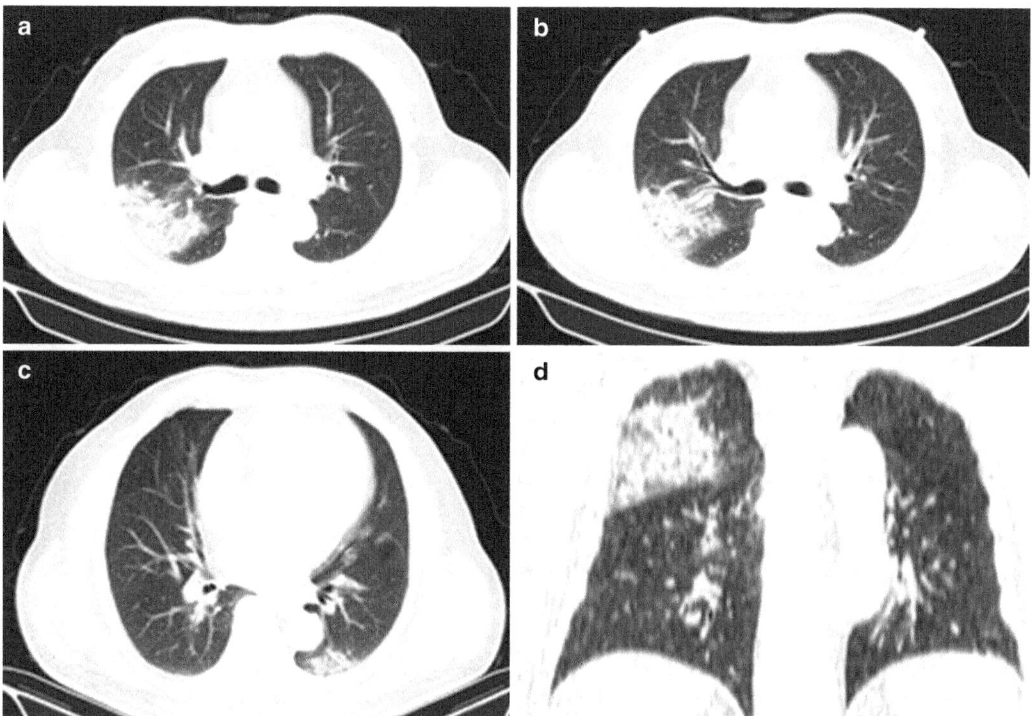

Fig. 5.20 Follow-up axial chest CT (**a**–**c**), reconstructed coronal (**d**) images 6 days after initial scan

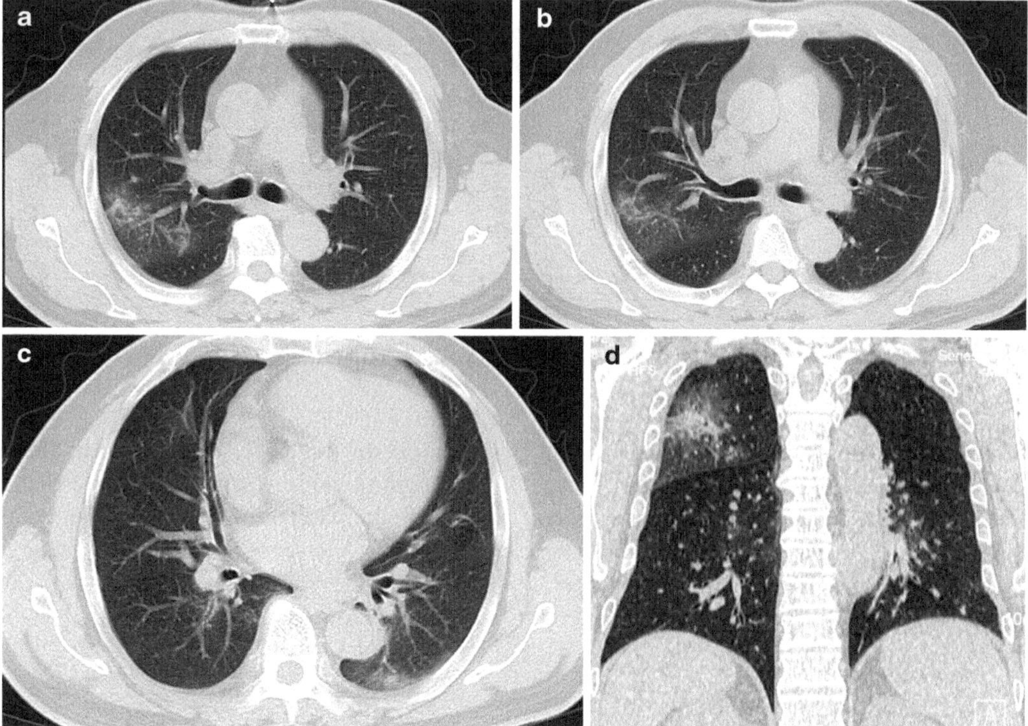

Fig. 5.21 Follow-up axial chest CT (**a**–**c**), reconstructed coronal (**d**) images 11 days after initial scan

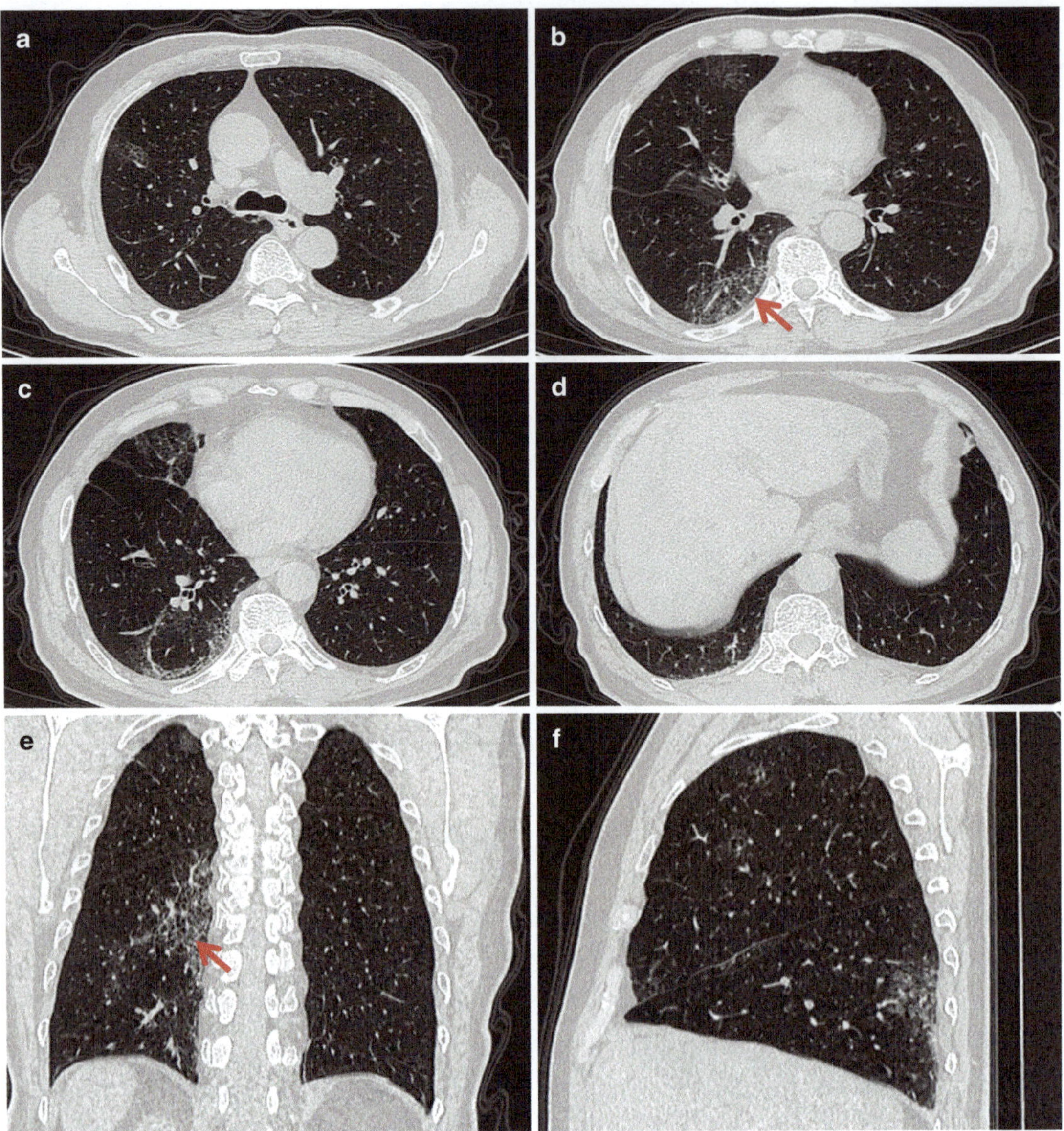

Fig. 5.22 Initial axial chest CT (**a–d**), reconstructed coronal (**e**) and sagittal (**f**) images of the patient

Comments: This is an elderly male patient, clinically classified as severe. At the early stage of the disease, the imaging manifestations were not serious, but there were multiple ground-glass shadows in the two lungs, while the reticular structure was obvious and there was no consolidation. In this case, the pulmonary lesions progressed obviously in a short period of time, and the main manifestation was still the reticular structure, but the scope was obviously enlarged. This may be the structural basis of lung in patients with clinical low oxygen saturation.

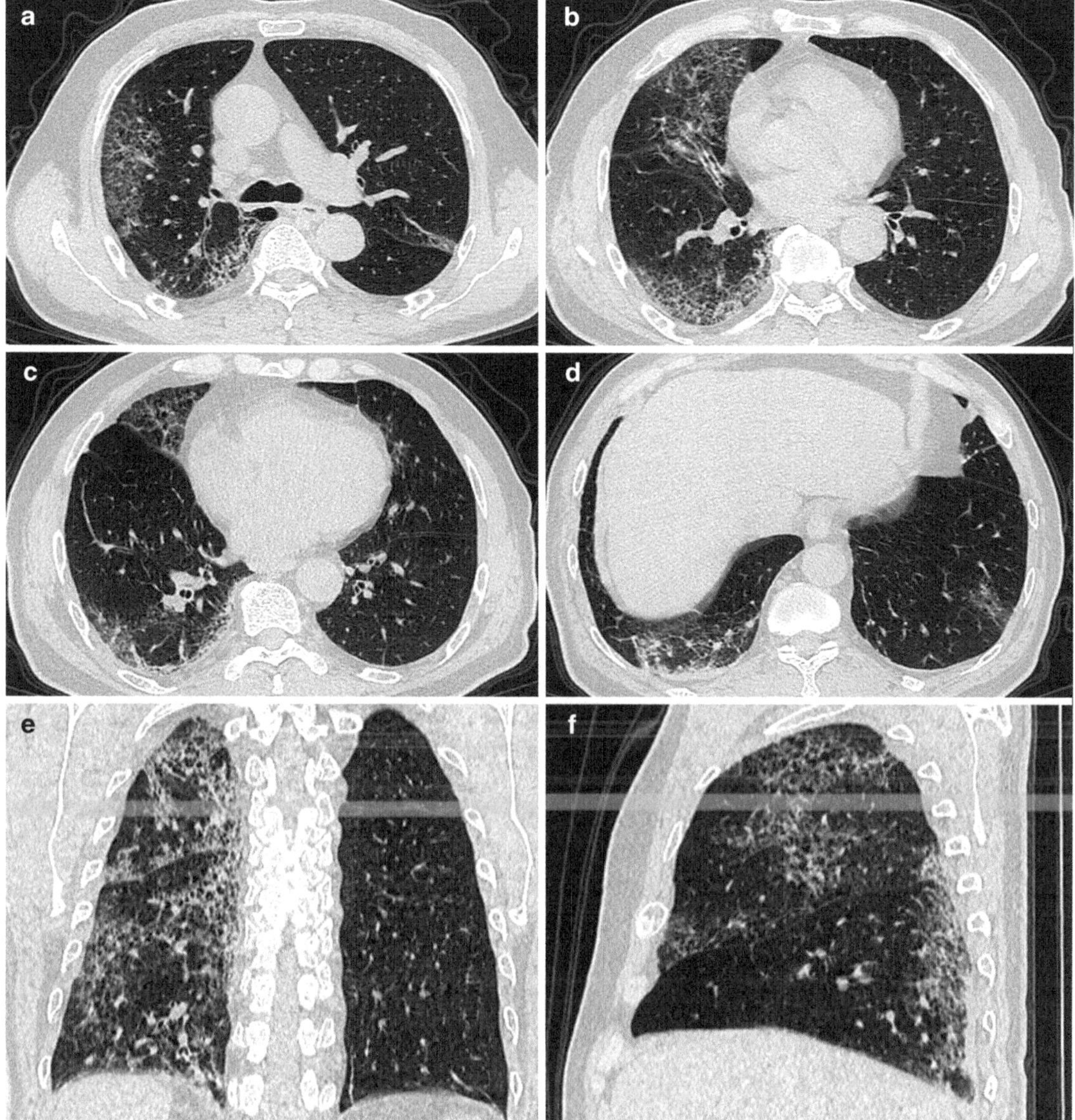

Fig. 5.23 Follow-up axial chest CT (**a–d**), reconstructed coronal (**e**) and sagittal (**f**) images 5 days after initial scan

References

1. Guan W, Ni Z, Hu Y, et al. Clinical characteristics of coronavirus disease 2019 in China. N Engl J Med. 2020;382(18):1708–20.
2. Liu K, Chen Y, Lin R, et al. Clinical features of COVID-19 in elderly patients: a comparison with young and middle-aged patients. J Infect. 2020;80(6):e14–8.
3. Wang L, He W, Yu X, et al. Coronavirus disease 2019 in elderly patients: characteristics and prognostic factors based on 4-week follow-up. J Infect. 2020;80(6):639–45.
4. Chen T, Wu D, Chen H, et al. Clinical characteristics of 113 deceased patients with coronavirus disease 2019: retrospective study. BMJ. 2020;368:m1091.
5. Zhu T, Wang Y, Zhou S, et al. A comparative study of chest computed tomography features in young and older adults with corona virus disease (COVID-19). J Thoracic Imaging. 2020;35(4):W97–W101.

Imaging Features of Familial Clustering of COVID-19

6

Zongyu Xie, Jian Wang, Cancan Zhao, Shuhua Li, Yuqing Gao, Tongtong Zhao, and Minming Zhang

COVID-19 has obvious family clustering, and clustering refers to the occurrence of 2 or more confirmed cases or asymptomatic infection in a small area within 14 days [1]. The clinical manifestations of familial clustering COVID-19 are related to exposure time, exposure degree, virus type, virus virulence, and patient age [2], which are mostly manifested as fever, chills, fatigue, occasional diarrhea, sore throat, or asymptomatic [3]. Symptoms are mild in children, and more severe in elderly or patients with chronic underlying diseases [4]. If there is an infected person in the family, it is easy to cause mutual infection; chest CT is helpful for the screening of suspected family cases, early diagnosis, early treatment, and early isolation. The CT findings of the family cluster COVID-19 cases are consistent with the typical manifestations of COVID-19. In the same group of family cases, the lesion density and degree are similar [5]. The number of lesions and the range of involvement of multi-generation infected persons are reduced compared with earlier generations. The chest CT of children may be negative, and the lung lesions of the elderly or patients with chronic underlying diseases may be more severe. In the follow-up after treatment, the vast majority of the lung lesions were absorbed to different degrees, and the residual shadows were mostly ground-glass opacities or fibrous shadows. The chest CT findings of most patients could finally return to normal.

6.1 Group 1 (Cases 1–3)

Case 1

Medical History and Clinical Manifestations

Patient A: A 33-year-old male was admitted in the hospital for 8 days with fever (highest body temperature: 38.6 °C), accompanied by chills and fatigue, and coughed for 1 day. Laboratory test results indicated decreased leukocyte count, normal lymphocyte count and percentage, and normal interleukin-6 (IL-6) and serum amyloid A (SAA). Exposure history: The patient had a close contacting history with a fitness coach from Wuhan, China 2 weeks before the onset of the disease. The SARS-CoV-2 nucleic acid test was positive 3 days after admission.

Z. Xie · C. Zhao · S. Li · Y. Gao
Department of Radiology, the First Affiliated Hospital of Bengbu Medical College, Bengbu, China

J. Wang
Department of Radiology, Tongde Hospital of Zhejiang Province, Hangzhou, China

T. Zhao
Department of Radiology, the Second People's Hospital of Fuyang City, Fuyang, China

M. Zhang (✉)
Department of Radiology, the Second Affiliated Hospital, Zhejiang University School of Medicine, Hangzhou, China
e-mail: zhangminming@zju.edu.cn

M. Zhang, B. Lin (eds.), *Diagnostic Imaging of Novel Coronavirus Pneumonia*,
https://doi.org/10.1007/978-981-15-5992-1_6

Imaging Features

Initial chest CT showed multiple localized ground-glass opacities in bilateral lungs with relative clear boundaries, which mainly distributed in the subpleural area and around the bronchovascular bundle. Vasodilation (**a**, **e**: red arrows) could be seen in the lesions (Fig. 6.1).

Follow-up chest CT (17 days after initial CT examination) showed multiple localized ground-glass opacities in both lungs, with clear bound-

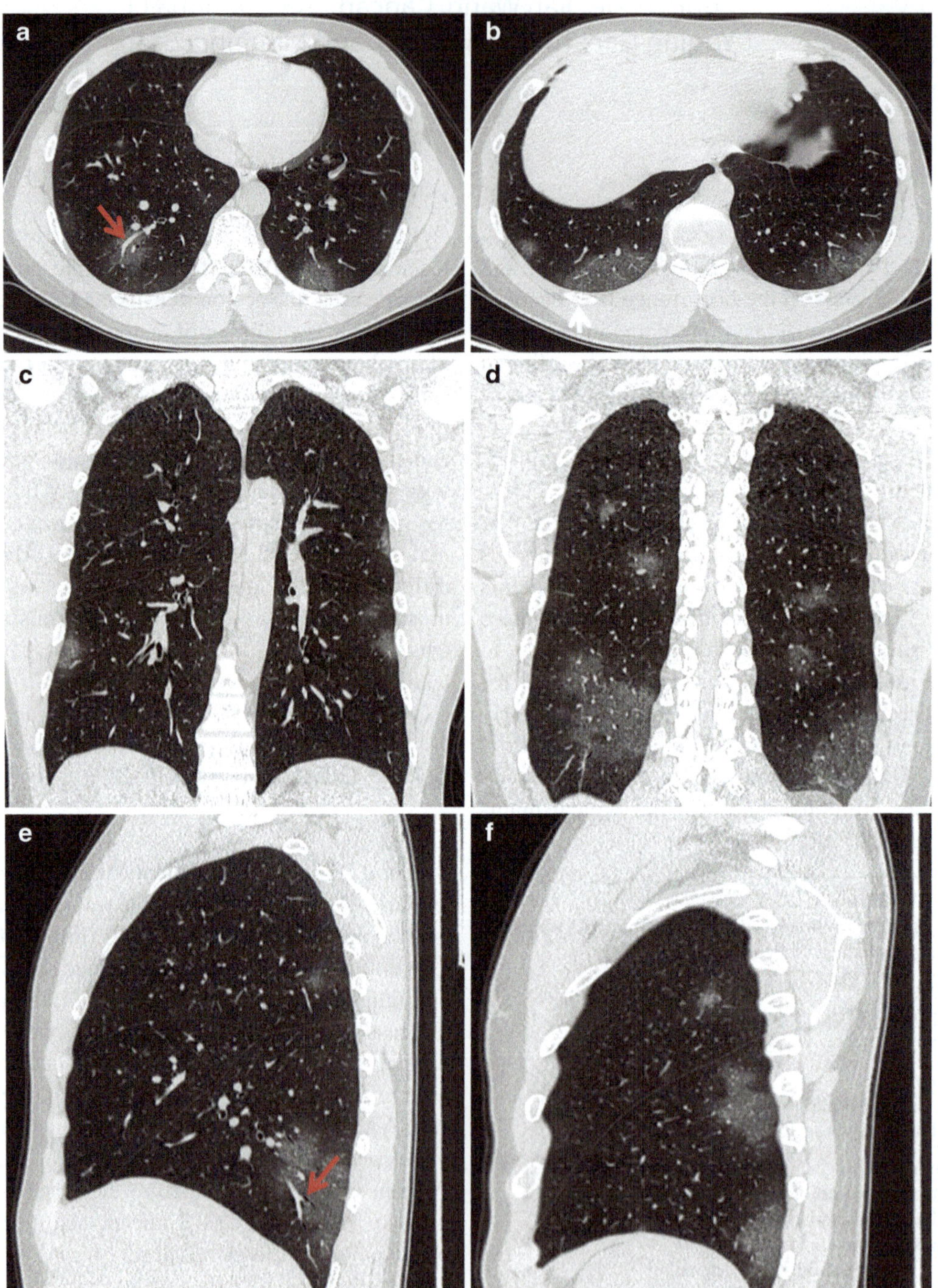

Fig. 6.1 Initial axial chest CT (**a**, **b**), reconstructed coronal (**c**, **d**) and sagittal (**e**, **f**) images of the patient

aries, which mainly distributed in the subpleural area and around the bronchovascular bundle. Vasodilation could be seen in the lesions. The lesions became smaller than before, and consolidation and linear opacities showed in some lesions (Fig. 6.2).

Follow-up chest CT (23 days after initial CT examination) showed multiple localized

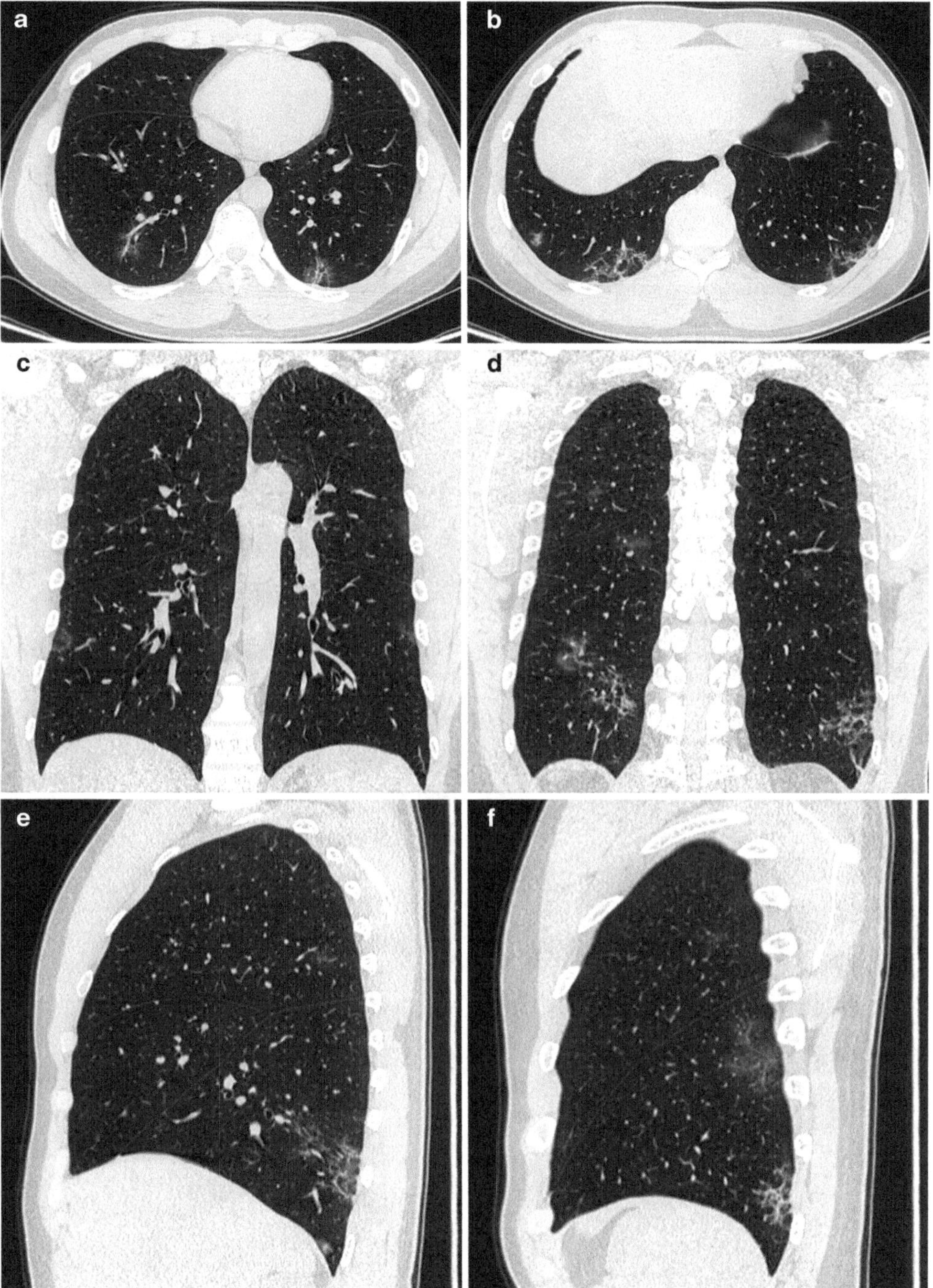

Fig. 6.2 Follow-up axial chest CT (**a**, **b**), reconstructed coronal (**c**, **d**) and sagittal (**e**, **f**) images 17 days after initial scan

ground-glass opacities in bilateral lungs, with much lower density than before. Linear opacities could be seen in some lesions, and the consolidation disappeared (Fig. 6.3).

On the 54th day, reexamination of chest CT showed that almost all the lesions were absorbed and improved, only a few fibrous foci remained (Fig. 6.4).

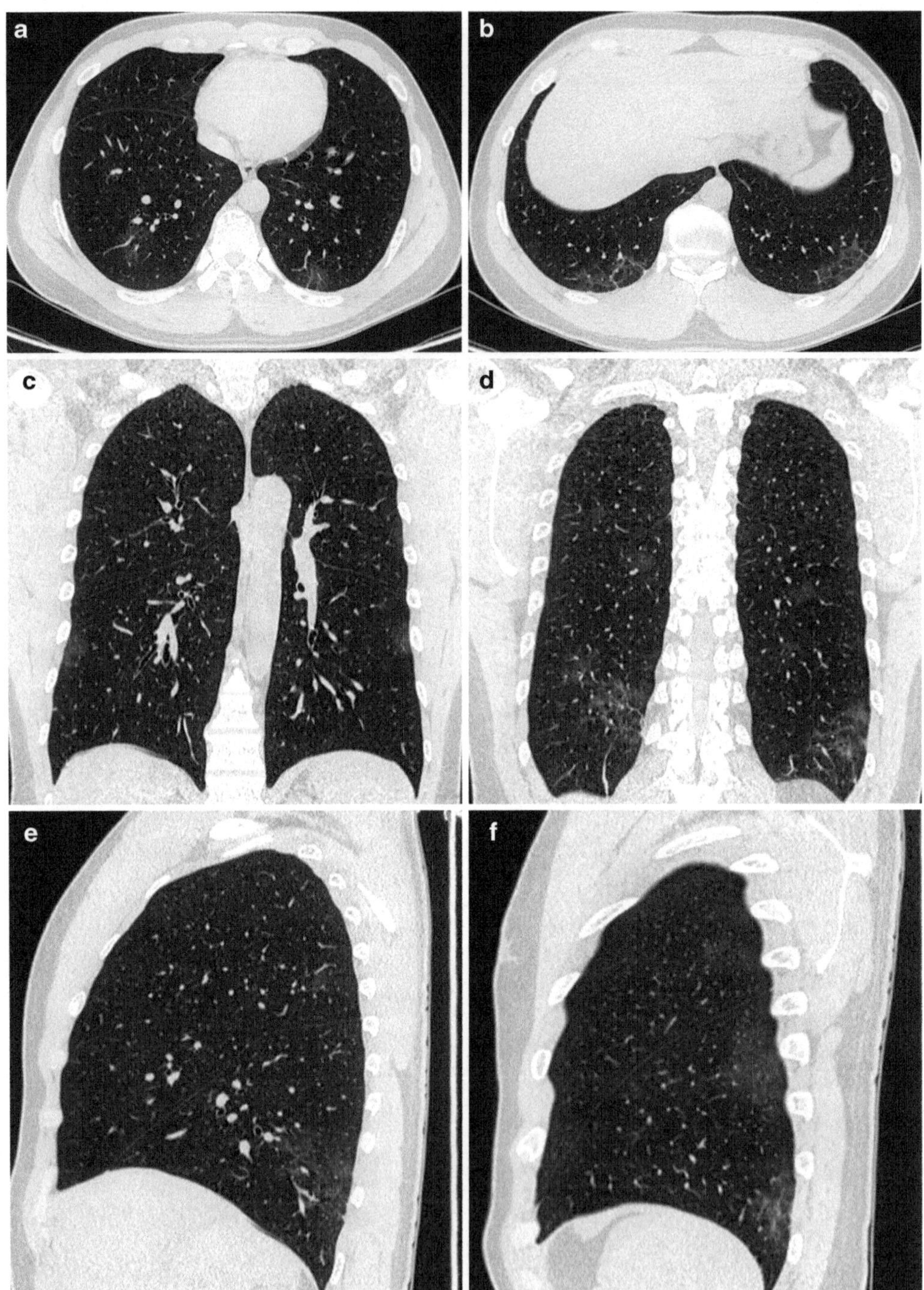

Fig. 6.3 Follow-up axial chest CT (**a**, **b**), reconstructed coronal (**c**, **d**) and sagittal (**e**, **f**) images 23 days after initial scan

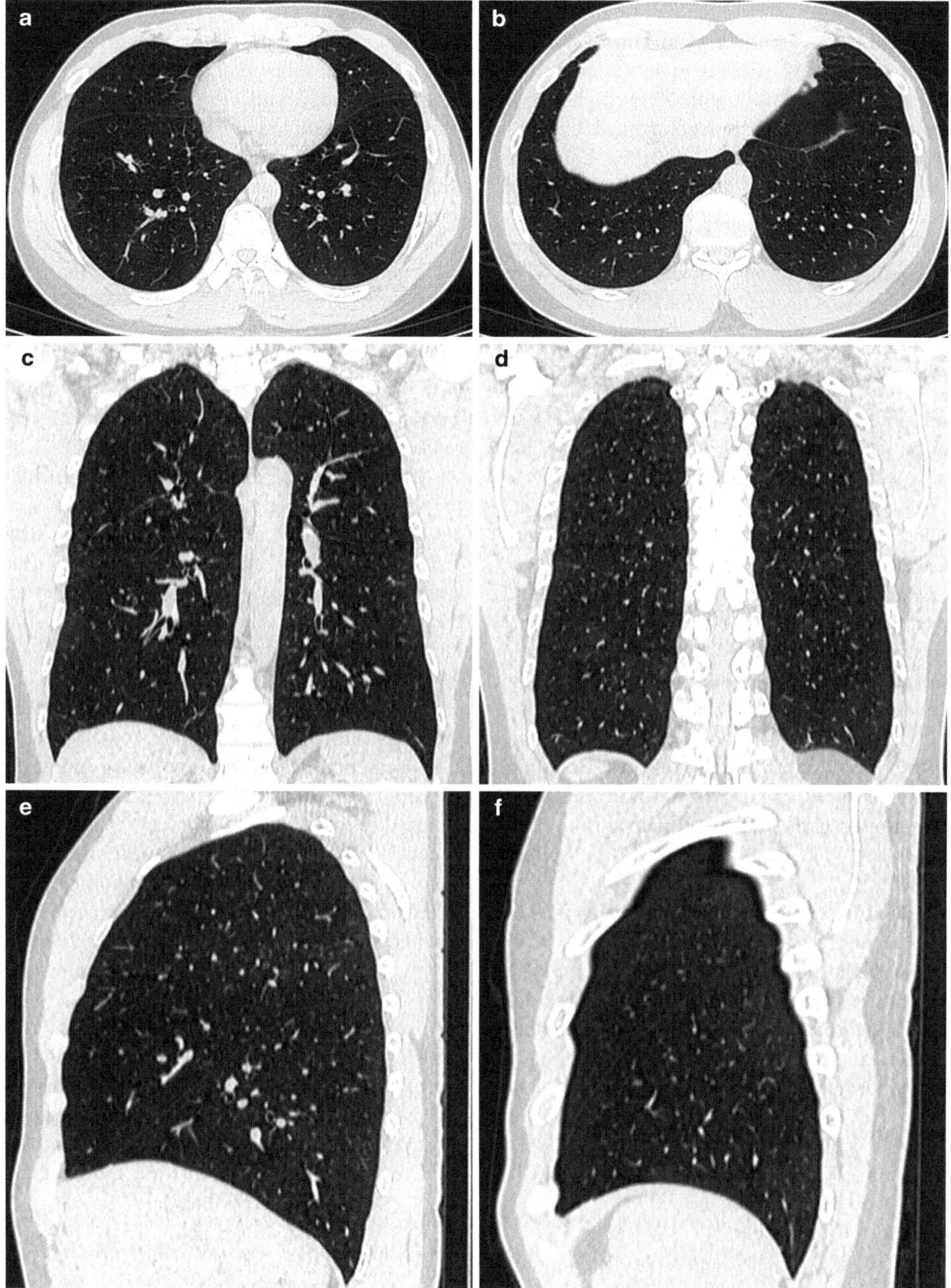

Fig. 6.4 Follow-up axial chest CT (**a**, **b**), reconstructed coronal (**c**, **d**) and sagittal (**e**, **f**) images 54 days after initial scan

Case 2

Medical History and Clinical Manifestations

Patient B: A 59-year-old male was admitted in the hospital for 8 days with fever (highest body temperature: 38.6 °C), accompanied by chills, runny nose, and occasional diarrhea. Laboratory test results indicated normal leukocyte count, normal lymphocyte count and percentage, normal IL-6, and elevated SAA. Exposure history: The patient is the father of the patient A with a clear exposure history. The SARS-CoV-2 nucleic acid test was positive 1 day after admission.

Imaging Features

Initial chest CT showed multiple ground-glass opacities in bilateral lungs, with blurred boundaries, which mainly distributed in the subpleural area and around the bronchovascular bundle, the left lung was obvious. Lesions contained dilated microvascular, with "halo sign" (red arrow) around (Fig. 6.5).

Follow-up chest CT (13 days after initial CT examination) showed that multiple ground-glass opacities lesions are smaller, the density become reduced. Linear opacities appeared in some lesions (Fig. 6.6).

After 42 days follow-up and reexamination, CT showed that most of the lesions were almost completely absorbed and improved, and a few thin ground-glass shadows remained (Fig. 6.7).

Case 3

Medical History and Clinical Manifestations

Patient C: A 54-year-old female was admitted in the hospital for 8 days with fever (highest body temperature: 39 °C), accompanied by chills and sore throat. Laboratory test results indicated decreased leukocyte count and lymphocyte count, elevated IL-6 and SAA. Exposure history: The patient is the mother of the patient A with a clear exposure history. The SARS-CoV-2 nucleic acid test was positive 1 day after admission.

Imaging Features

Initial chest CT showed patchy ground-glass opacities in the subpleural area of the lower lobe of the left lung, with clear boundaries. In the lesion, there were linear opacities, focal consolidation (**f**: red arrow), microvascular thickening (**b**: red arrow), and grid-like "crazy-paving pattern" (**e**: red arrow) (Fig. 6.8).

Follow-up chest CT (15 days after the initial CT examination) showed that most of the multiple localized patchy ground-glass opacities in both lungs were narrow in scope and low in density. At the same time, some new lesions (**a**: red arrow) appeared in both lungs, some of which were solid (**f**: red arrow) or linear structures (**c**: red arrow) (Fig. 6.9).

After 28 days of follow-up, CT showed that the ground-glass opacity in patchy area was obviously weakened or disappeared, and the new lesions were absorbed completely. The linear structure also disappeared completely, suggesting that this kind of linear structure is not fibrotic, but may be caused by lobular atelectasis (Fig. 6.10).

Follow-up chest CT (73 days after initial CT examination) showed no obvious abnormality in the lungs (Fig. 6.11).

Comments: This is a group of typical cases of familial aggregation of COVID-19. All the patients were common clinical types. Only patient A has a clear epidemiological history and is considered as the second generation of virus infection. The other two family members, the parents of the patients, were three generations of people infected with the virus. Fever was the first symptom in all the patients. The initial CT findings were consistent with the typical change of COVID-19. The main lesions were ground-glass opacities. In the follow-up CT images, most of the lesions were improved in different degrees, some lesion progressed to consolidation, and the final remaining lesions were thin ground-glass opacity or completely normal.

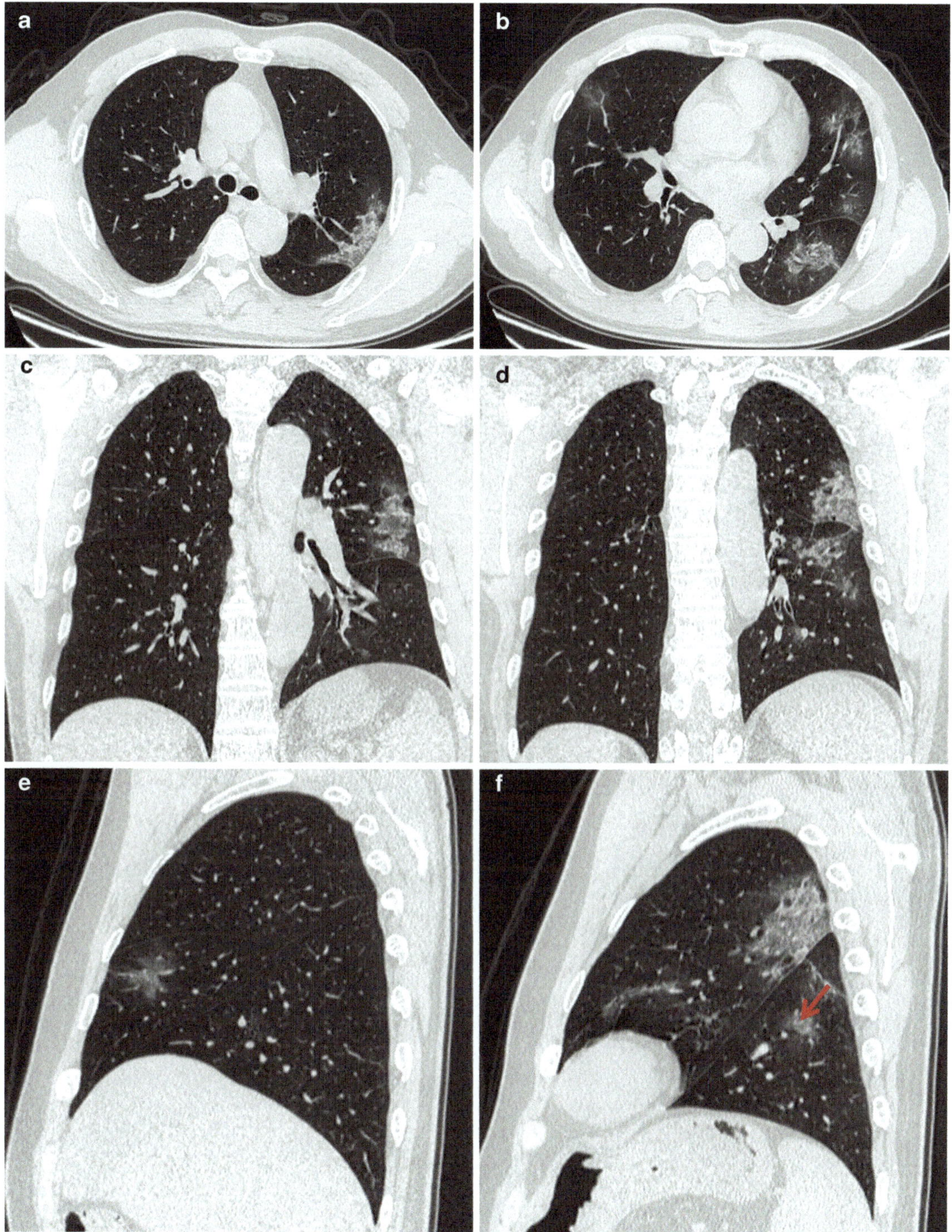

Fig. 6.5 Initial axial chest CT (**a**, **b**), reconstructed coronal (**c**, **d**) and sagittal (**e**, **f**) images of the patient

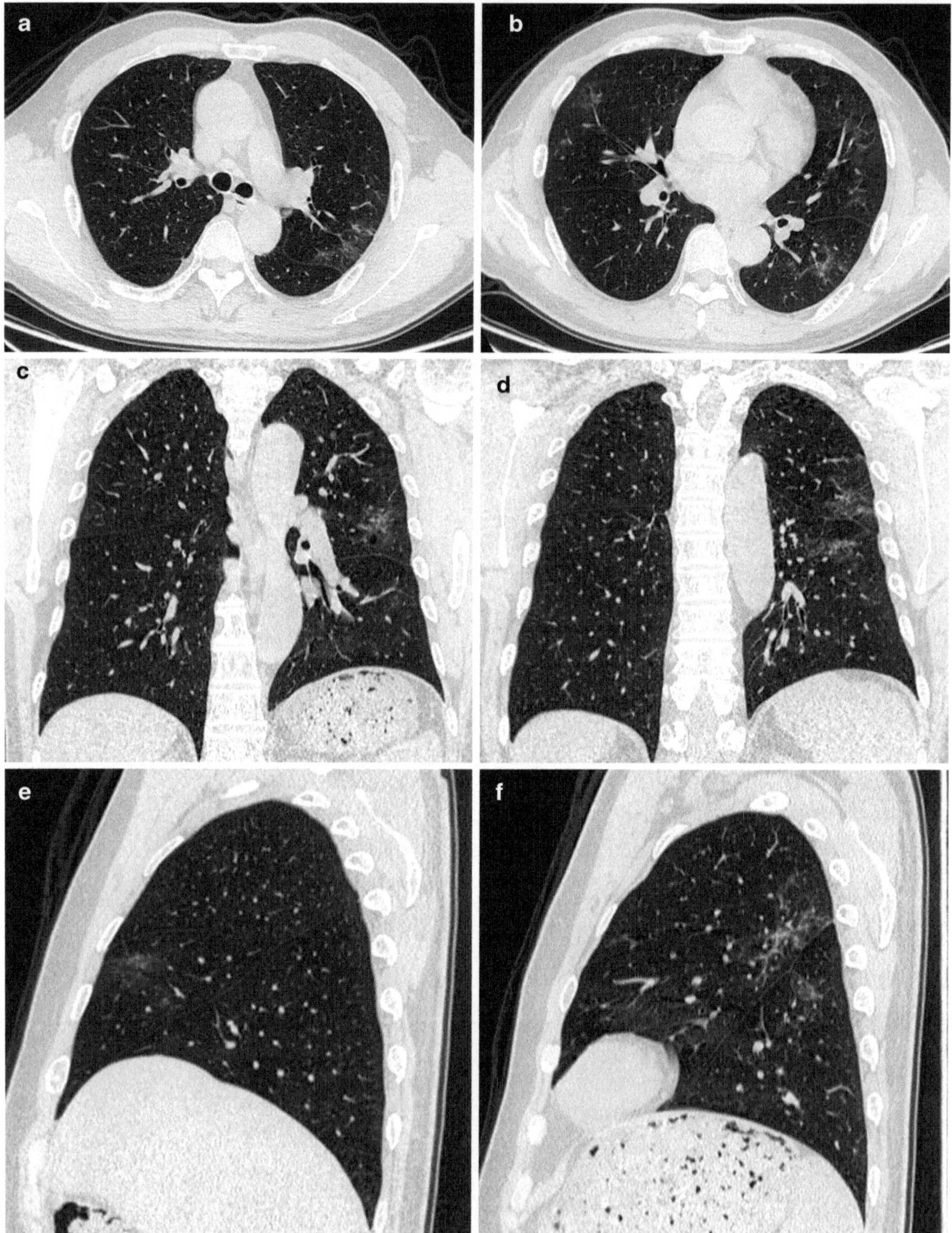

Fig. 6.6 Chest CT (**a**, **b**), reconstructed coronal (**c**, **d**) and sagittal (**e**, **f**) images of the patient 13 days after initial scan

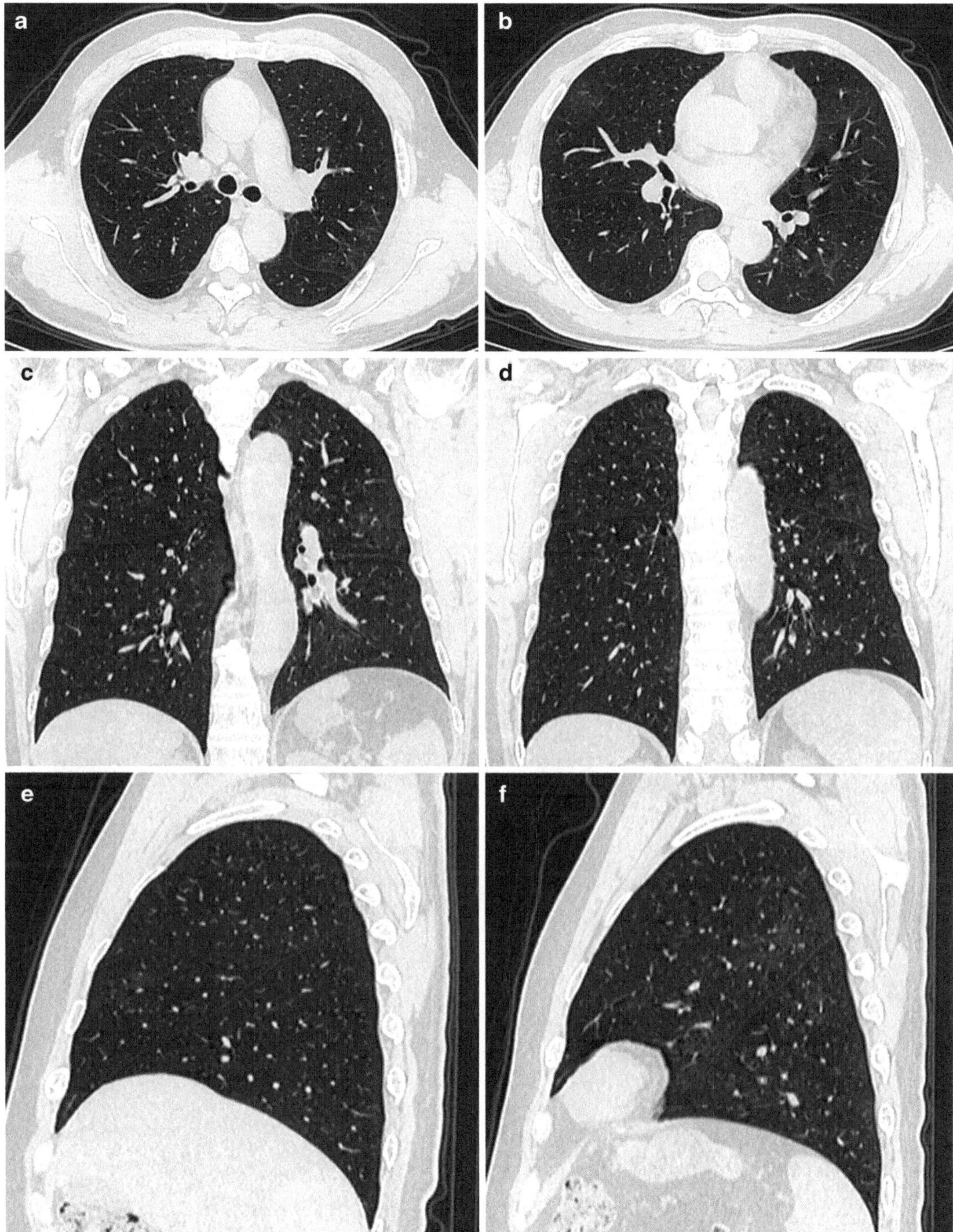

Fig. 6.7 Chest CT (**a**, **b**), reconstructed coronal (**c**, **d**) and sagittal (**e**, **f**) images of the patient 42 days after initial scan

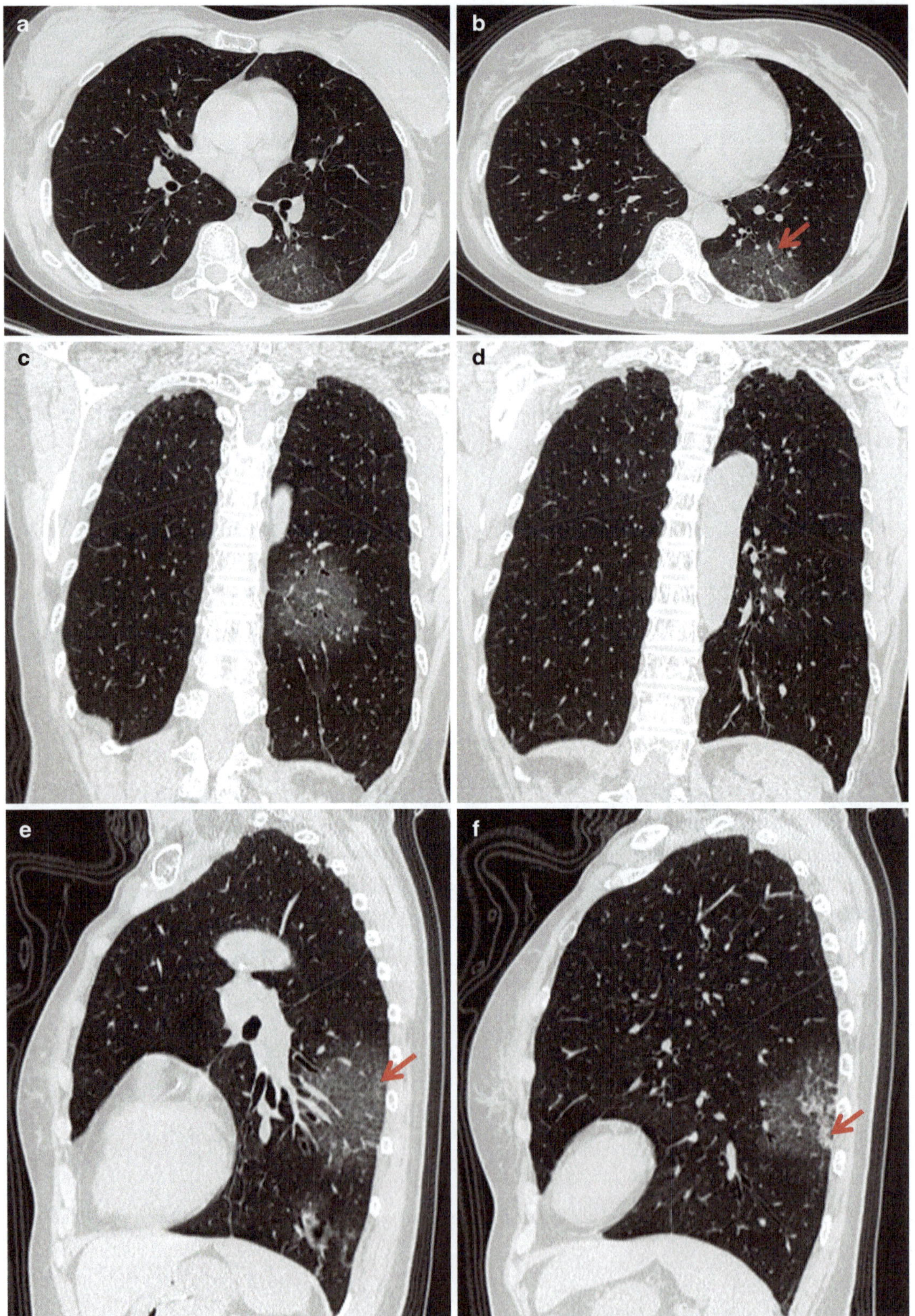

Fig. 6.8 Initial chest CT (**a**, **b**), reconstructed coronal (**c**, **d**) and sagittal (**e**, **f**) images of the patient

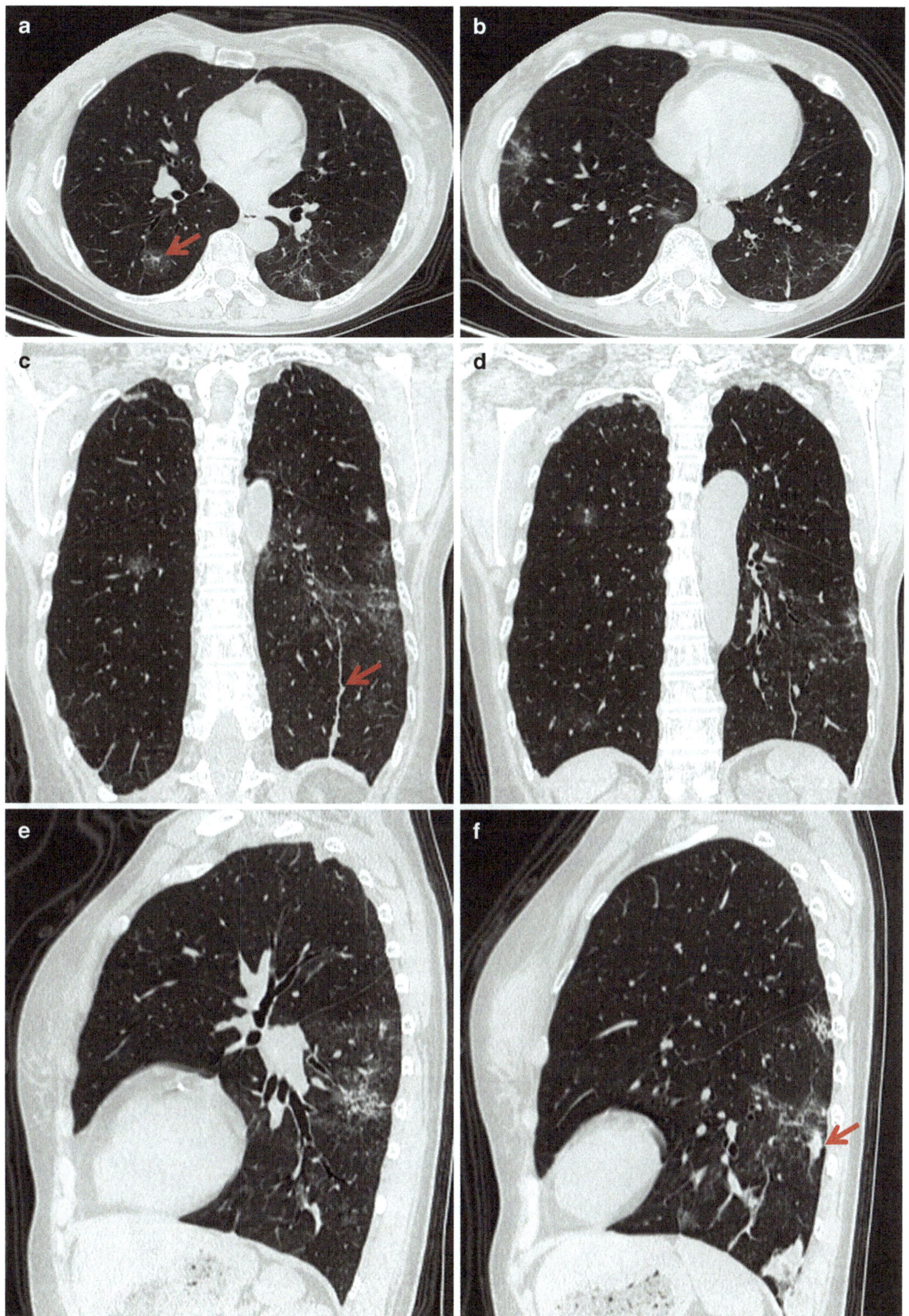

Fig. 6.9 Follow-up chest CT (**a**, **b**), reconstructed coronal (**c**, **d**) and sagittal (**e**, **f**) images of the patient 15 days after initial scan

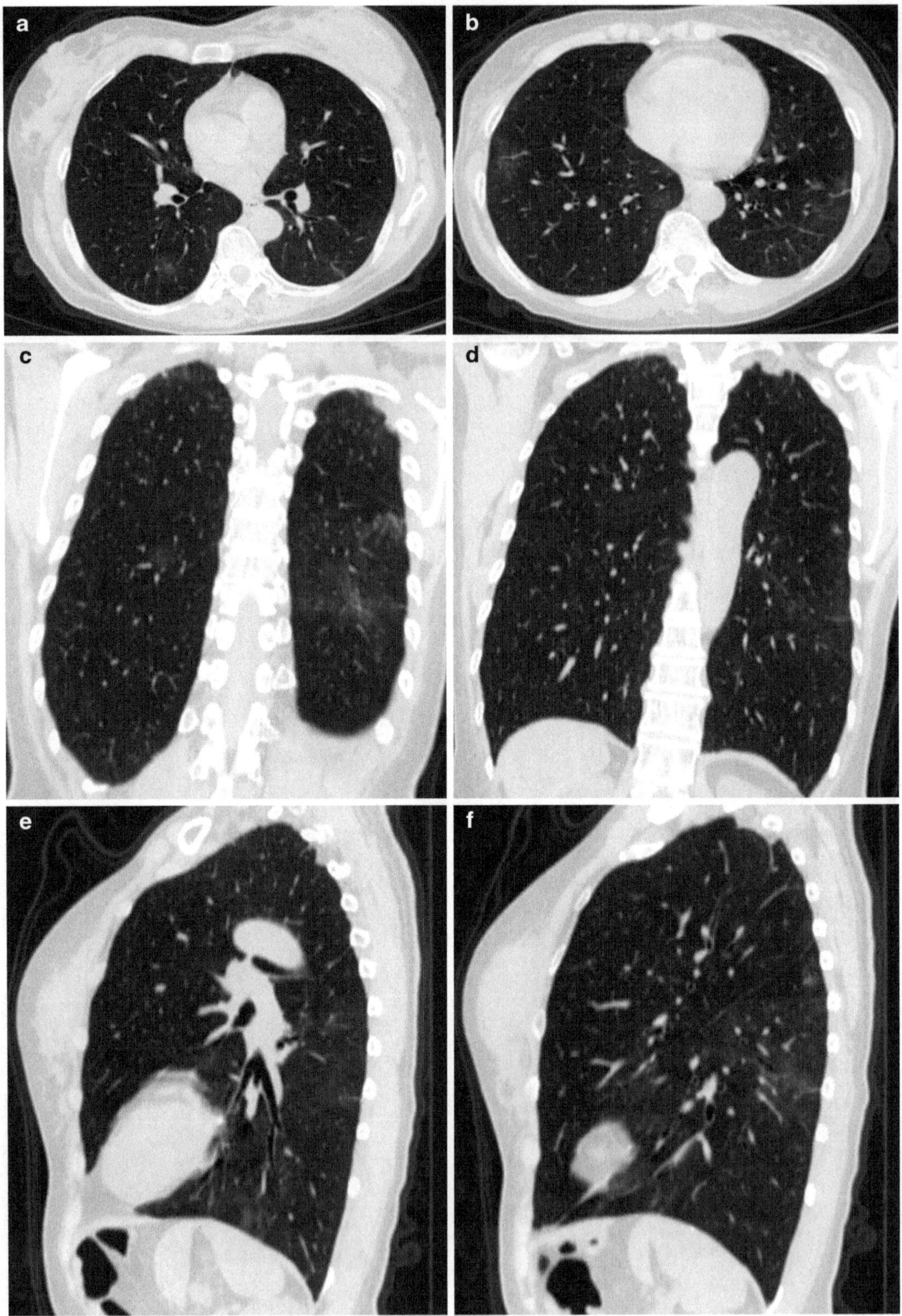

Fig. 6.10 Follow-up chest CT (**a**, **b**), reconstructed coronal (**c**, **d**) and sagittal (**e**, **f**) images of the patient 28 days after initial scan

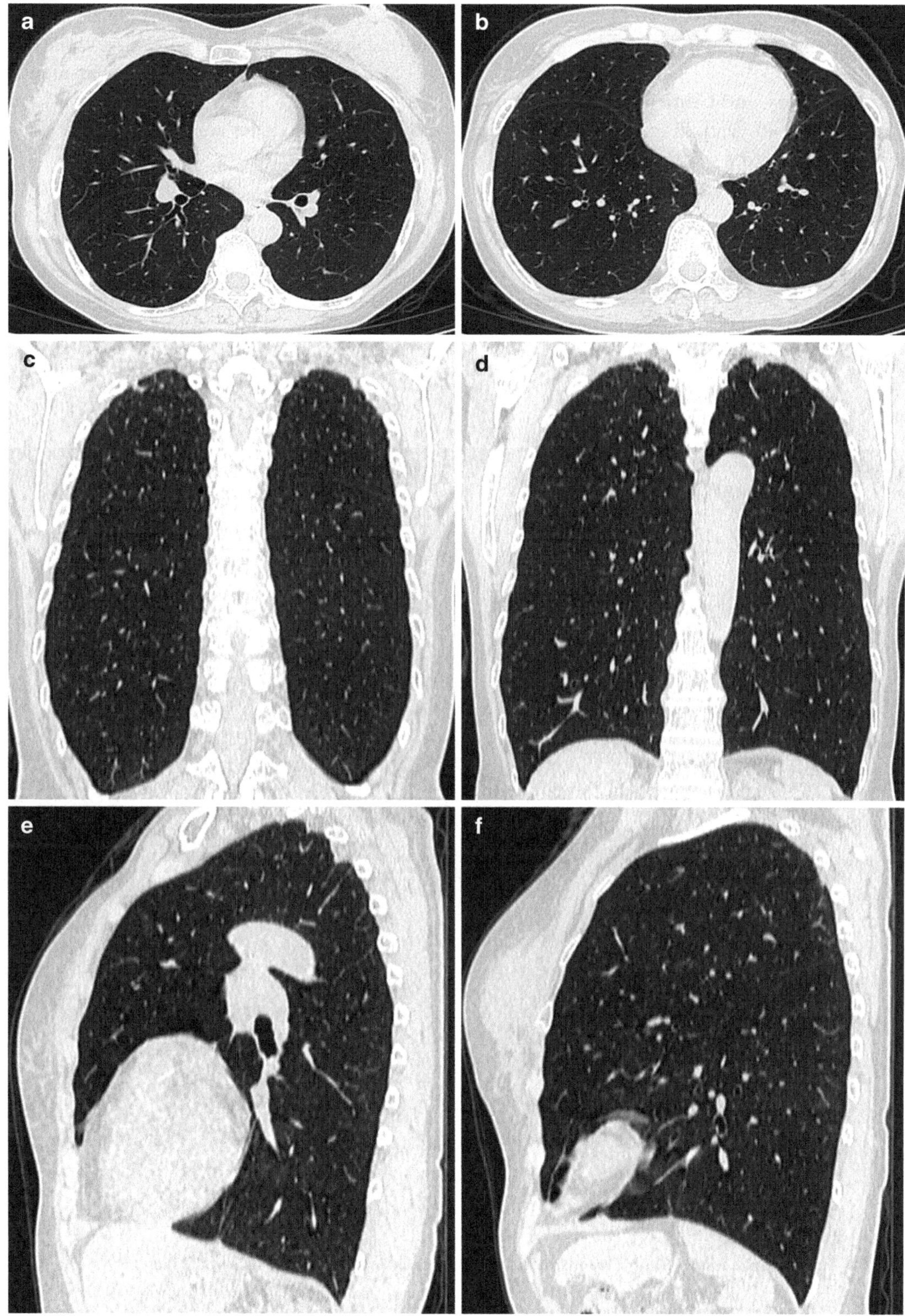

Fig. 6.11 Follow-up chest CT (**a**, **b**), reconstructed coronal (**c**, **d**) and sagittal (**e**, **f**) images of the patient 73 days after initial scan

6.2 Group 2 (Cases 4–7)

Case 4

Medical History and Clinical Manifestations

Patient A: A 48-year-old male was admitted in the hospital for 3 days with fever (highest body temperature: 39 °C) without obvious inducement, accompanied by cough, mainly dry cough. Laboratory test results indicated normal leukocyte count and lymphocyte counts, normal IL-6, and increased CRP and SAA. Exposure history: The patient, his wife, and son drove back home from Wuhan, China 5 days prior to symptom onset. At present, his wife and younger daughter were hospitalized in the local hospital, and his son and elder daughter were isolated at home after visiting the local hospital. The SARS-CoV-2 nucleic acid test was positive 1 day after admission.

Imaging Features

Initial chest CT showed multiple patchy ground-glass opacities in bilateral lungs with some consolidation in a predominantly subpleural distribution. Some lesions showed grid changes (**c**: red arrow). The mediastinal window showed a mild local thickening of the right pleura (**b**: red arrow) (Fig. 6.12).

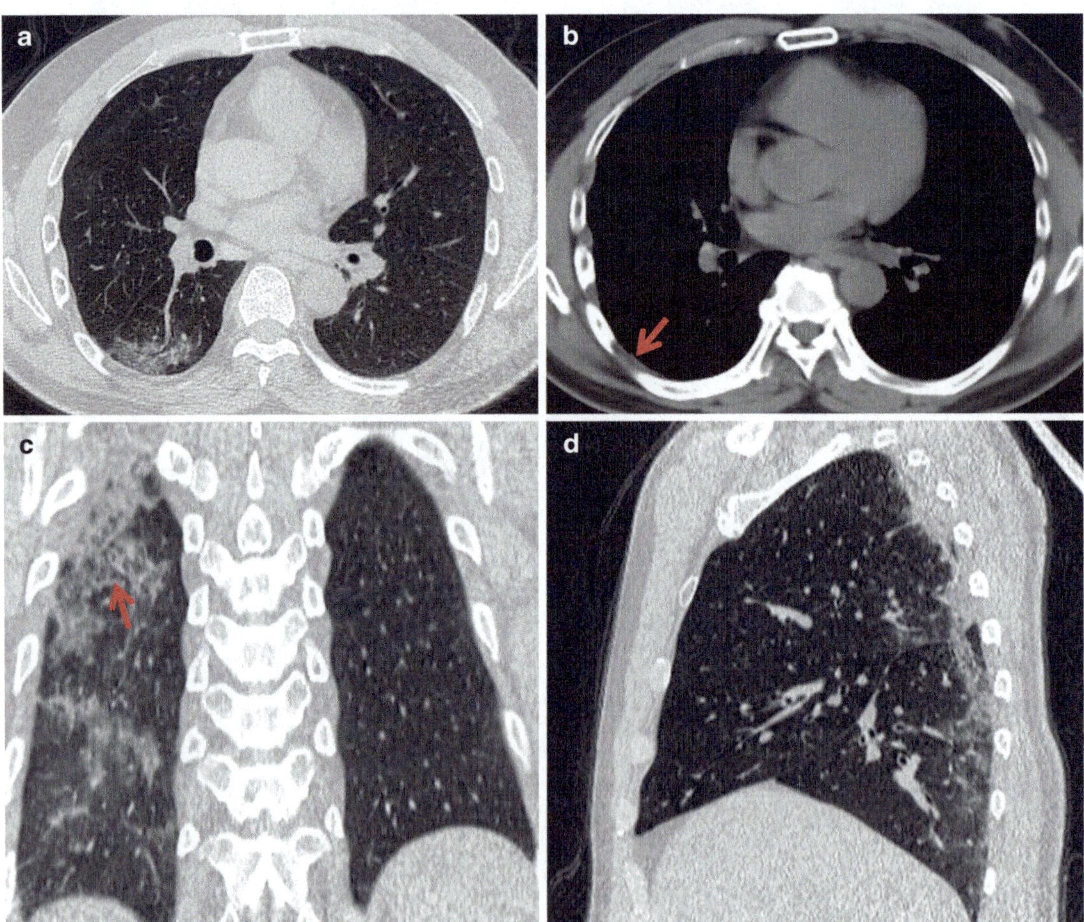

Fig. 6.12 Initial axial chest CT (**a**, **b**), reconstructed coronal (**c**) and sagittal (**d**) images of the patient

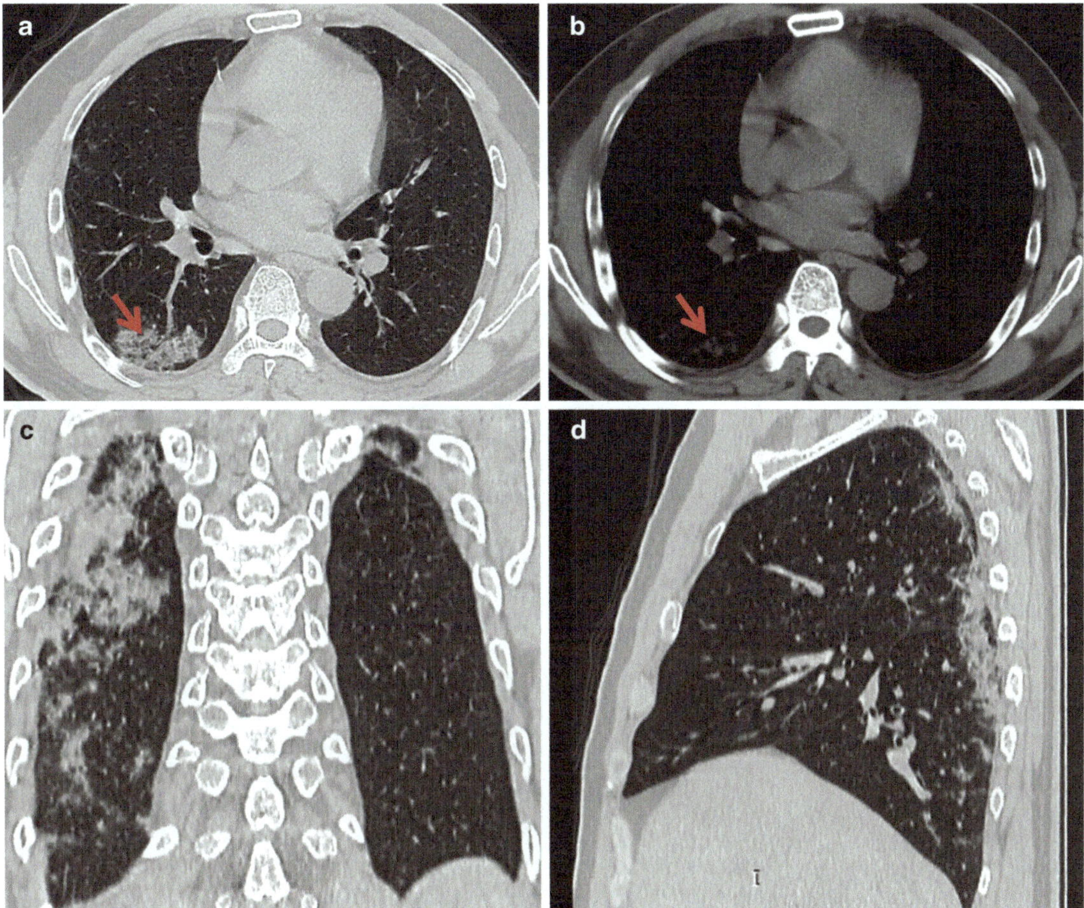

Fig. 6.13 Follow-up axial chest CT (**a**, **b**), reconstructed coronal (**c**) and sagittal (**d**) images 4 days after initial scan

Follow-up chest CT (4 days after initial CT examination) showed the lesions were slight progressed compared with the previous CT imaging. Partial lesions consolidation can be clearly seen in the right lower lobe (**a**, **b**: red arrows) (Fig. 6.13).

Follow-up chest CT (15 days after initial CT examination) showed the lesion was further absorbed and the subpleural line became thin (**d**: red arrow) (Fig. 6.14).

Follow-up chest CT (34 days after initial CT examination) showed the patchy shadows of the lungs were basically absorbed and tended to fibrosis. The sagittal image showed that subpleural line was basic disappearance (**d**: red arrows) (Fig. 6.15).

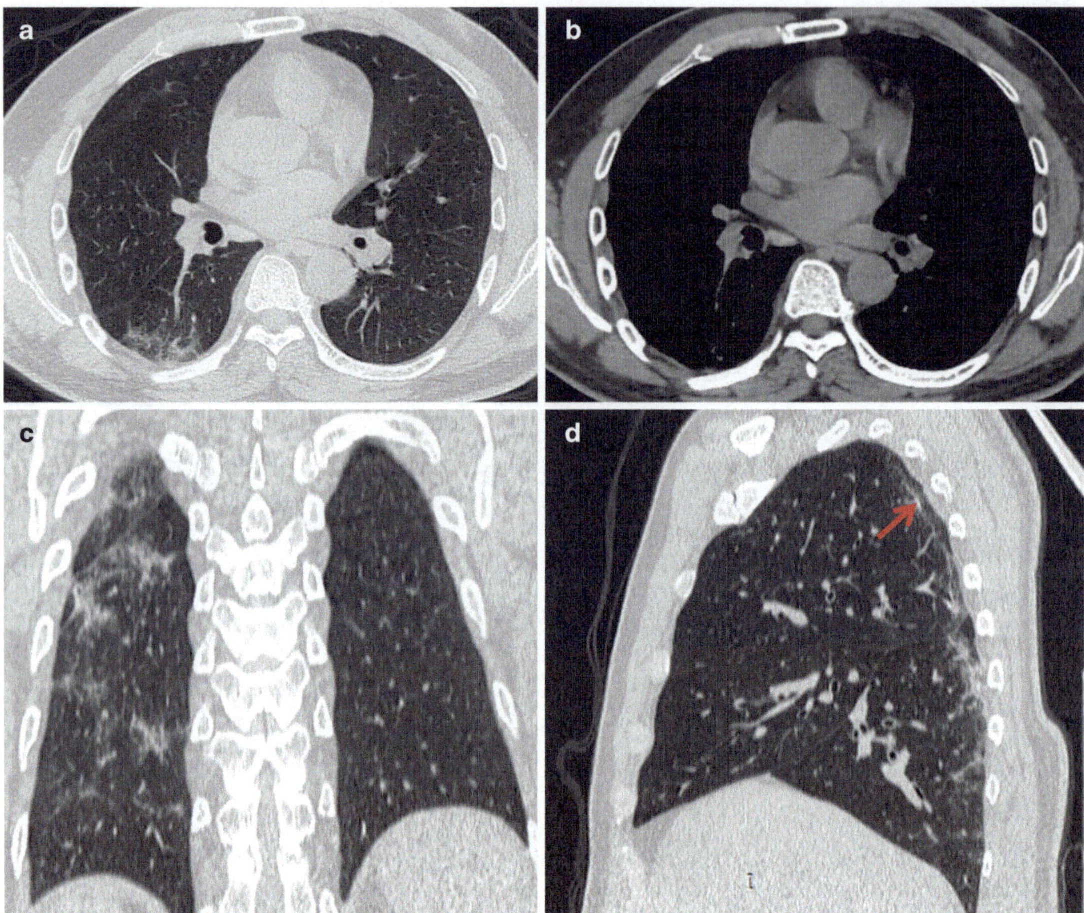

Fig. 6.14 Follow-up axial chest CT (**a**, **b**), reconstructed coronal (**c**) and sagittal (**d**) images 15 days after initial scan

Case 5

Medical History and Clinical Manifestations

Patient B: A 49-year-old female was admitted in the hospital for 3 days with fever (highest body temperature: 39 °C) without obvious inducement, accompanied by chills and cough, a small amount of white sputum. Laboratory test results indicated normal leukocyte count and lymphocyte counts, normal IL-6, and increased CRP and SAA. Exposure history: The patient, his husband, and son drove back home from Wuhan, China 5 days prior to symptom onset. The SARS-CoV-2 nucleic acid test was positive 1 day after admission. The patient had diabetes for more than 4 years and hypertension for more than 6 years.

Imaging Features

Initial chest CT showed multiple patchy high-density shadows in both lungs and some consolidation mainly distributed in the both

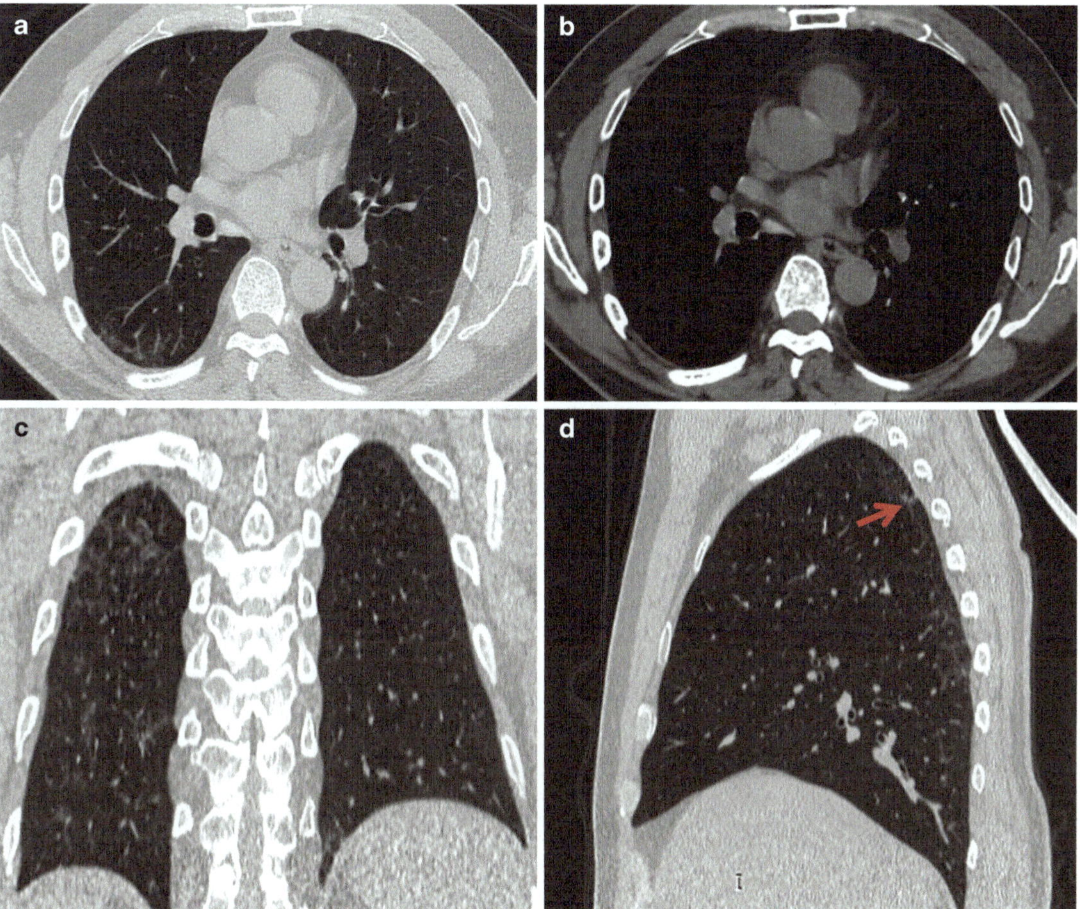

Fig. 6.15 Follow-up axial chest CT (**a**, **b**), reconstructed coronal (**c**) and sagittal (**d**) images 34 days after initial scan

lower lobes. Some lesions showed "crazy-paving pattern" (**c**: red arrow) and "halo signs." Mediastinal window demonstrated partial consolidation of lesions in the both lower lobes (**b**: red arrows) (Fig. 6.16).

Follow-up chest CT (4 days after initial CT examination) showed the lesions were significantly increased and expanded than before, "crazy-paving pattern," "microvascular thickening" (**a**: red arrow), "halo signs," and "reversed halo signs" (**c**, **d**: red arrow) were seen (Fig. 6.17).

Follow-up chest CT (8 days after initial CT examination) showed the lesions of the bilateral lung became more solid and the density increased. Some lesions showed linear opacities. Mediastinal window demonstrated consolidation of lesions in the both lower lobes (**a**, **b**: red arrows) (Fig. 6.18).

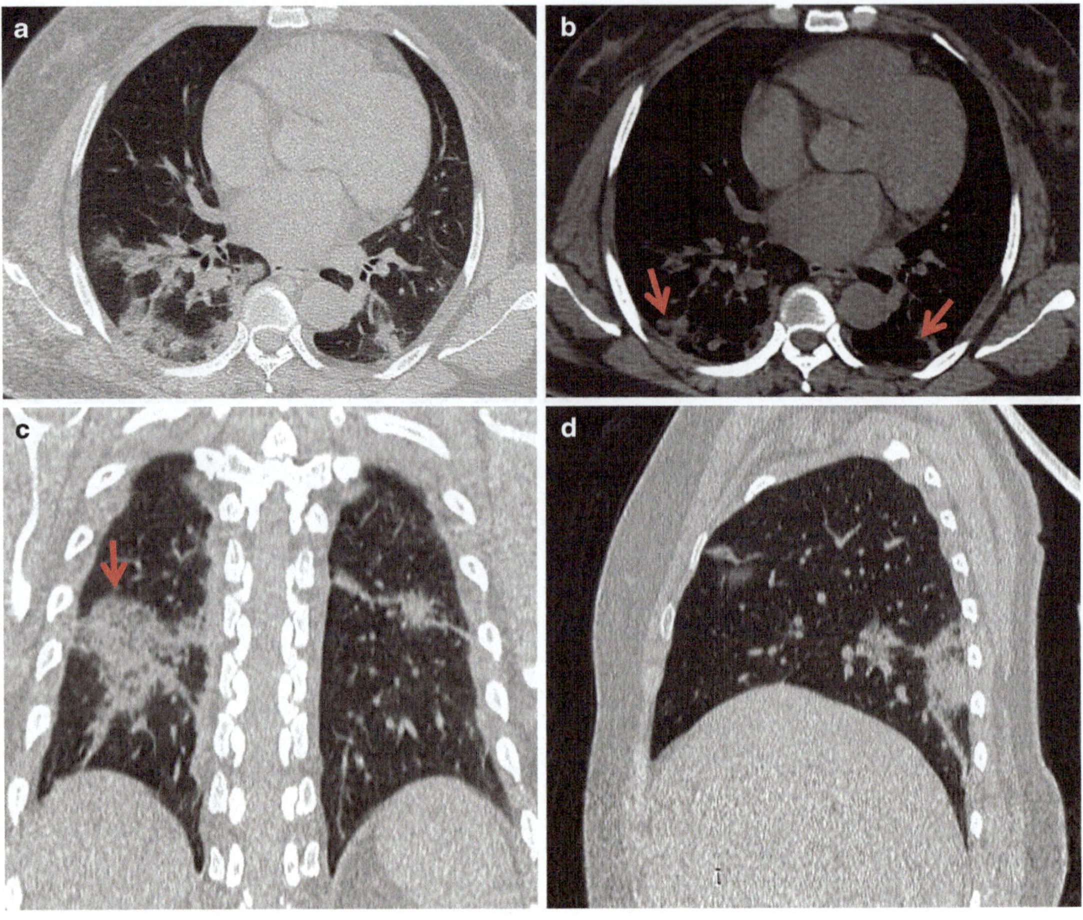

Fig. 6.16 Initial axial chest CT (**a**, **b**), reconstructed coronal (**c**) and sagittal (**d**) images of the patient

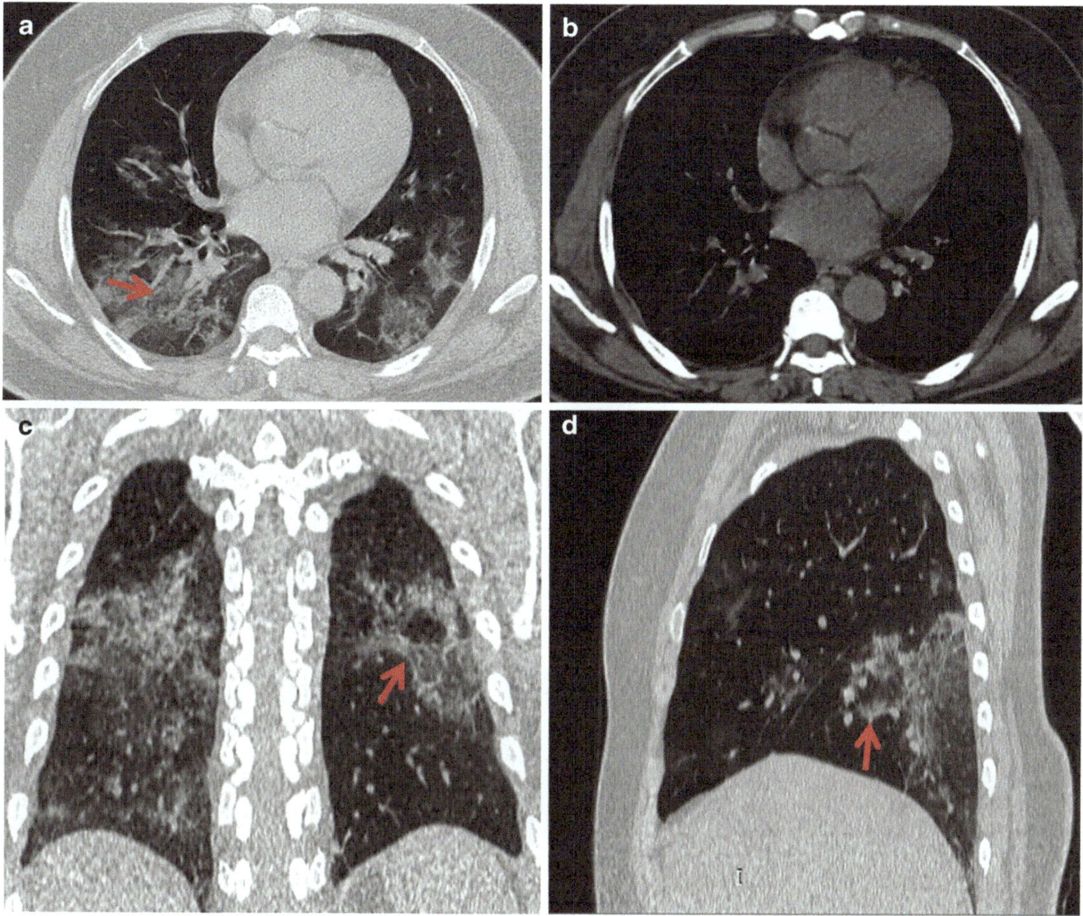

Fig. 6.17 Follow-up axial chest CT (**a**, **b**), reconstructed coronal (**c**) and sagittal (**d**) images 4 days after initial scan

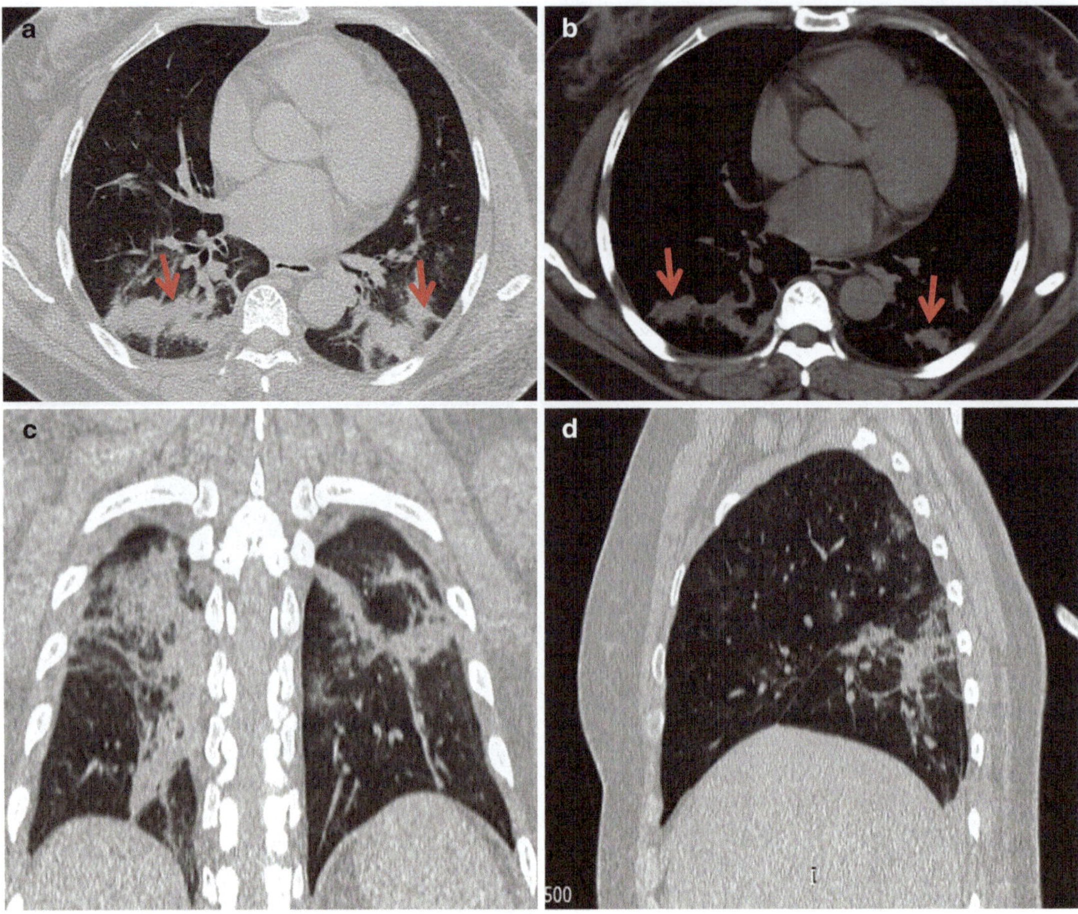

Fig. 6.18 Follow-up axial chest CT (**a**, **b**), reconstructed coronal (**c**) and sagittal (**d**) images 8 days after initial scan

Follow-up chest CT (19 days after initial CT examination) showed the lesions were further absorbed in two lungs compared with the previous CT imaging (Fig. 6.19).

Follow-up chest CT (37 days after initial CT examination) showed the lesions were significantly absorbed and tended to dissipate (Fig. 6.20).

Case 6

Medical History and Clinical Manifestations

Patient C: A 21-year-old female was admitted in the hospital for 2 days with low fever (highest body temperature: 37.5 °C). Laboratory test results indicated normal leukocyte count and lymphocyte counts, normal IL-6, normal CRP,

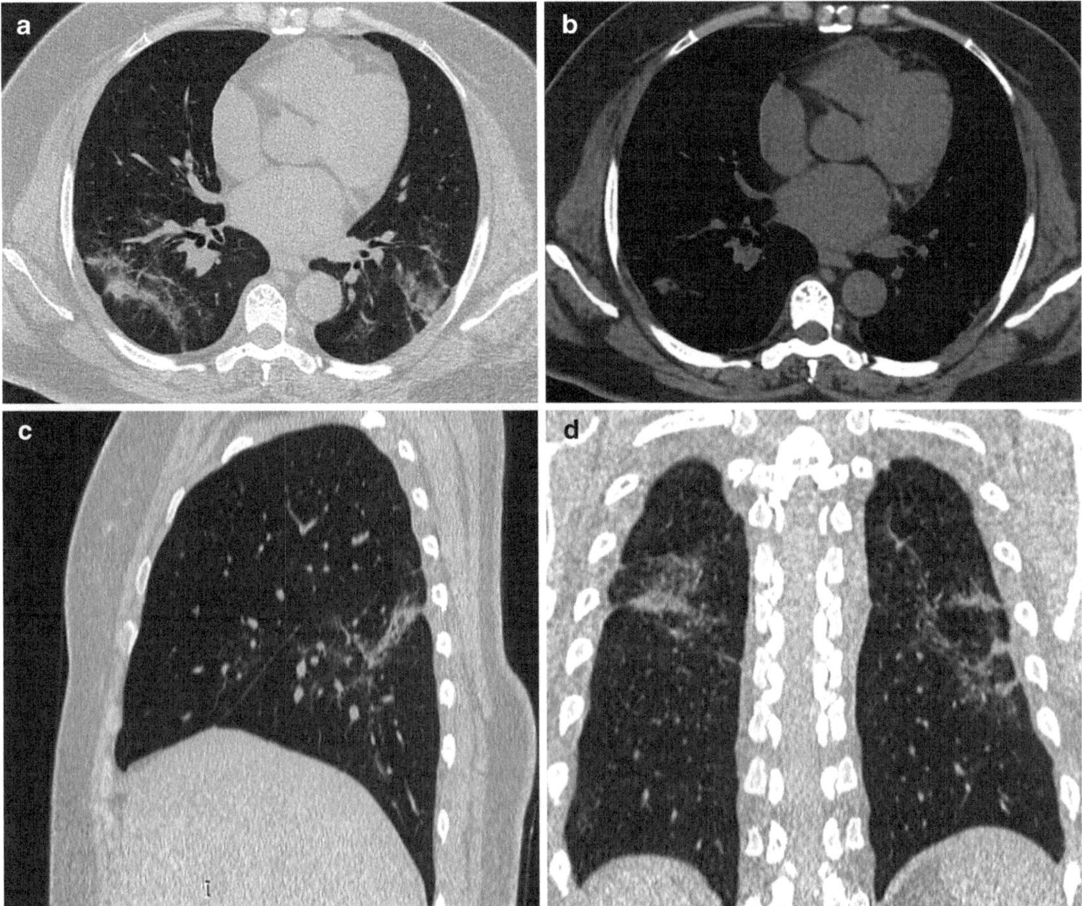

Fig. 6.19 Follow-up axial chest CT (**a**, **b**), reconstructed coronal (**c**) and sagittal (**d**) images 19 days after initial scan

and SAA. Exposure history: The patient's parents lived in Wuhan, China. Her parents and brother drove back home from Wuhan 6 days prior to symptom onset. The SARS-CoV-2 nucleic acid test was positive 2 days after admission.

Imaging Features

Initial chest CT showed a patchy ground-glass shadow under the pleura of the right lower lobe of the lung. "Halo signs" (**a**, **d**: red arrows) were visible (Fig. 6.21).

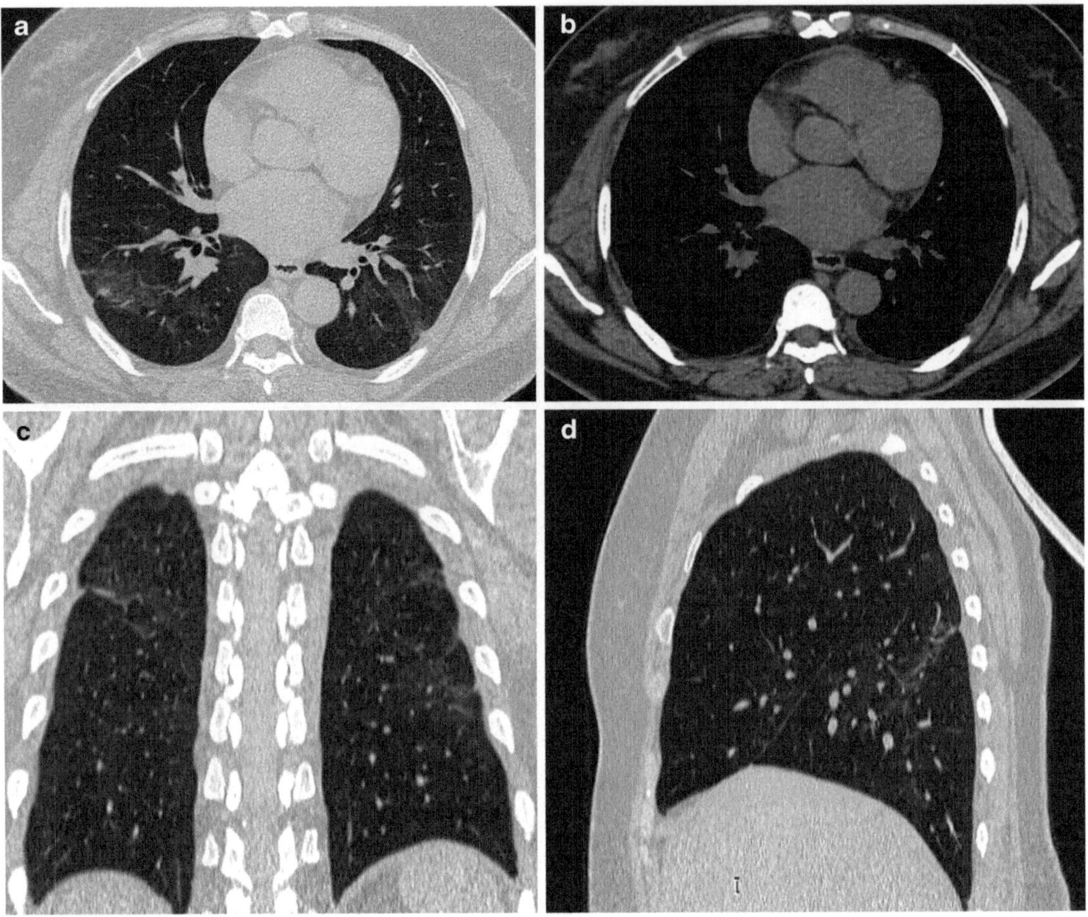

Fig. 6.20 Follow-up axial chest CT (**a**, **b**), reconstructed coronal (**c**) and sagittal (**d**) images 37 days after initial scan

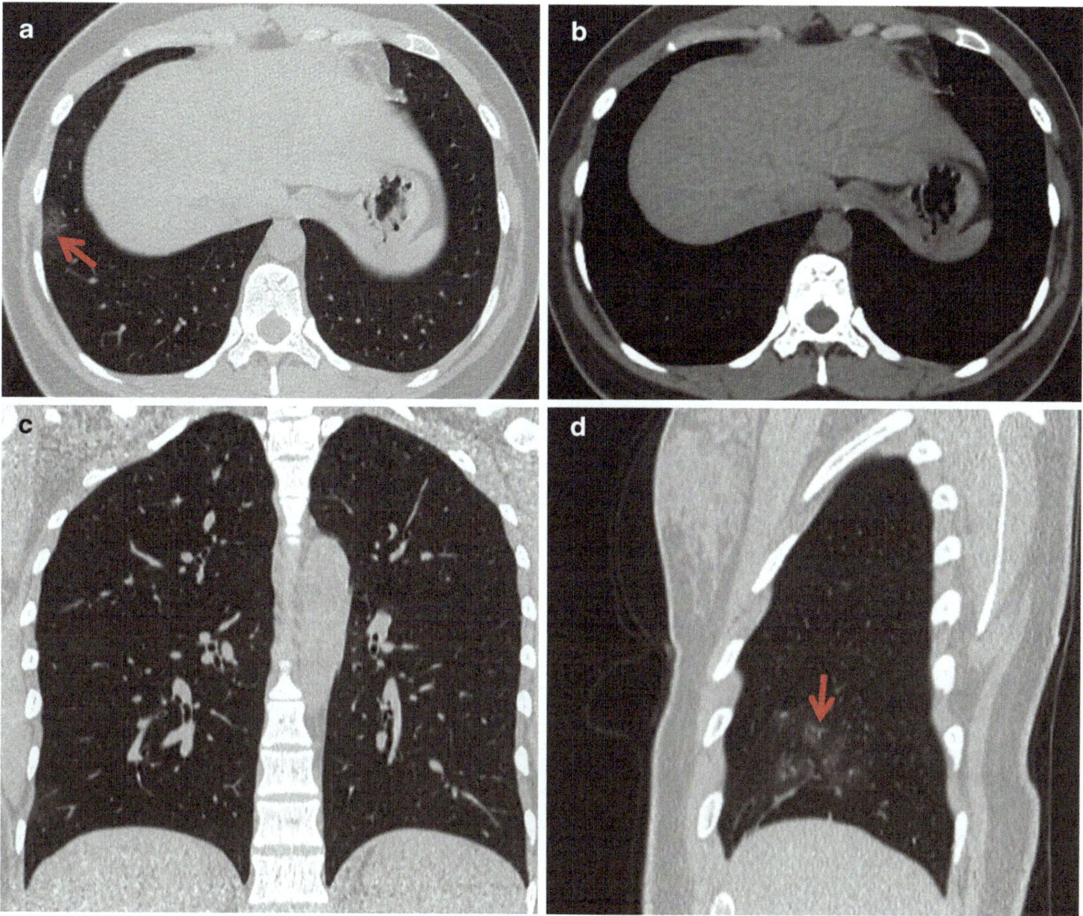

Fig. 6.21 Initial axial chest CT (**a**, **b**), reconstructed coronal (**c**) and sagittal (**d**) images of the patient

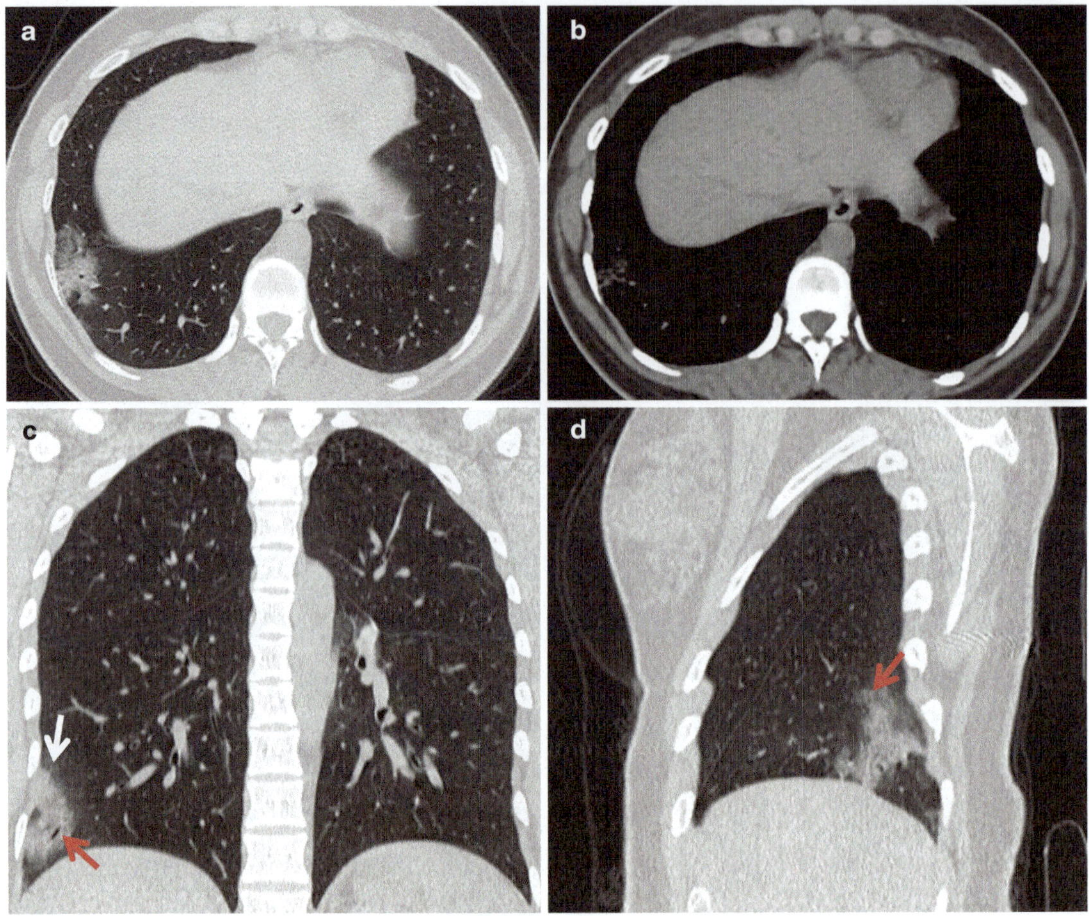

Fig. 6.22 Follow-up axial chest CT (**a**, **b**), reconstructed coronal (**c**) and sagittal (**d**) images 5 days after initial scan

Follow-up chest CT (5 days after initial CT examination) showed lesions in the lower lobe of the right lung were enlarged, and the density expanded. "Microvascular thickening," "paving stone sign," and "air bronchogram" (**c**: red arrow) were seen inside, and "halo sign" (**c**: white arrow) was seen around. A new lesion appeared in the lower lobe of the right lung and the previous lesions were completely absorbed (**d**: red arrow) (Fig. 6.22).

Follow-up chest CT (8 days after initial CT examination) showed the lesion in the lower lobe of the right lung was absorbed and density decreased (Fig. 6.23).

Follow-up chest CT (32 days after initial CT examination) showed the lesion in the lower lobe

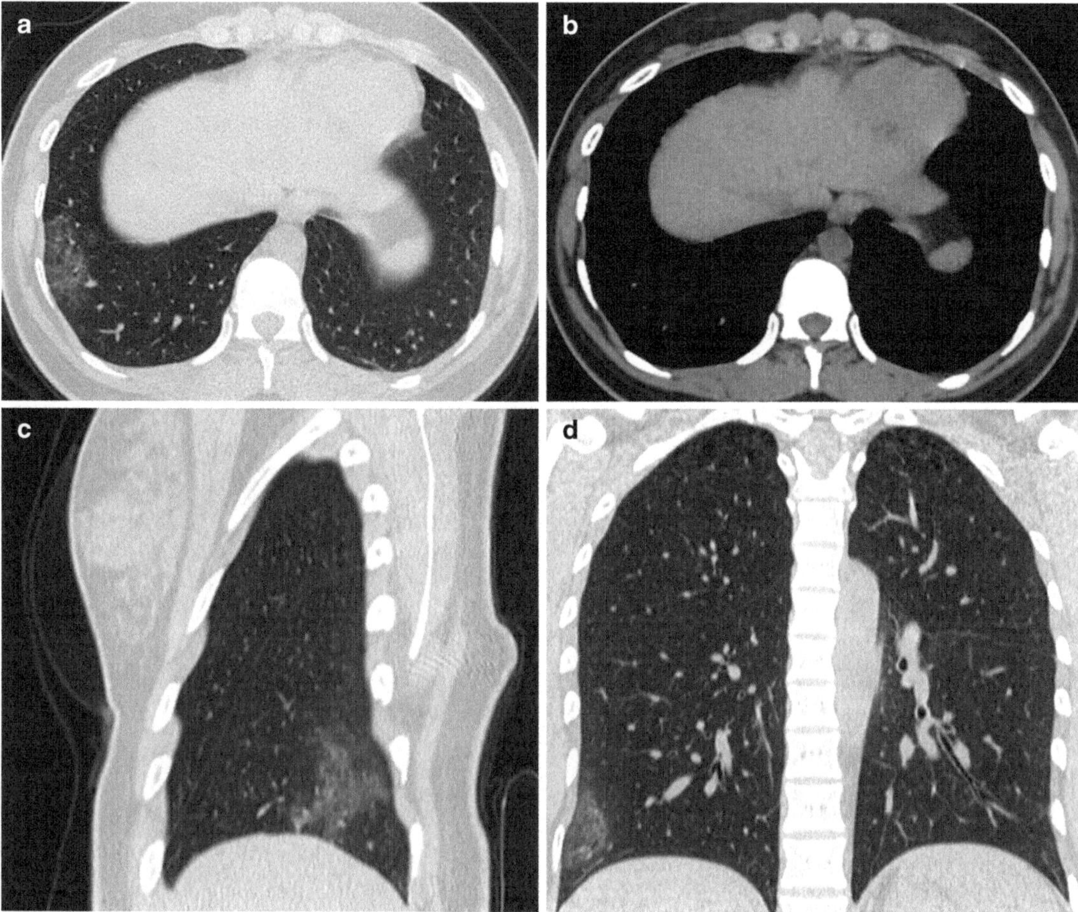

Fig. 6.23 Follow-up axial chest CT (**a**, **b**), reconstructed coronal (**c**) and sagittal (**d**) images 8 days after initial scan

of the right lung was completely absorbed and dissipated (Fig. 6.24).

Case 7

Medical History and Clinical Manifestations

Patient D: A 14-year-old girl was admitted in the hospital for 3 days with fever (highest body temperature: 39 °C) accompanied by fatigue and cough. Laboratory test results indicated normal leukocyte count and lymphocyte counts, normal IL-6 and CRP, and increased SAA. Exposure history: The parents of the patient lived in Wuhan, China. Her parents and brother drove back home from Wuhan, China 5 days prior to symptom onset. The SARS-CoV-2 nucleic acid test was positive 2 days after admission.

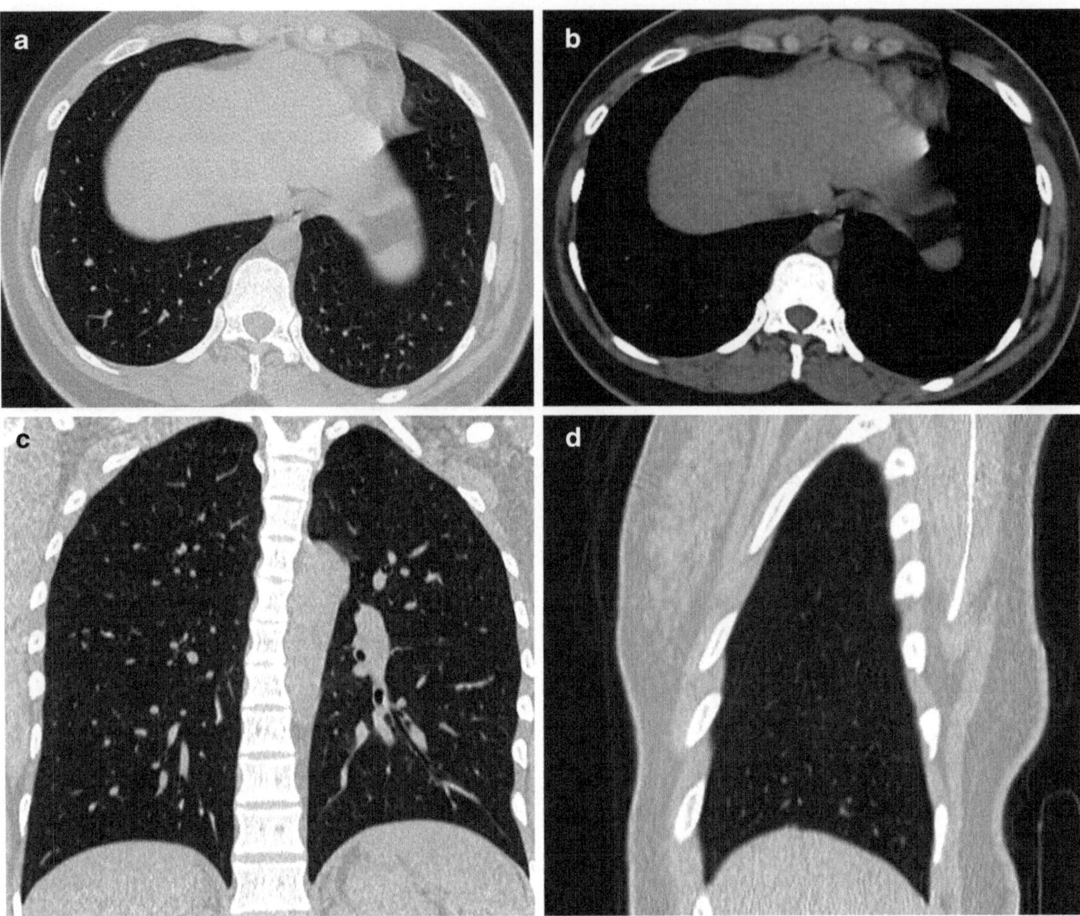

Fig. 6.24 Follow-up axial chest CT (**a**, **b**), reconstructed coronal (**c**) and sagittal (**d**) images 32 days after initial scan

Imaging Features

Initial chest CT showed patchy, nodular high-density shadows under the pleura of the lower lobe of bilateral lungs. "Microvascular thickening" (**a**: red arrow), "crazy-paving pattern" (**c**: red arrow), and "halo sign" were showed in lesions. Mediastinal window showed partial consolidation of the lesion (**b**: red arrow) (Fig. 6.25).

Follow-up chest CT (6 days after initial CT examination) showed that density of lesions in the lower lobe of both lungs was further increased and lesions became consolidated, and the range was not significantly expanded. Mediastinal window showed obvious change in consolidated lesion (**b**: red arrow) (Fig. 6.26).

Follow-up chest CT (10 days after initial CT examination) showed the scope of lesions in the

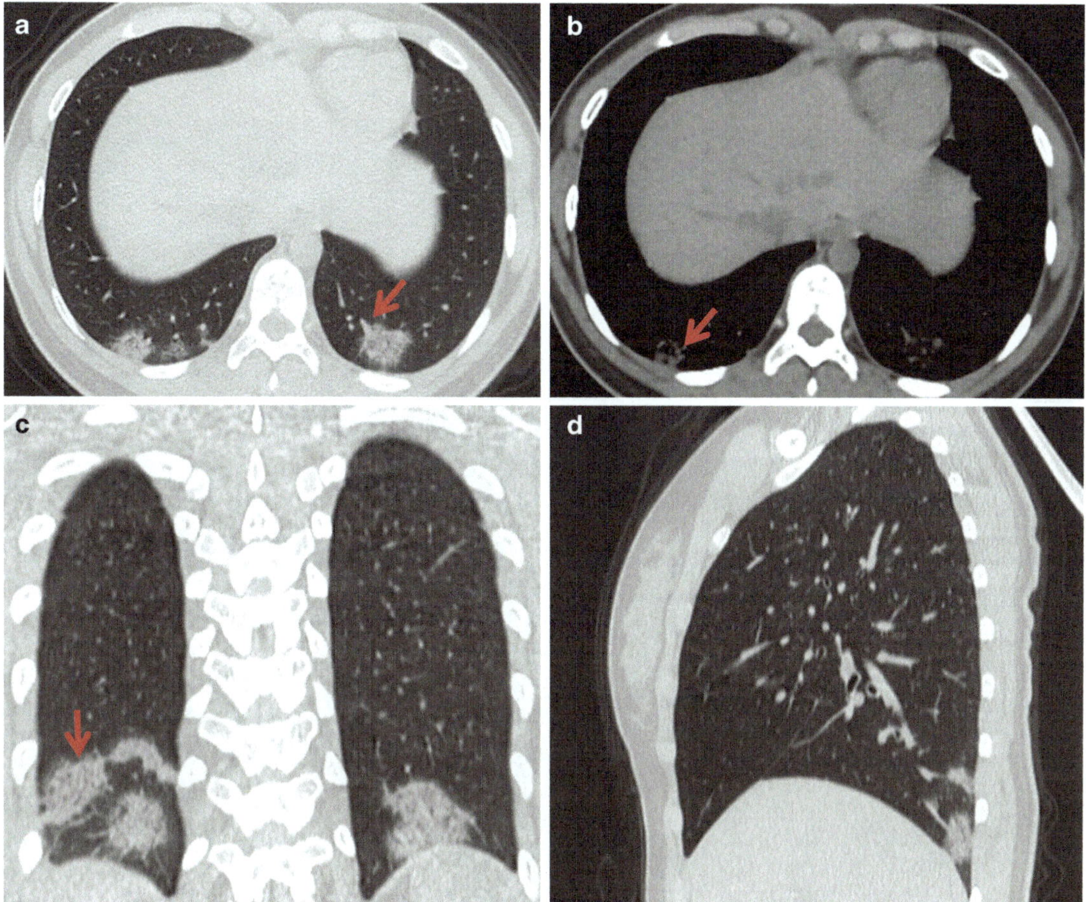

Fig. 6.25 Initial axial chest CT (**a**, **b**), reconstructed coronal (**c**) and sagittal (**d**) images of the patient

lower lobe of both lungs decreased. Mediastinal window showed obvious absorption (**b**: red arrow) (Fig. 6.27).

Follow-up chest CT (35 days after initial CT examination) showed the lesions in the lower lobe of the bilateral lungs were basically absorbed compared with the previous CT imaging (Fig. 6.28).

Comments: This is a group of typical cases of familial aggregation of COVID-19. All the patients were common clinical types except for patient B. Patient B had previous basic diseases of hypertension and diabetes; her clinical classification was severe type. Patients A and B were the earliest to develop the disease, and had a clear history of residence in Wuhan, China. It was con-

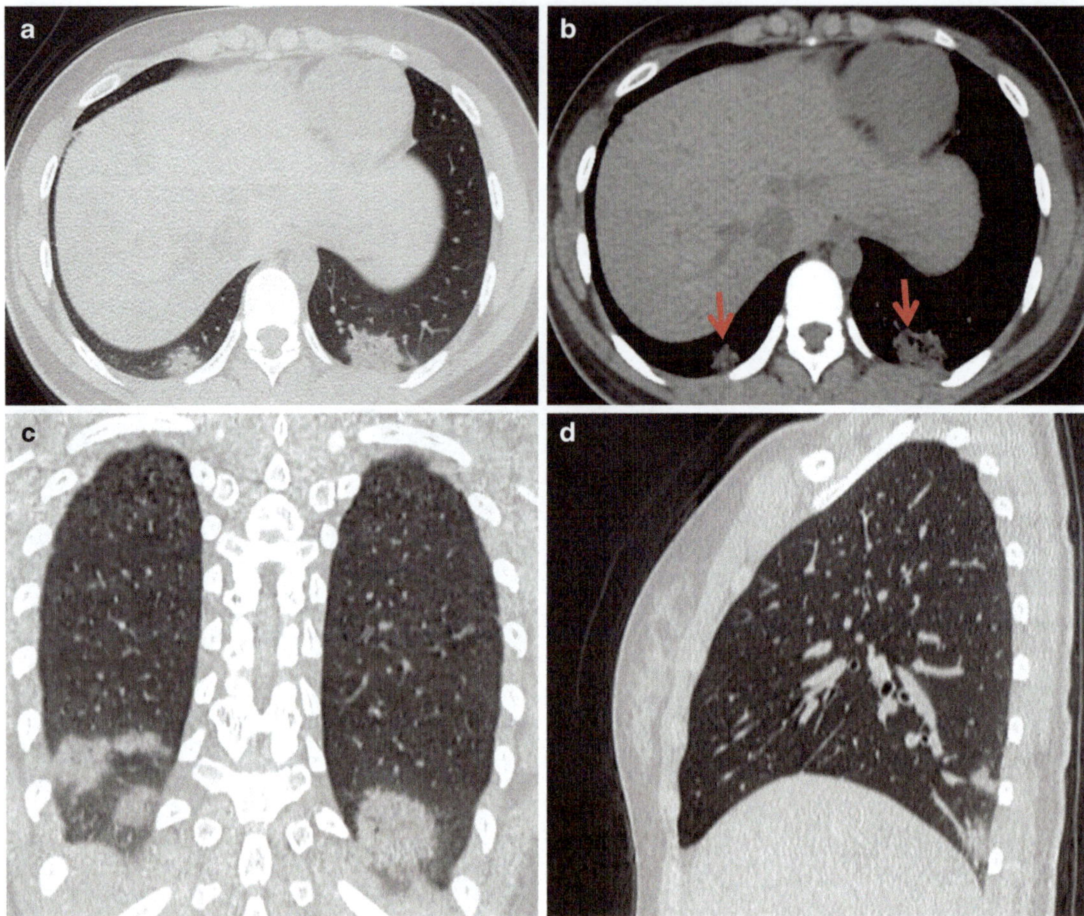

Fig. 6.26 Follow-up axial chest CT (**a**, **b**), reconstructed coronal (**c**) and sagittal (**d**) images 6 days after initial scan

sidered as the first-generation case. The other two family members, the children of the patients, were second generations of people infected with the SARS-CoV-2. Fever was the first symptom in all the patients. The first CT findings were consistent with the typical change of COVID-19 disease; the main lesion was multiple patchy ground-glass opacities. In the follow-up CT images, which showed the dynamic change process of the lesion, most of the lesions were improved in different degrees, some lesion progressed to consolidation, and the final remaining lesions were thin ground-glass opacity or completely normal.

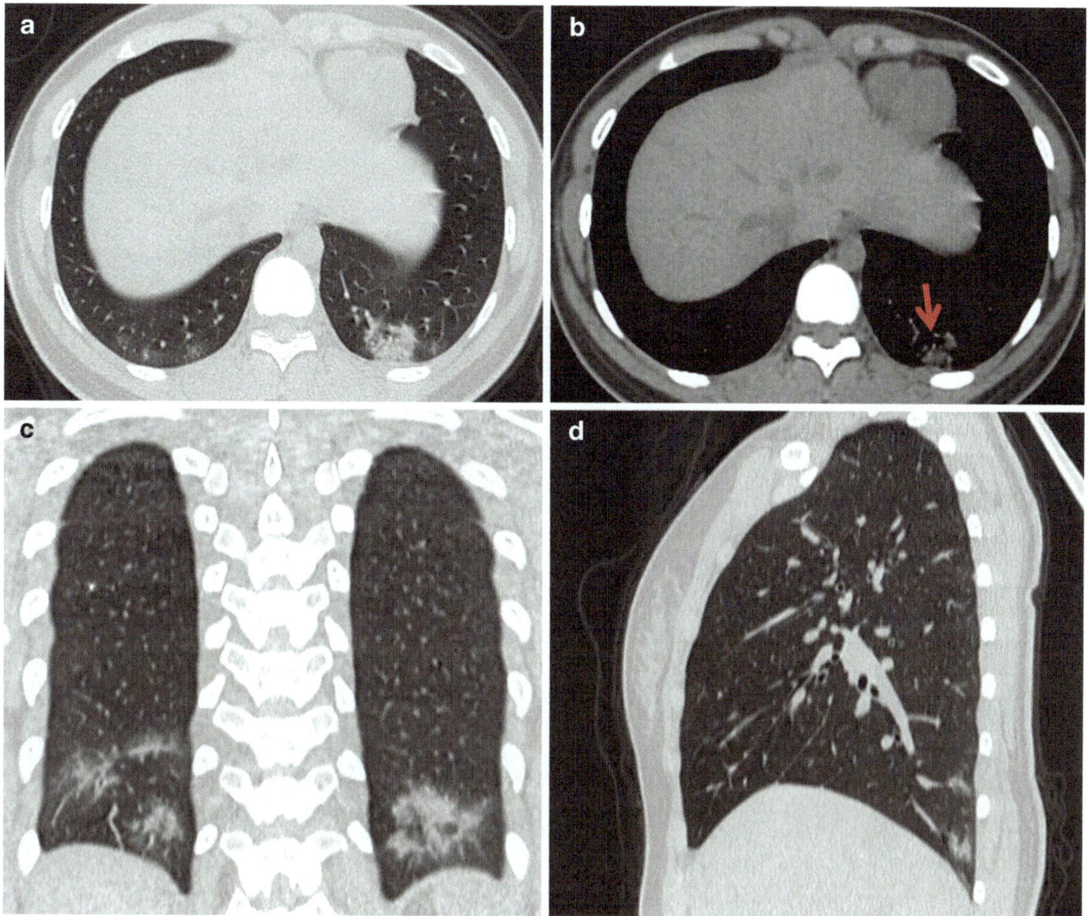

Fig. 6.27 Follow-up axial chest CT (**a**, **b**), reconstructed coronal (**c**) and sagittal (**d**) images 10 days after initial scan

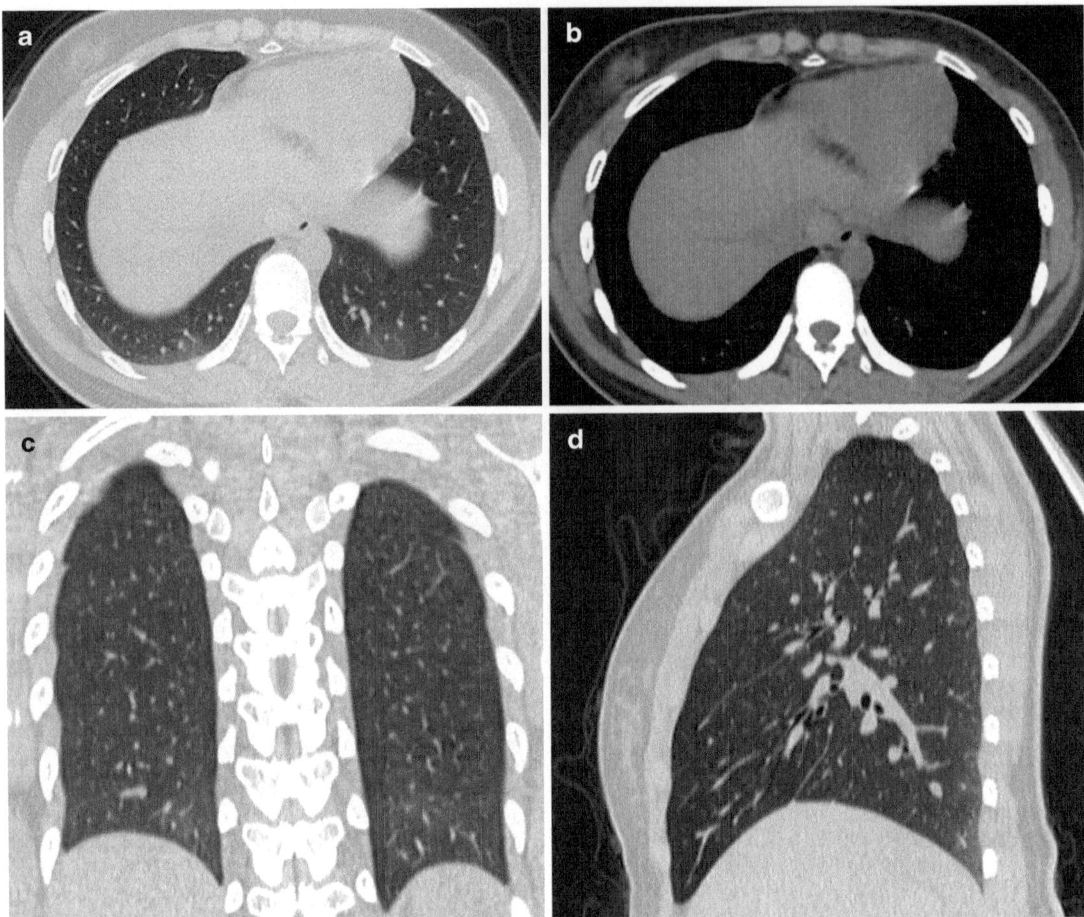

Fig. 6.28 Follow-up axial chest CT (**a**, **b**), reconstructed coronal (**c**) and sagittal (**d**) images 35 days after initial scan

6.3 Group 3 (Cases 8–11)

Case 8
Medical History and Clinical Manifestations

Patient A: A 43-year-old female was admitted in the hospital for 17 days with lower fever (highest body temperature: 37.5 °C) accompanied by cough, sputum and white sputum, and slight symptoms of chest tightness, which were aggravated after activity. Laboratory test results indicated normal leukocyte, neutrophil count, lymphocyte count, lymphocyte percentage, increased IL-6, and normal SAA. Exposure history: The patient returned home from Xi'an, China, by train 1 day prior to symptom onset. The SARS-CoV-2 nucleic acid test was positive on the day of admission.

Imaging Features

Initial chest CT showed multiple patchy ground-glass opacities in bilateral lungs, small patchy consolidation shadows (**a**, **b**: red arrows) were seen locally, and the boundary of the lesions

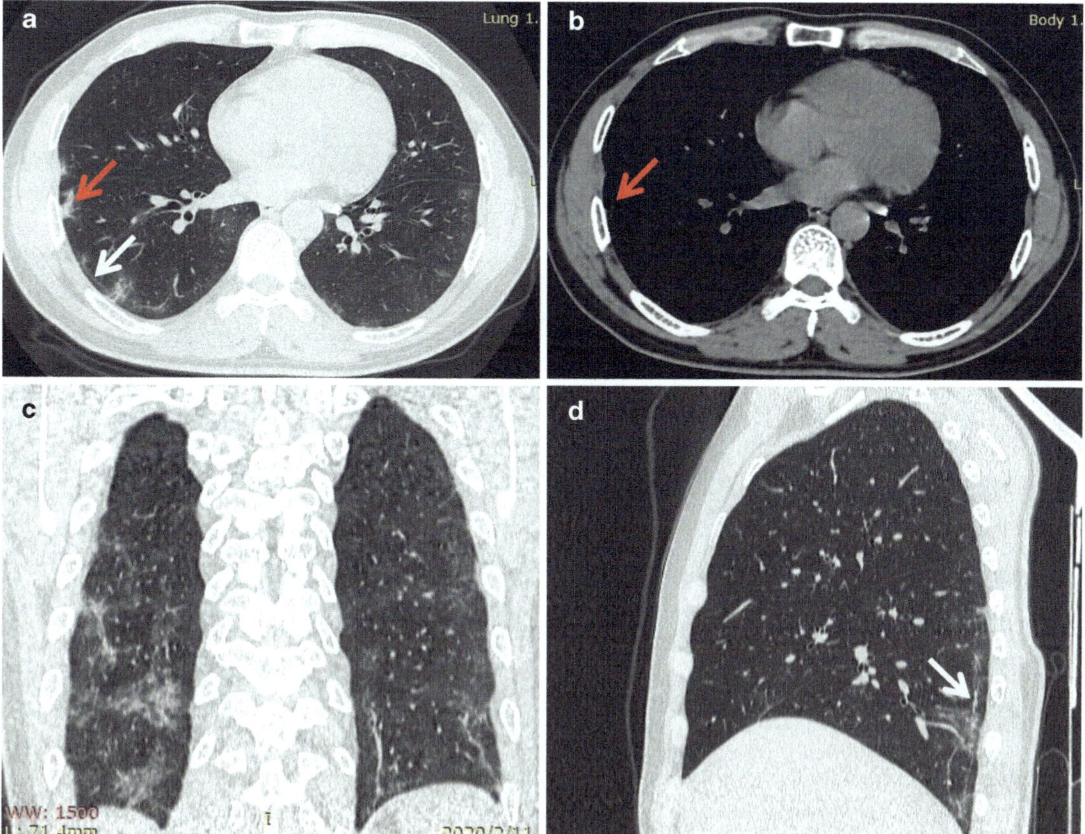

Fig. 6.29 Initial axial chest CT (**a**, **b**), reconstructed coronal (**c**) and sagittal (**d**) images of the patient

was blurred, which was mainly distributed under the pleura. "Halo sign" was seen, and the subpleural curve density increased shadow, namely the subpleural line (**a**, **d**: white arrows). The mediastinal window demonstrated a partial lesion in the right lower lobe of the lung (Fig. 6.29).

Follow-up chest CT (6 days after initial CT examination) showed the subpleural line (**a**, **d**: red arrows) was visible, and the lesion density was decreased and the extent was narrowed. The right lower lobe consolidation disappeared in the mediastinal window (Fig. 6.30).

Follow-up chest CT (11 days after initial CT examination) showed the lesion in both lungs was further absorbed, the density decreased, and the range reduced (Fig. 6.31).

Follow-up chest CT (25 days after initial CT examination) showed complete absorption of the lesions in both lungs (Fig. 6.32).

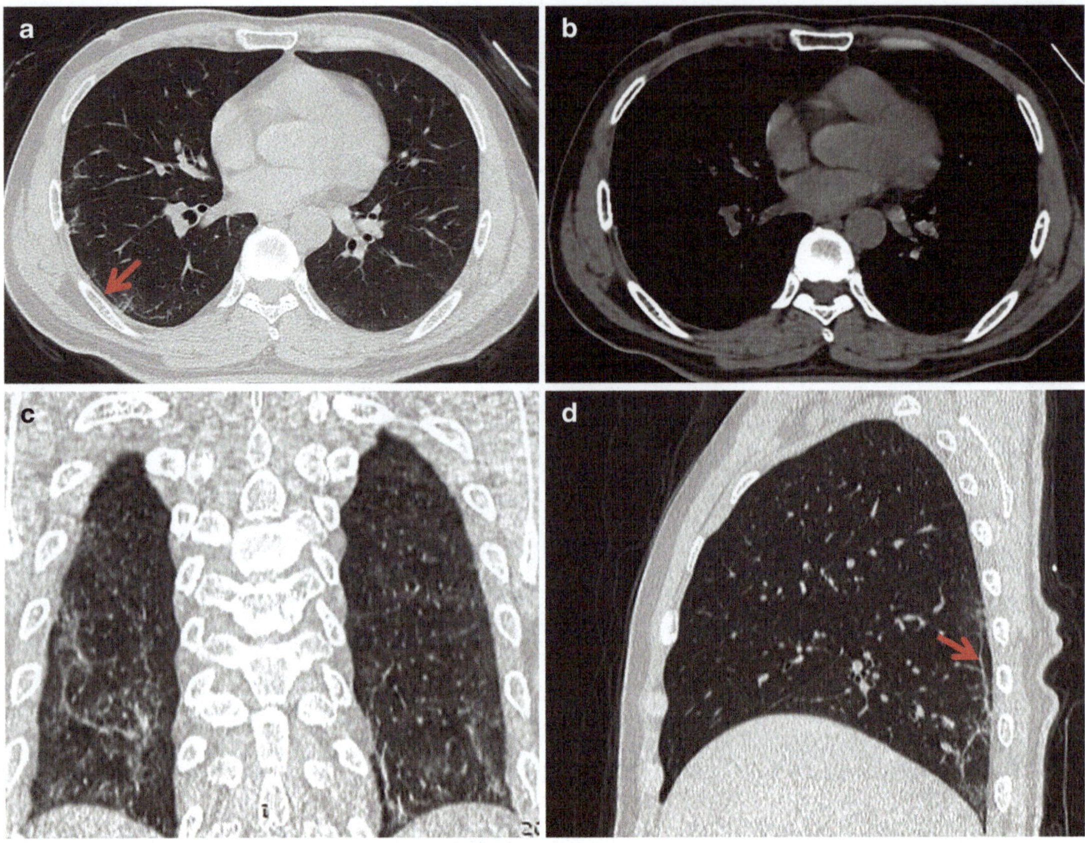

Fig. 6.30 Follow-up axial chest CT (**a**, **b**), reconstructed coronal (**c**) and sagittal (**d**) images 6 days after initial scan

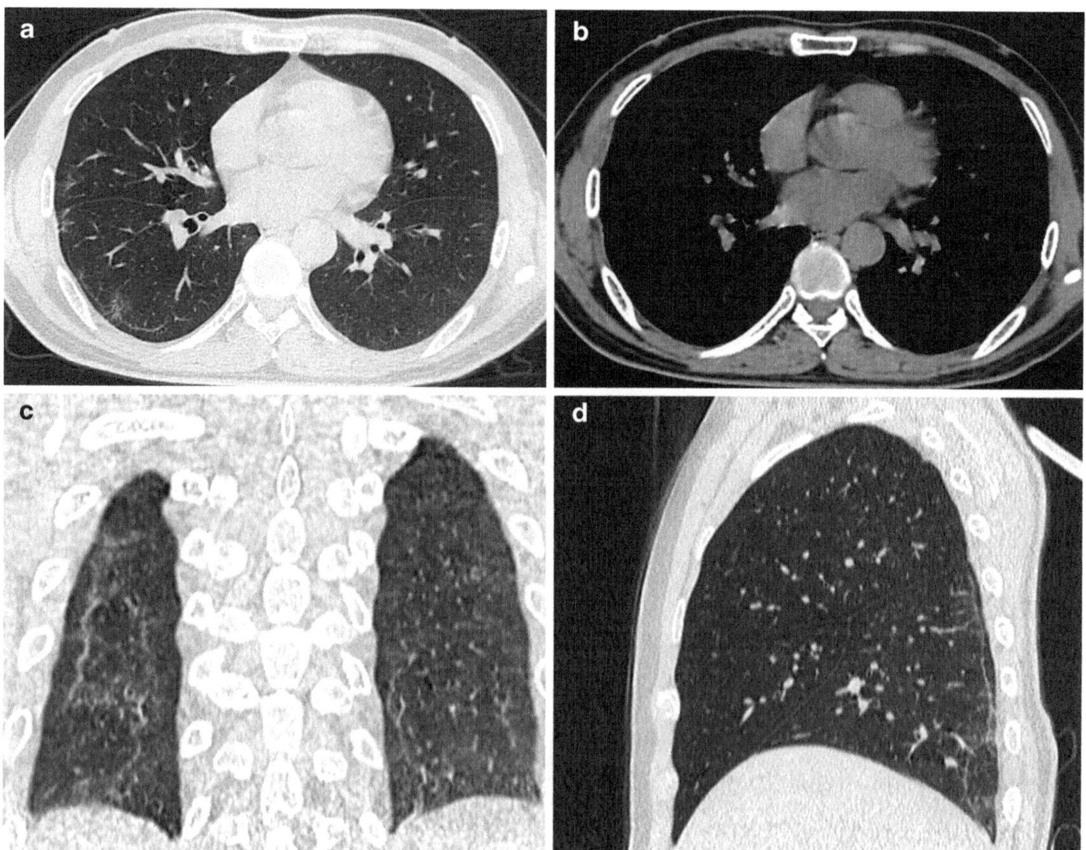

Fig. 6.31 Follow-up axial chest CT (**a**, **b**), reconstructed coronal (**c**) and sagittal (**d**) images 11 days after initial scan

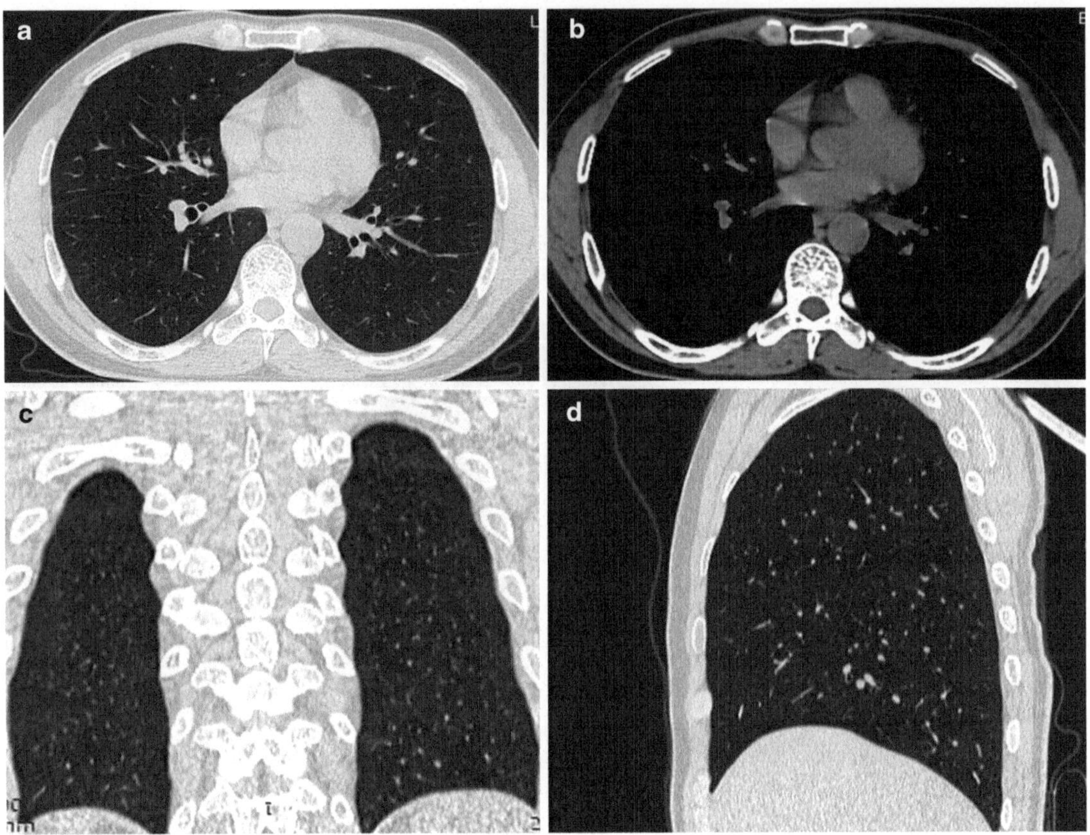

Fig. 6.32 Follow-up axial chest CT (**a**, **b**), reconstructed coronal (**c**) and sagittal (**d**) images 25 days after initial scan

Case 9

Medical History and Clinical Manifestations

Patient B: A 38-year-old female was admitted in the hospital for 1 day with dry cough accompanied by pharyngeal discomfort. Laboratory test results indicated normal leukocyte count, neutrophil count, lymphocyte count, lymphocyte percentage, normal IL-6, except an increased SAA. Exposure history: The patient returned home from Xi'an, Shanxi Province, China by train 5 days prior to symptom onset. Her husband, brother, and father-in-law were all confirmed COVID-19. The SARS-CoV-2 nucleic acid test was positive after admission.

Imaging Features

Initial chest CT showed multiple patchy ground-glass opacities (**a**: red arrow) in the left lung, blurred boundary of lesions, mainly distrib-

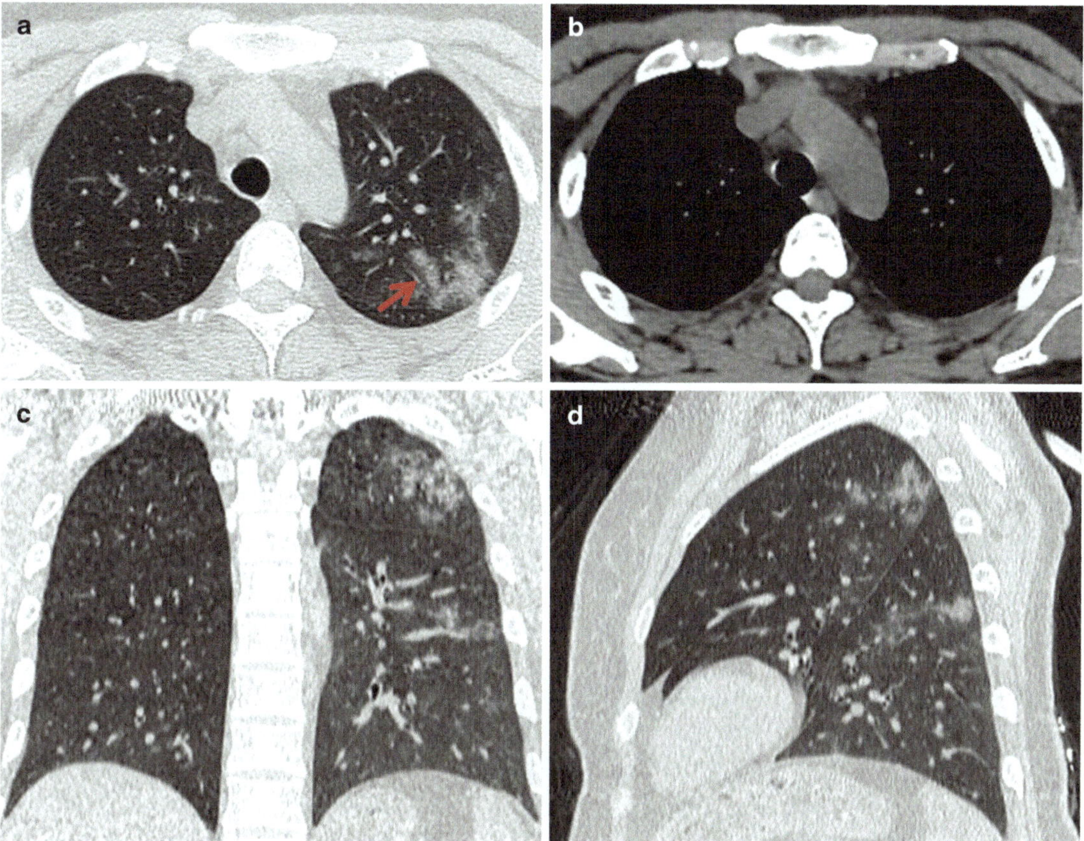

Fig. 6.33 Initial axial chest CT (**a**, **b**), reconstructed coronal (**c**) and sagittal (**d**) images of the patient

uted under the pleura of the left lung, and "halo sign" was seen (Fig. 6.33).

Follow-up chest CT (4 days after initial CT examination) showed that the density of the lesions was decreased than before, the extent was narrowed, and the lesion in the lower lobe of left lung was absorbed (Fig. 6.34).

Follow-up chest CT (17 days after initial CT examination) showed complete absorption of the lesions in bilateral lungs (Fig. 6.35).

Follow-up chest CT (28 days after initial CT examination) showed no obvious abnormalities in both lungs (Fig. 6.36).

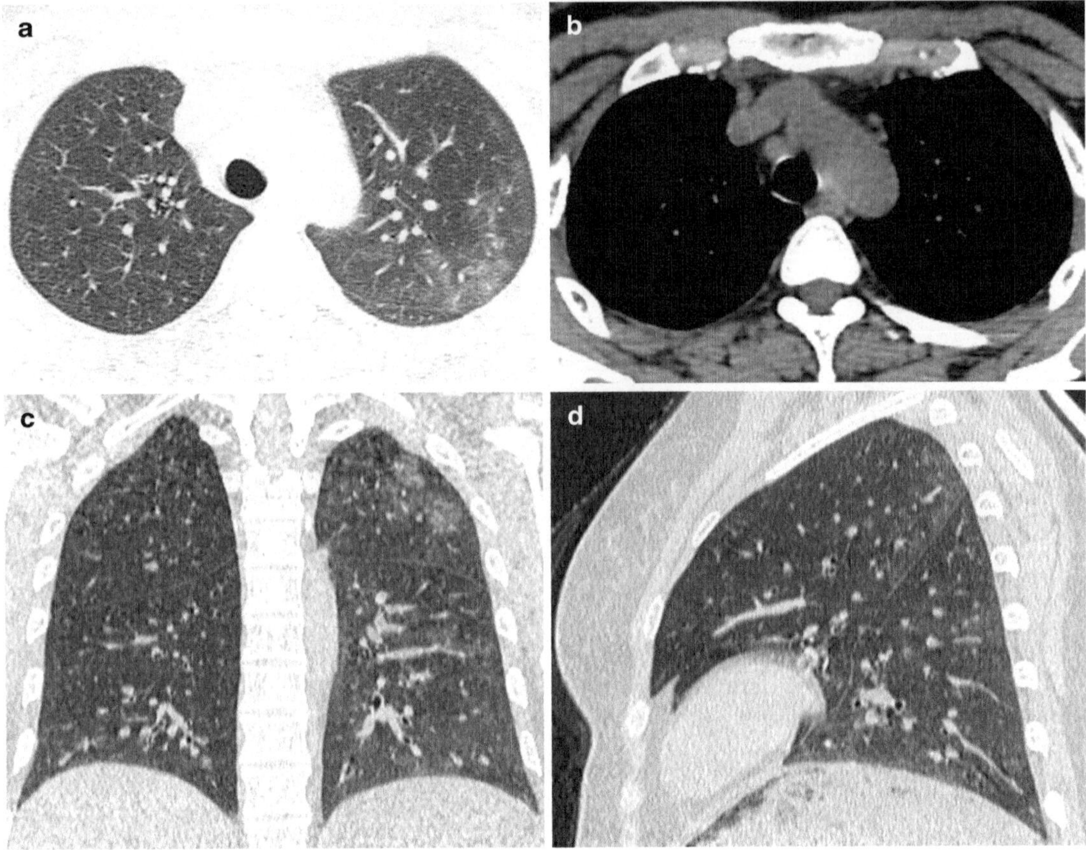

Fig. 6.34 Follow-up axial chest CT (**a**, **b**), reconstructed coronal (**c**) and sagittal (**d**) images 4 days after initial scan

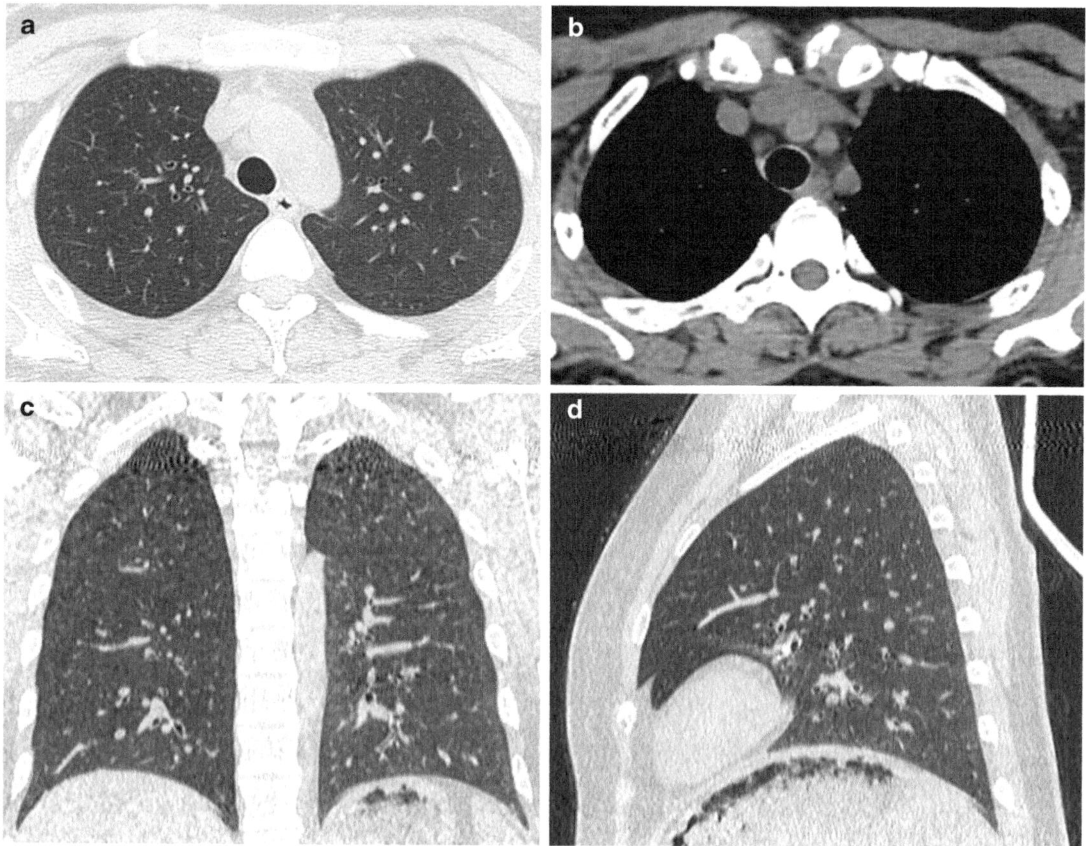

Fig. 6.35 Follow-up axial chest CT (**a**, **b**), reconstructed coronal (**c**) and sagittal (**d**) images 17 days after initial scan

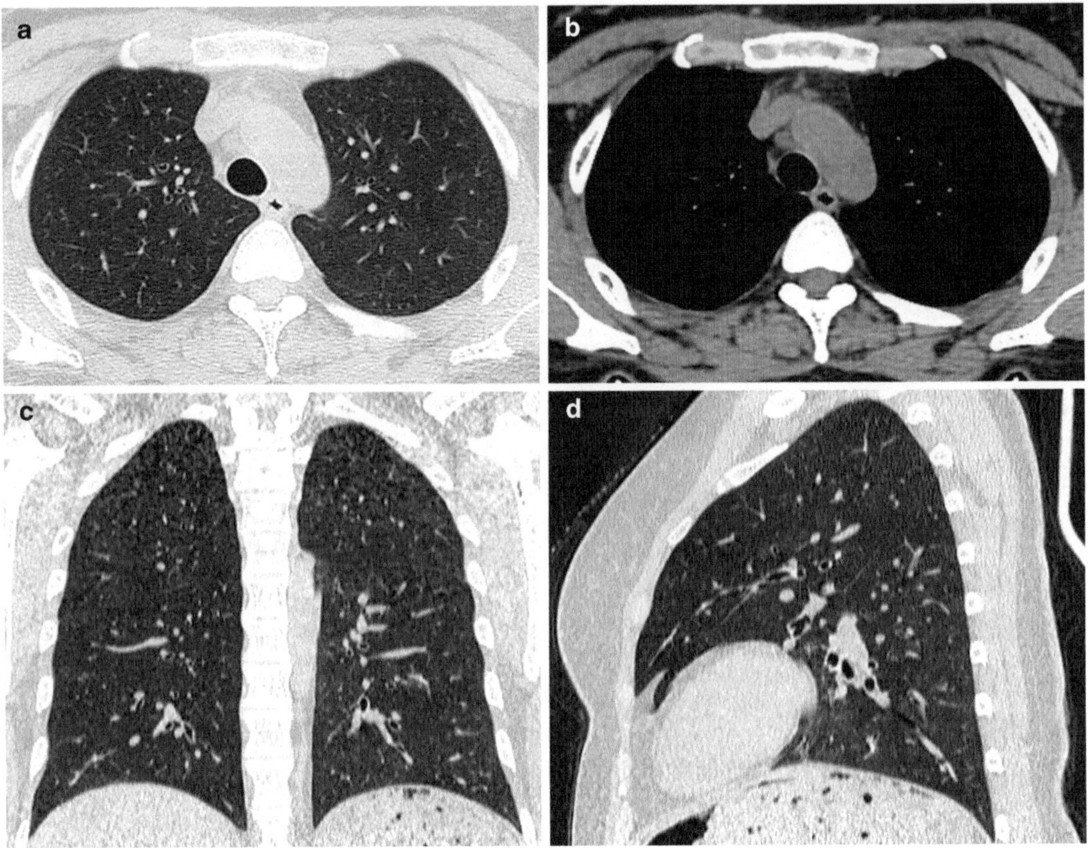

Fig. 6.36 Follow-up axial chest CT (**a**, **b**), reconstructed coronal (**c**) and sagittal (**d**) images 28 days after initial scan

Case 10

Medical History and Clinical Manifestations

Patient C: A 39-year-old male was admitted in the hospital for 1 day with fatigue. Laboratory test results indicated normal leukocyte count, neutrophil count, lymphocyte count, lymphocyte percentage, normal IL-6, except increased SAA. Exposure history: His father was confirmed COVID-19. The SARS-CoV-2 nucleic acid test was positive after admission.

Imaging Features

Initial chest CT showed patchy ground-glass opacities and linear opacities in the subpleural of the upper lobe of the right lung and the lower lobe of the left lung, small focal consolidation (**a**, **b**: red arrows). The boundary of the lesion was blurred, and the "halo sign" was seen. Part of the lesion in the lower lobe of the left lung was shown in the mediastinal window (Fig. 6.37).

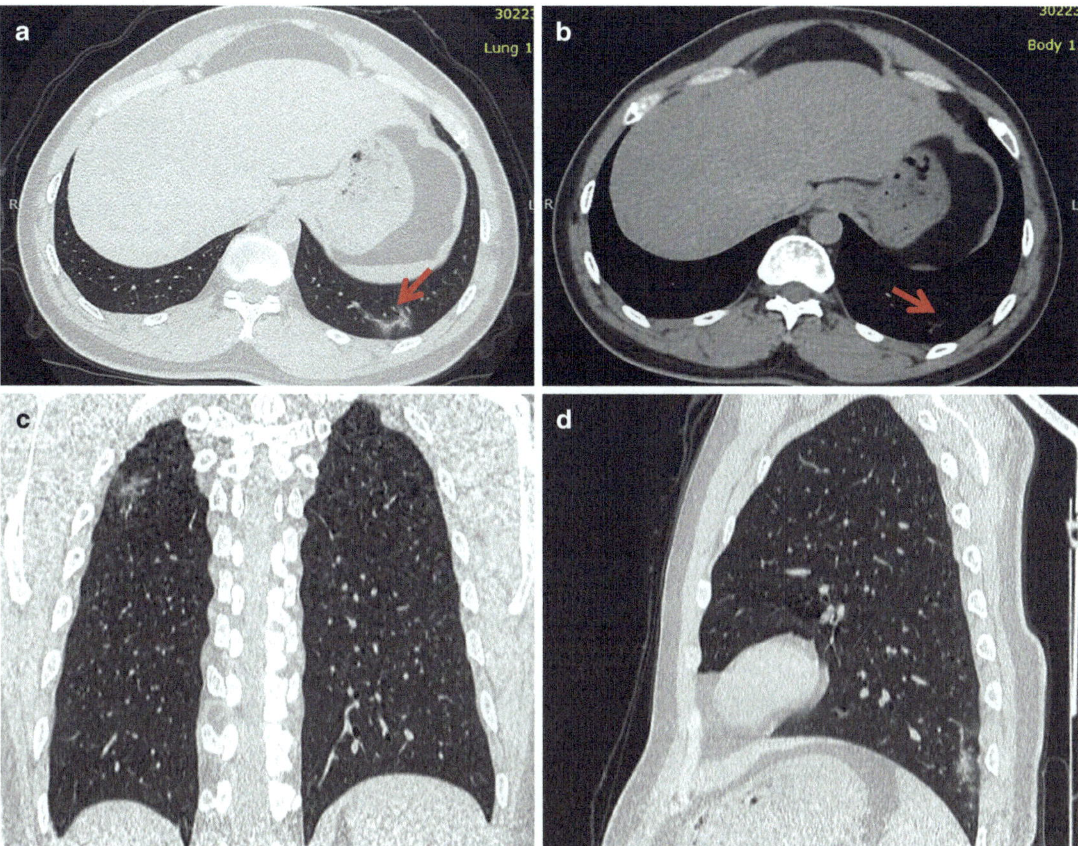

Fig. 6.37 Initial axial chest CT (**a**, **b**), reconstructed coronal (**c**) and sagittal (**d**) images of the patient

Follow-up chest CT (5 days after initial CT examination) showed that the density of the lesion was decreased than before (**b**: red arrow). Consolidation of the lower lobe of the left lung disappeared in the mediastinal window (red arrow) (Fig. 6.38).

Follow-up chest CT (18 days after initial CT examination) showed further absorption of the lesion in the lower lobe of the left lung, with a few residual linear opacities and patchy light ground-glass opacities. The lesion in the upper lobe of the right lung was completely absorbed (Fig. 6.39).

Follow-up chest CT (29 days after initial CT examination) showed further absorption of the lesion in the lower lobe of the left lung, with a few remaining linear opacities (**d**: red arrow) (Fig. 6.40).

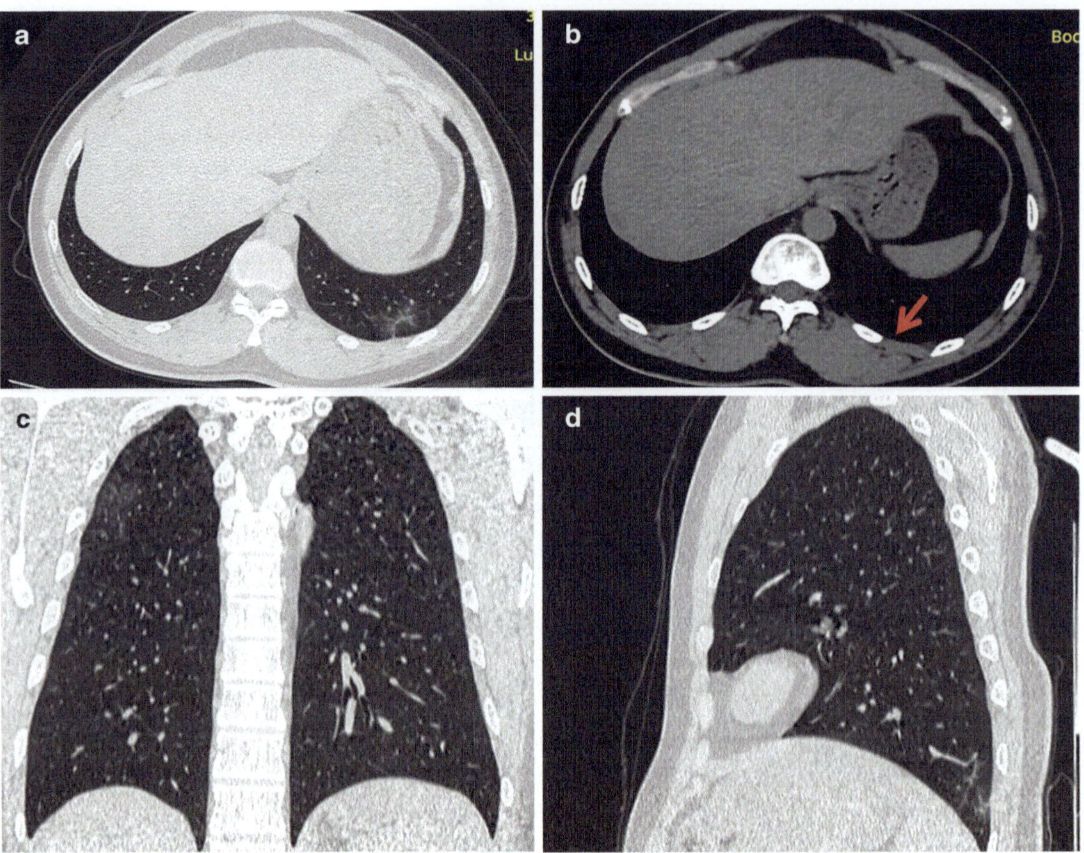

Fig. 6.38 Follow-up axial chest CT (**a**, **b**), reconstructed coronal (**c**) and sagittal (**d**) images 5 days after initial scan

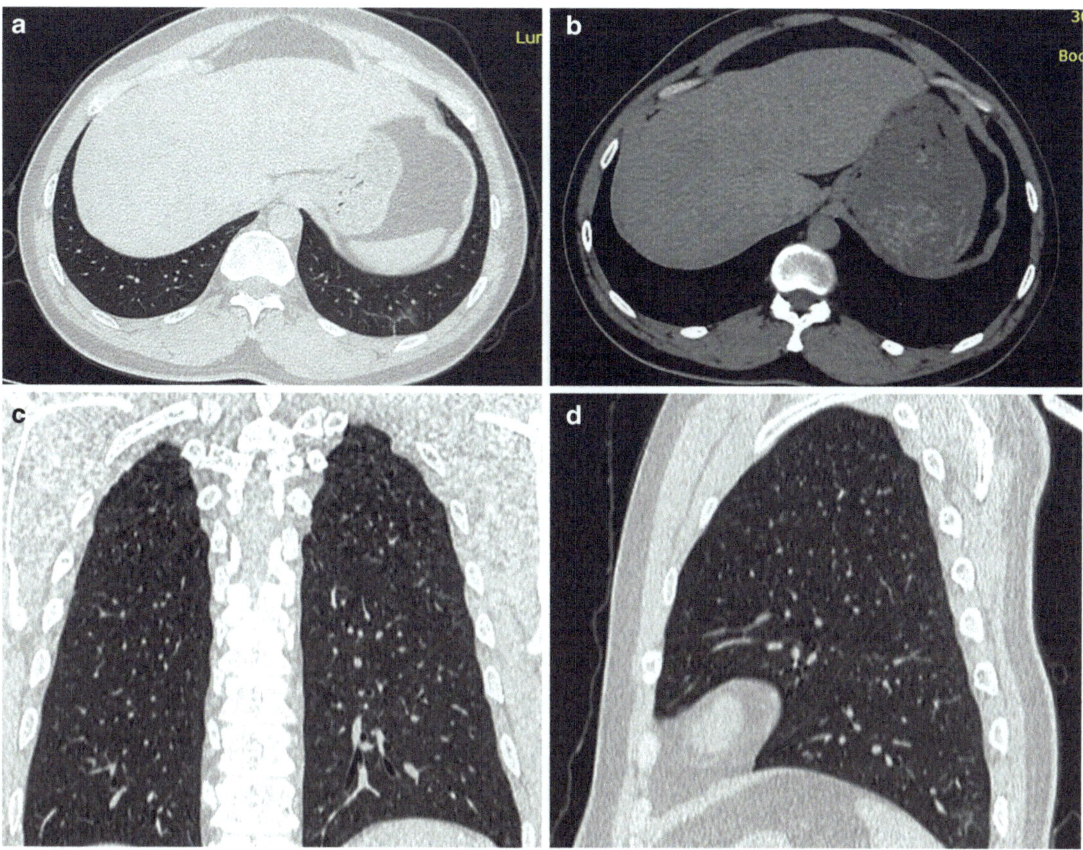

Fig. 6.39 Follow-up axial chest CT (**a**, **b**), reconstructed coronal (**c**) and sagittal (**d**) images 18 days after initial scan

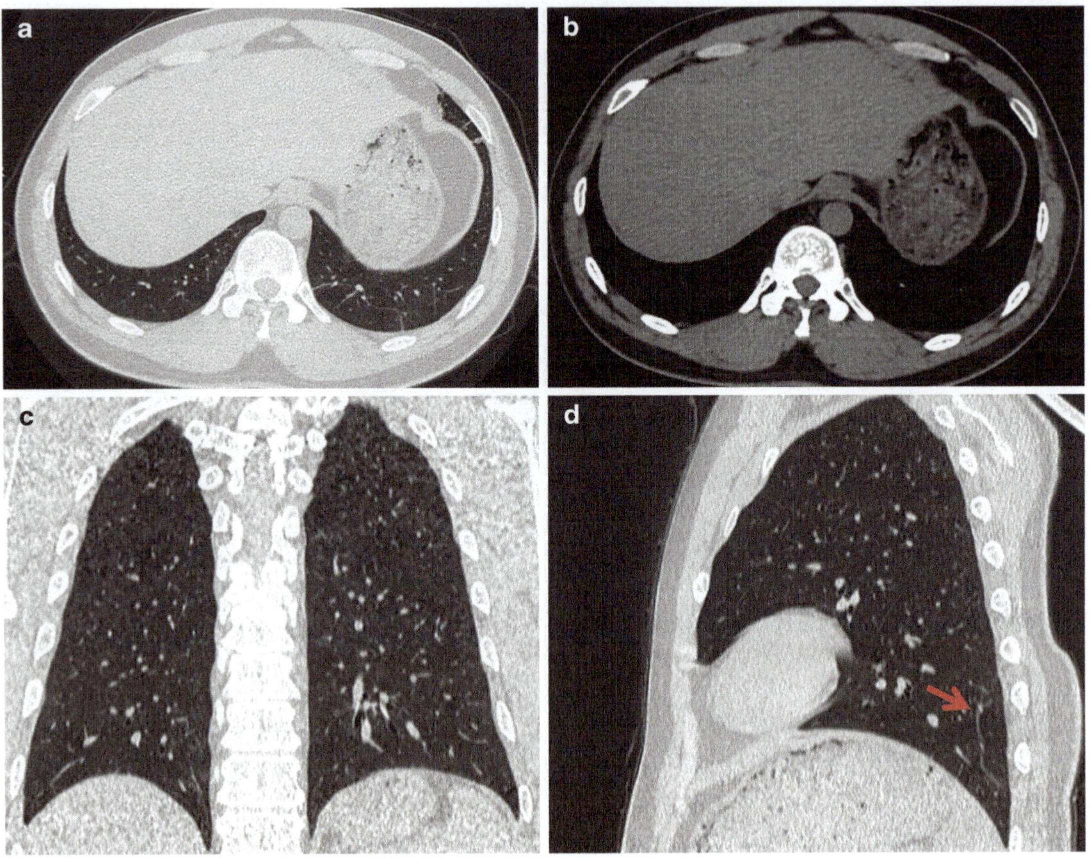

Fig. 6.40 Follow-up axial chest CT (**a**, **b**), reconstructed coronal (**c**) and sagittal (**d**) images 29 days after initial scan

Case 11

Medical History and Clinical Manifestations

Patient D: A 69-year-old female was admitted in the hospital for 7 days with fever (highest body temperature: 40 °C) after suffering from cold accompanied by chills, shiver, chest tightness, asthma, and coughed with white phlegm. Laboratory test results indicated increased leukocyte count, decreased lymphocyte percentage, and increased C-reactive protein, IL-6, and SAA. Exposure history: Two sons of the patient returned from Guizhou province, China and Xi'an, Shaanxi Province, China, respectively. The patient D had a history of contact with his two sons. The SARS-CoV-2 nucleic acid test was positive on the day of admission. The patient had type 2 diabetes and grade 3 hypertension.

Imaging Features

Initial chest CT showed multiple patchy and large patchy ground-glass opacities in bilateral lungs, some of which were accompanied by consolidation shadows. The boundary of the lesions was blurred. "Air bronchogram" (**a**: red arrow) and "mosaic signs" were visible. The coronal image showed honeycombed changes in both lungs (**c**: red arrow). Lesions in the lower lobes of both lungs could be seen in the mediastinal window (Fig. 6.41).

Follow-up chest CT (7 days after initial CT examination) showed multiple flaky consolidation shadows in both lungs, mainly distributed in the dorsal part of the lower lobe of both lungs. These lesions were more progressive than before, with increased density and consolidation. The

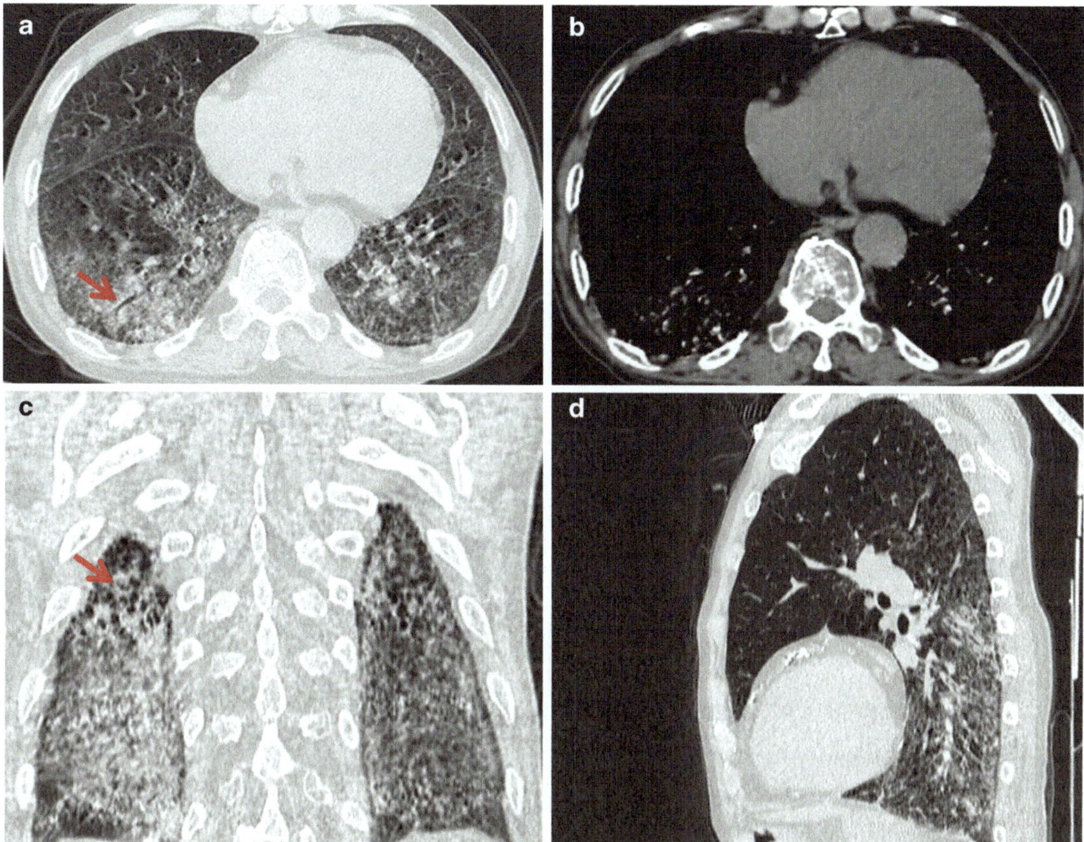

Fig. 6.41 Initial axial chest CT (**a**, **b**), reconstructed coronal (**c**) and sagittal (**d**) images of the patient

mediastinal window demonstrates lesions in the lower lobes of both lungs, with small amount of pleural effusion on both sides (**b**: red arrows) (Fig. 6.42).

Follow-up chest CT (17 days after initial CT examination) showed multiple consolidations in bilateral lungs, mainly distributed in the dorsal part of the lower lobe of both lungs, increased number of honeycomb signs in the right lung (**c**: red arrow), and advanced lesions in the lower lobe of both lungs. Thickening pleura at the mediastinal window was showed. Small amount of pleural effusion at the left side was absorbed than before (Fig. 6.43).

Comments: Among the familial aggregation cases in this group, patient A was firstly developed, and he returned home from other province by train, which was considered to be the first-generation viral infection. CT finding was typical, showing multiple patchy ground-glass opacities in the subpleural area of bilateral lungs, accompanied by partial consolidation. Patients B, C, and D were members of his family and had contact history with patient A, which was considered as second-generation viral infection. Patients A, B, and C were all middle-aged patients with no underlying disease, and the clinical analysis showed that they were all the common type with good prognosis. Among them, the pulmonary lesions of patients A and B were completely absorbed, and there was a little residual fibrosis in the lungs of patient C. Patient D was an elderly male with previous underlying diseases of hypertension and diabetes. His clinical classification was severe and he had a bad prognosis.

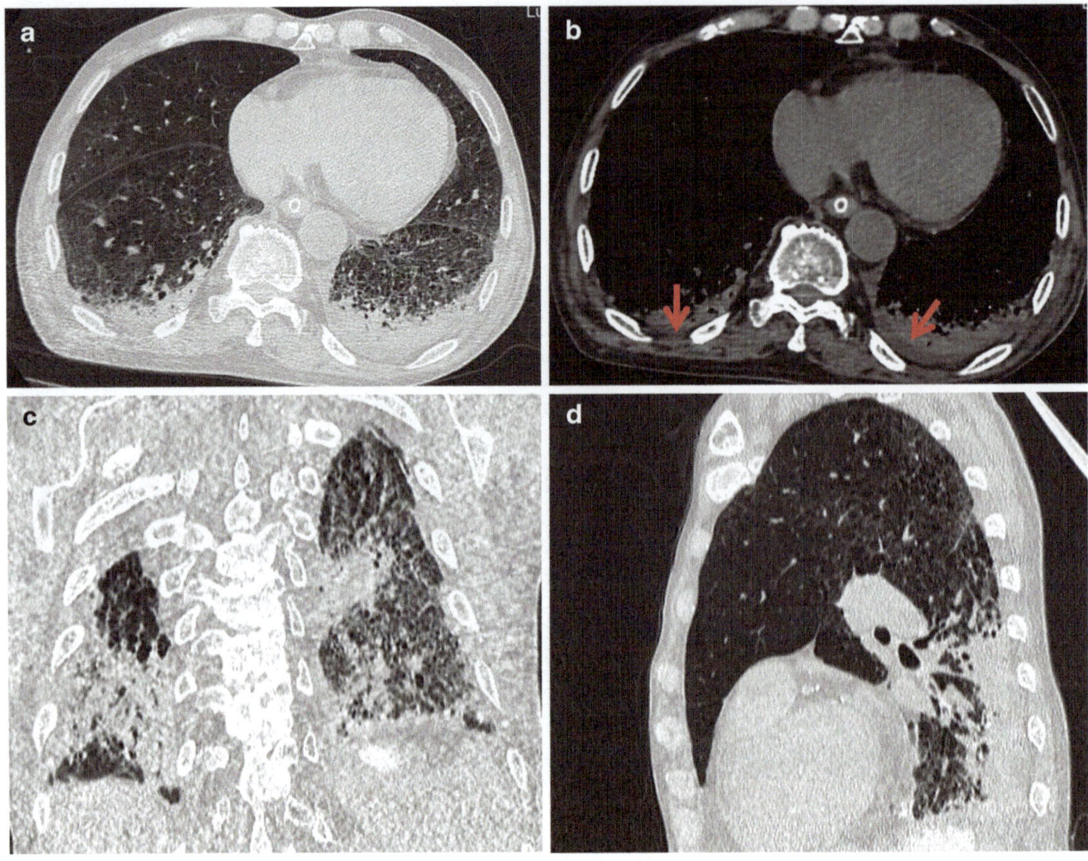

Fig. 6.42 Follow-up axial chest CT (**a**, **b**), reconstructed coronal (**c**) and sagittal (**d**) images 7 days after initial scan

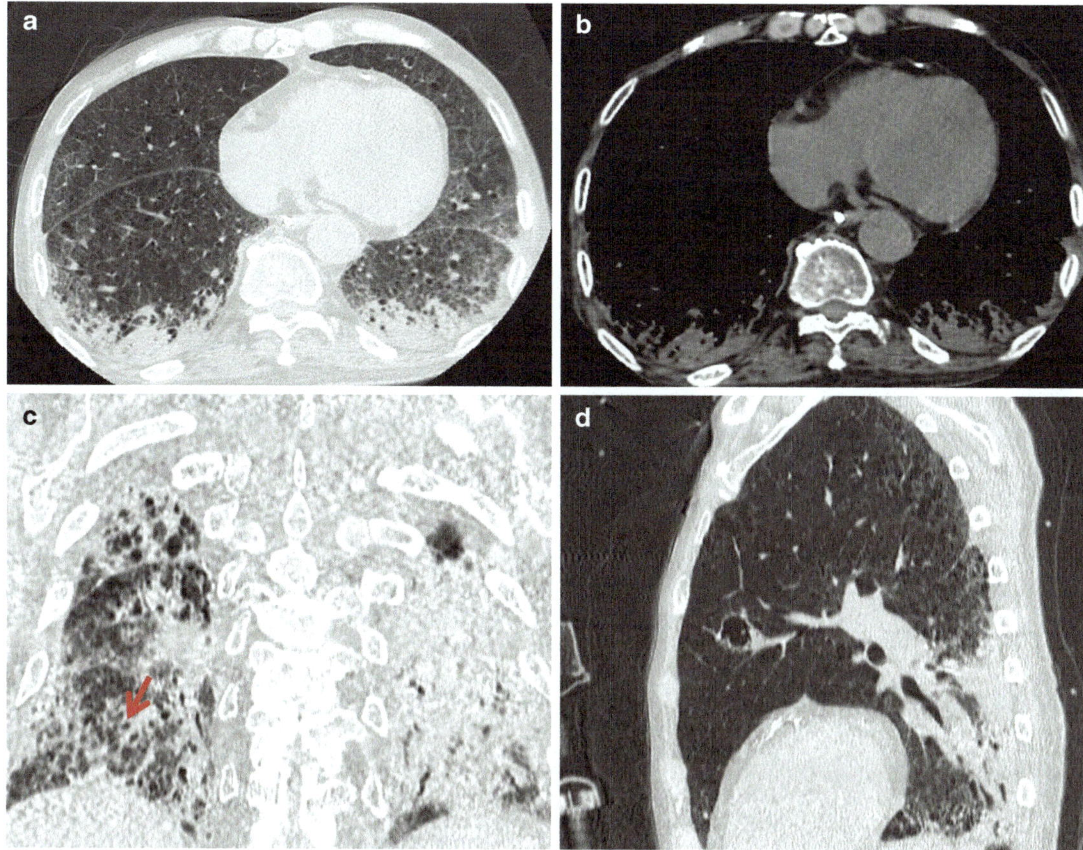

Fig. 6.43 Follow-up axial chest CT (**a**, **b**), reconstructed coronal (**c**) and sagittal (**d**) images 17 days after initial scan

References

1. Epidemiology Working Group, Strategy and Policy Working Group for NCIP Epidemic Response, Chinese Center for Disease Control and Prevention. Cluster Investigation Technical Guideline for the 2019 Novel Coronavirus Pneumonia (COVID-19), China (1st Trial Version). Chin J Epidemiol. 2020;41(03):293–5.
2. Yang H, Xu J, Yan L, et al. The preliminary analysis on the characteristics of the cluster for the corona virus disease. Chin J Epidemiol. 2020;41:623–8.
3. Zhang J, Tian S, Lou J, et al. Familial cluster of COVID-19 infection from an asymptomatic. Crit Care. 2020;24(1):119.
4. Guan WJ, Ni ZY, Hu Y, et al. Clinical characteristics of coronavirus disease 2019 in China. N Engl J Med. 2020;NEJMoa2002032.
5. Cao l, Li w, Yu h, et al. Clinical and imaging manifestations of familial clustering corona virus disease 2019. Chin J Med Imaging Technol. 2020;36(3):415–9.

7 Imaging Features of COVID-19 in Children

Bin Lin and Minming Zhang

The incidence rate of SARS-CoV-2 (the virus name of COVID-19) infection for children is significantly lower than that for adults with clear characteristic of clustering in terms of the incidence rate of such disease. A definite history of aggregation in infected families can be found for most children who are suffering from such disease [1–5]. Comparing with the clinical characteristics of adult patients, the clinical symptoms of the confirmed child cases are relatively mild with fast recovery, shorter detoxification time, and favorable prognosis. Most child patients only show the symptoms of upper respiratory tract infection and are also self-limiting, while for some children and newborn babies, their symptoms may not typical, including emesis, diarrhea, etc., the symptoms of digestive tract, or merely weak in spirit and tachypnea [6]. An epidemiologic study of 2135 cases of children (less than 18 years old) infected with COVID-19 has found that more than 90% of the child patients are either patients with no symptom or patients with mild to average symptoms, wherein the asymptomatic cases account for about 13% [5]. Though the incidence rate of severe or critical case is low for children, the pediatricians still need to attach importance to and have close monitoring of it, especially for child patients with certain underlying medical conditions, efforts should be made to ensure early identification and timely medical treatment.

Compared with adults, the imaging findings of the children infected with COVID-19 are mild and not typical, which suggests that CT may be used for imaging screening of suspected children with contact history in epidemic area or contact history with confirmed patients, while we should be careful of the impact of ionizing radiation on children. Negative results are often found in the CT imaging examined for children in an early stage since their infection with the COVID-19.

As the disease develops, lesions gradually appear. The lesion locations on the patients are more commonly found under the external pleurae of both lungs, and multiple lesions may also be found. In comparison with the distribution of the lesion locations on adults infected with COVID-19, the lesions on child patients are relatively confined to a certain location, with relatively less diffuse distribution. Also the ground-glass opacity is also less typical than that of adults since the lesions on child patients are comparatively less in size and some appear in a form of "thin clouds."

Case 1

Medical History and Clinical Manifestations

A 15-year-old boy was admitted in the hospital for 5 days with fever (highest body temperature: 38.5 °C), dry cough, and chest congestion.

B. Lin · M. Zhang (✉)
Department of Radiology, the Second Affiliated Hospital, Zhejiang University School of Medicine, Hangzhou, China
e-mail: zjdxlinbin@zju.edu.cn; zhangminming@zju.edu.cn

M. Zhang, B. Lin (eds.), *Diagnostic Imaging of Novel Coronavirus Pneumonia*,
https://doi.org/10.1007/978-981-15-5992-1_7

Laboratory test results indicated that the neutrophilic granulocyte count, neutrophilic granulocyte percentage, lymphocyte percentage, and C-reactive protein were elevated. The patient came from Hubei Province, China to visit his local relatives. He was tested positive for nucleic acid of the SARS-CoV-2 on the day of admission.

Imaging Features

Initial chest CT showed the existence of multiple patchy consolidation opacities in two lungs with visible ground-glass shadows found around the lesions, which mainly distributed around subpleural locations and bronchovascular bundles. Thickened blood vessel shadows can be found in the lesions. Air bronchogram could be seen in some lesions (Fig. 7.1).

By following up chest CT (2 days after the first CT examination), we could find the dynamic changes of multiple patchy lesions in bilateral lungs. The area of GGOs in the upper lung field was enlarged, and the density of lesions in the lower lung field was increased (red frame) (Fig. 7.2).

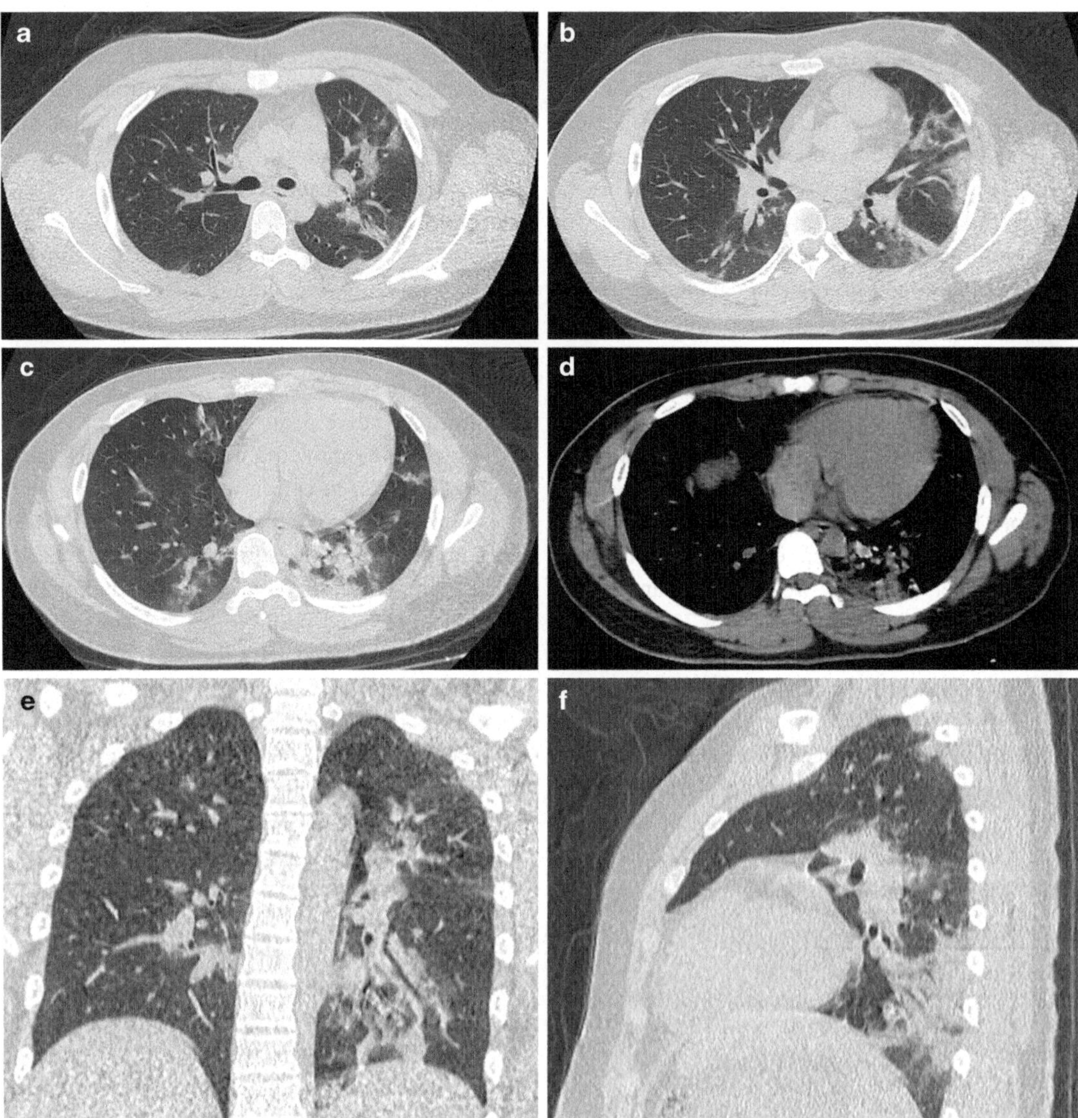

Fig. 7.1 Initial chest CT (**a**–**d**), reconstructed coronal (**e**) and sagittal (**f**) images of the patient

Follow-up chest CT (4 days after the first CT examination) showed that the density of all lesions became lighter and the range was narrowed (Fig. 7.3).

Follow-up chest CT (8 days after the first CT examination) showed that the focus was almost completely absorbed, and only slight ground-glass shadow remained (Fig. 7.4).

Comments: The CT manifestations of this child patient were typical, but the dynamic changes were rapid and the recovery was fast.

Case 2

Medical History and Clinical Manifestation

A 14-year-old girl was admitted in the hospital for 5 days with fever (highest body temperature: 39 °C), fatigue, and cough. Her parents all had a fever one after another on one night. Laboratory test results indicated that blood routine examination and blood biochemical examination were normal. The parents of the patient were permanent residents of Wuhan, China. They drove back home from Wuhan 4 days prior to symptom onset. She was tested negative for nucleic acid of the

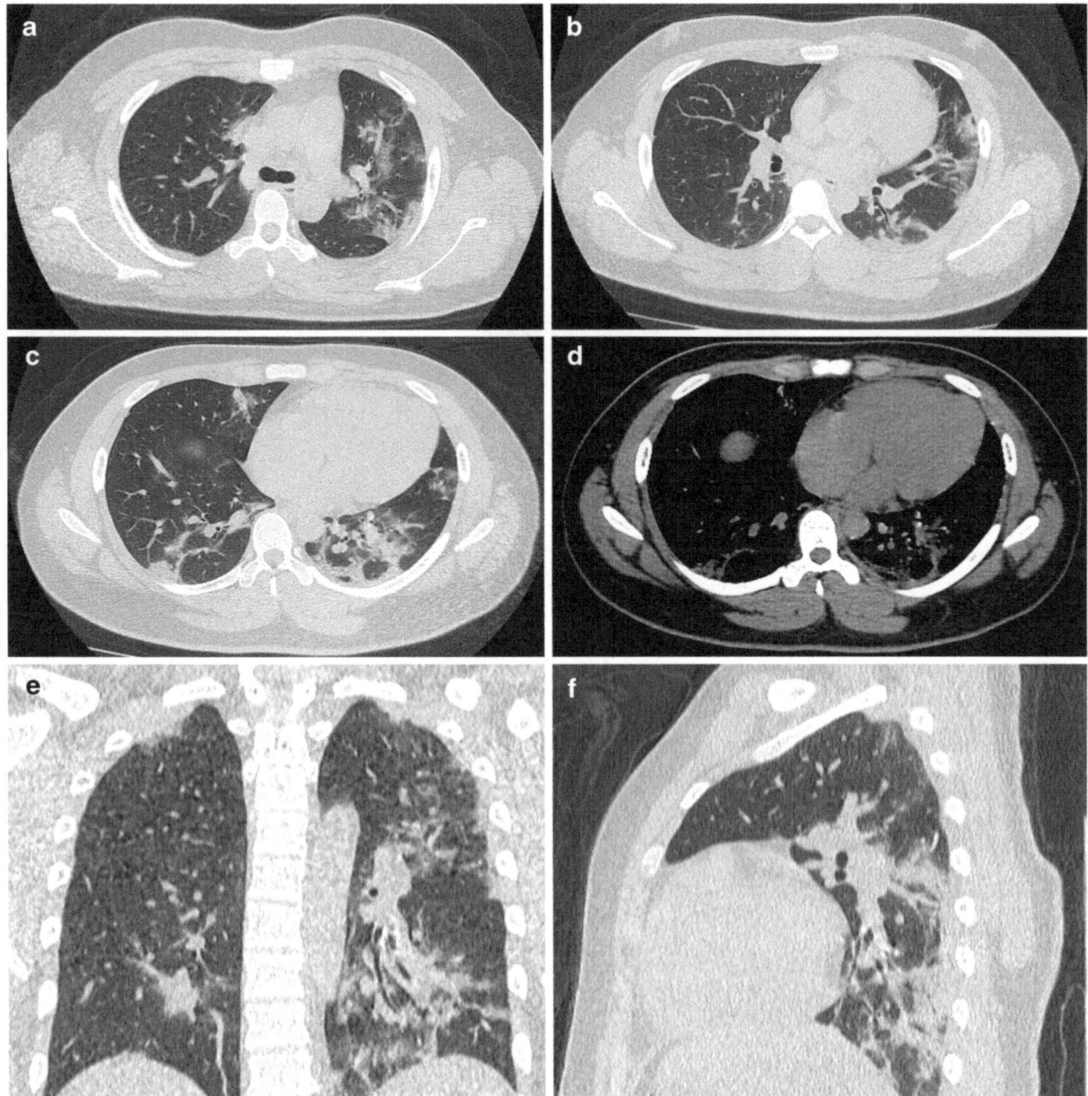

Fig. 7.2 Follow-up axial chest CT (**a**–**d**), reconstructed coronal (**e**) and sagittal (**f**) images 2 days after initial scan

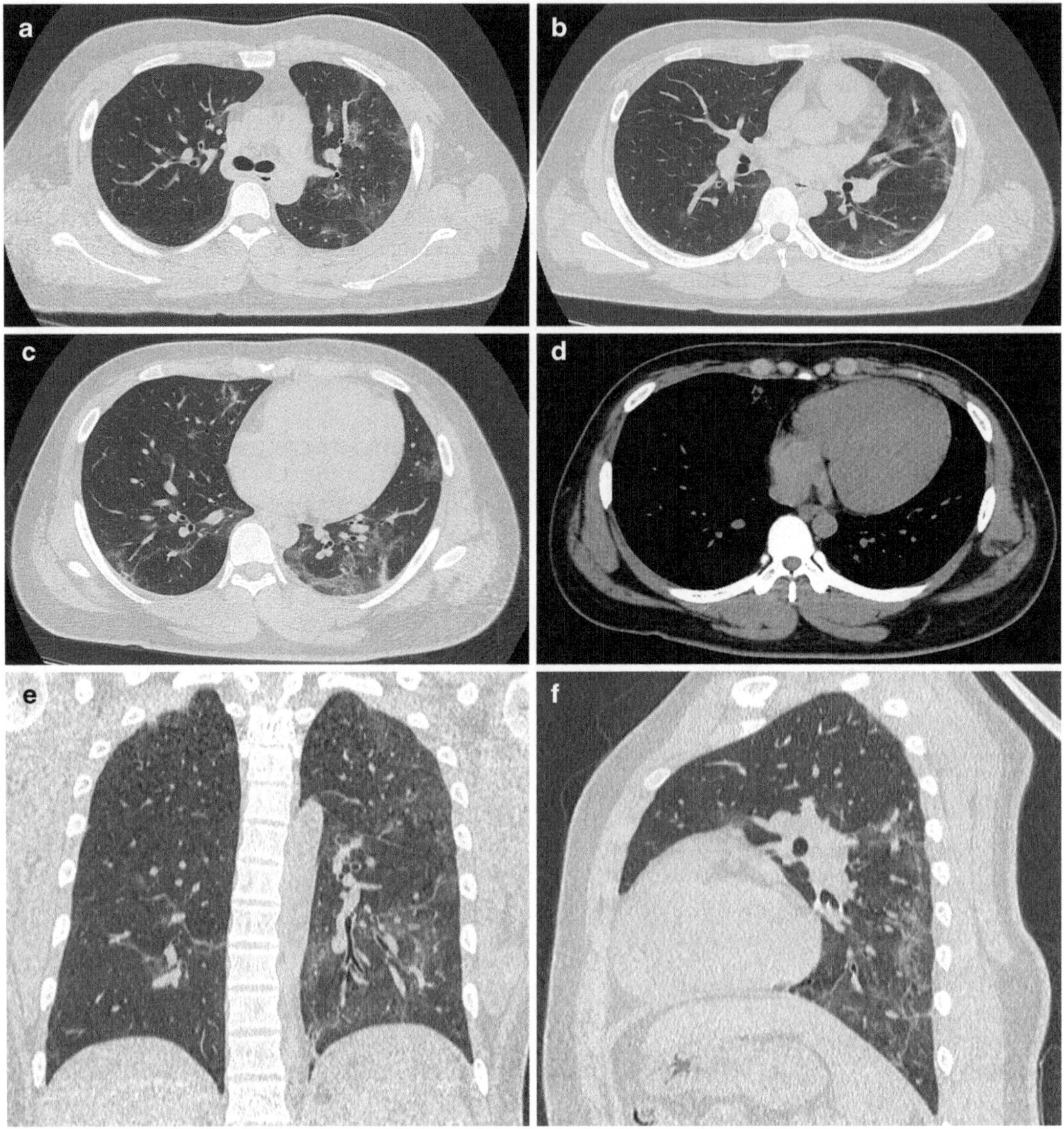

Fig. 7.3 Follow-up axial chest CT (**a**–**d**), reconstructed coronal (**e**) and sagittal (**f**) images 4 days after initial scan

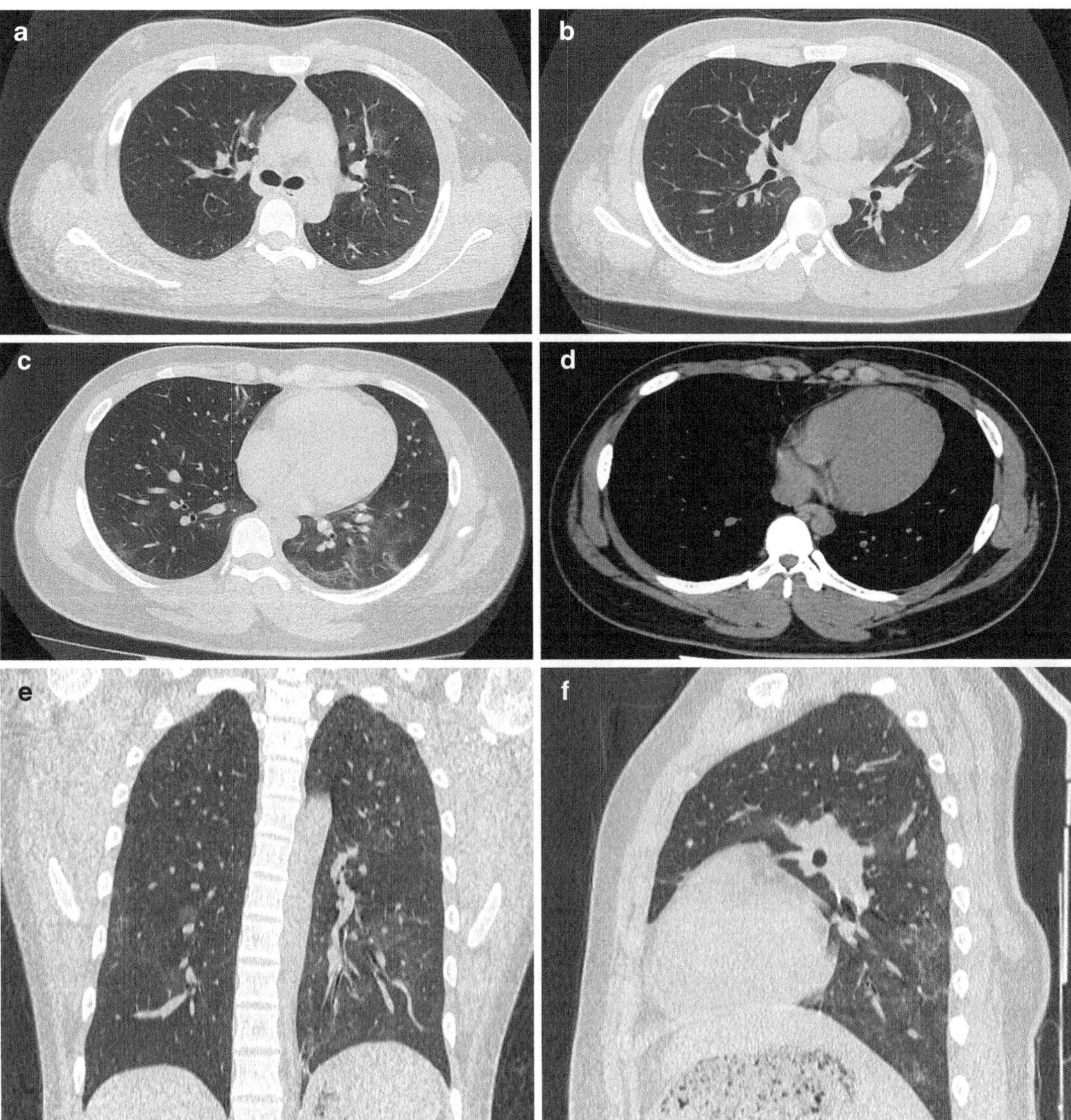

Fig. 7.4 Follow-up axial chest CT (**a–d**), reconstructed coronal (**e**) and sagittal (**f**) images 8 days after initial scan

SARS-CoV-2 on the day of admission, then 2 days later, the test turned to be positive.

Imaging Features

Chest CT showed patchy shadows with grid-like structure in the subpleural areas of the posterior basal segments of the lower lobes of the two lungs. Small nodular GGO was found in the upper lobe of the right lung (Fig. 7.5).

Follow-up chest CT (3 days after Initial CT examination) showed that the density of the

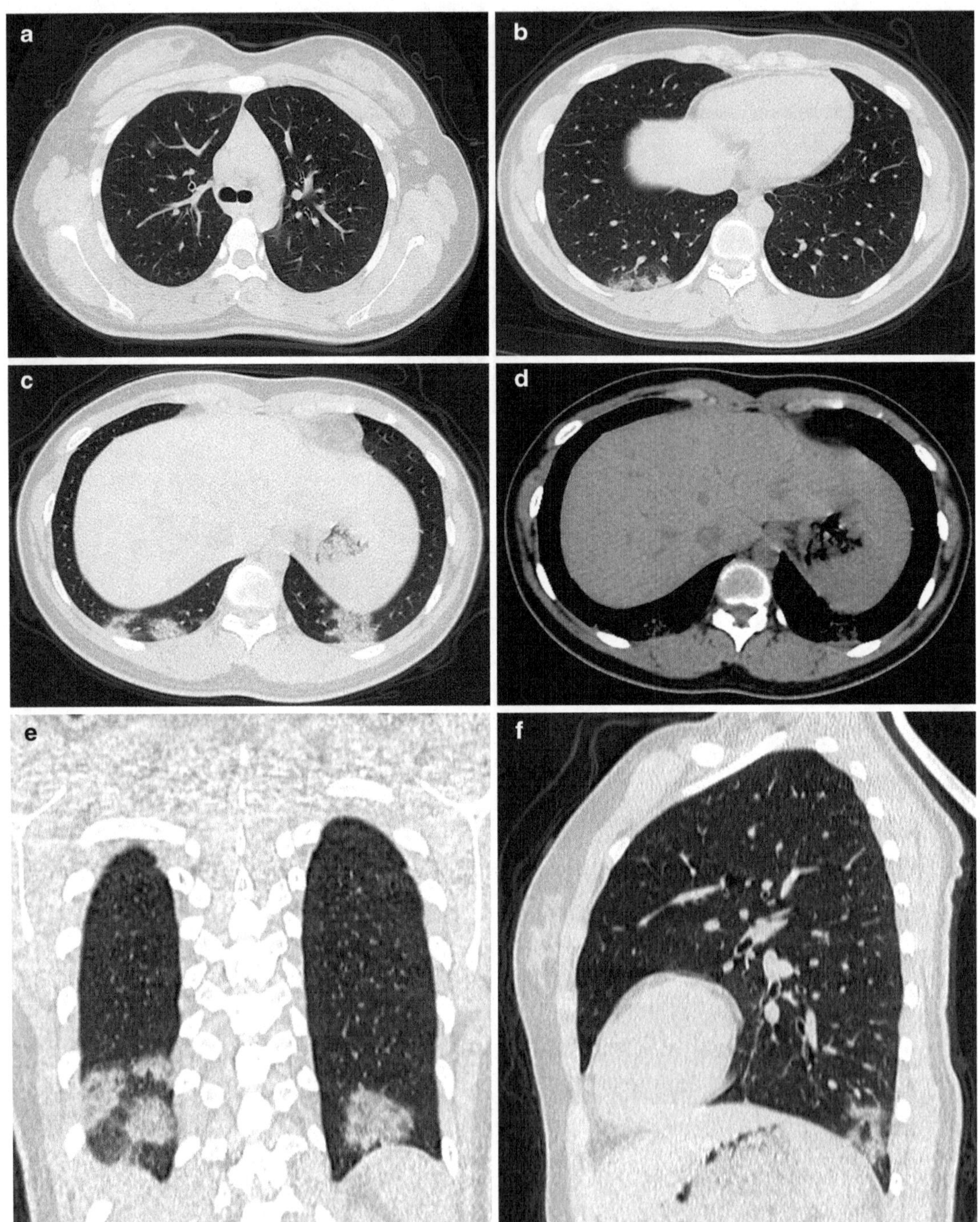

Fig. 7.5 Initial chest CT (**a**–**d**), reconstructed coronal (**e**) and sagittal (**f**) images of the patient

lesions fades out a bit compared with the earlier image (Fig. 7.6).

Follow-up chest CT (6 days after Initial CT examination) showed a reduction in the scope of the lesions and the density of the lesions decreased (Fig. 7.7).

Follow-up chest CT (10 days after initial CT examination) showed lesions of both lungs were further absorbed (Fig. 7.8).

Comments: The child patient had a definite history of aggregation in an infected family. She was tested negative first and then positive in the

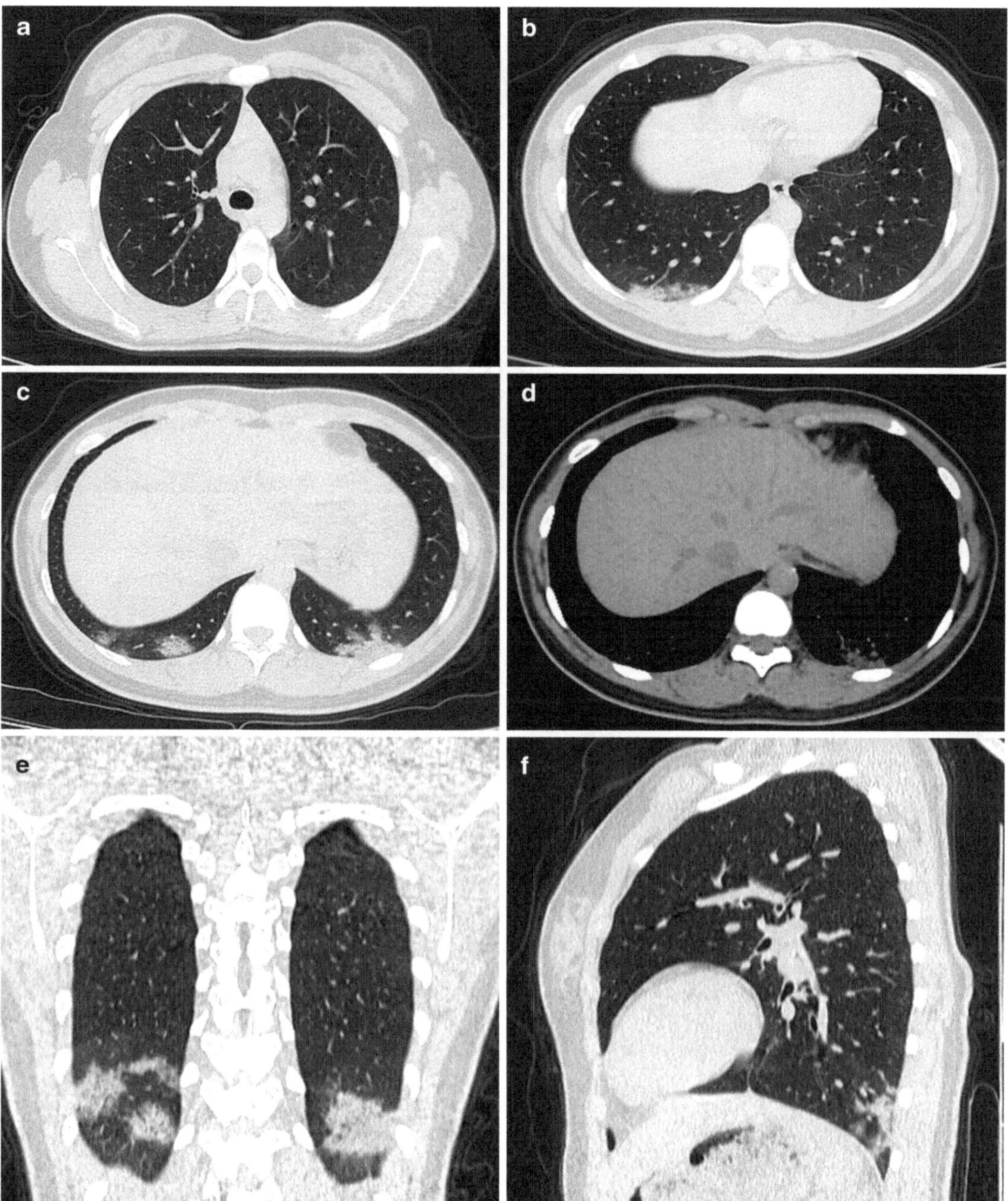

Fig. 7.6 Follow-up axial chest CT (**a**–**d**), reconstructed coronal (**e**) and sagittal (**f**) images 3 days after initial scan

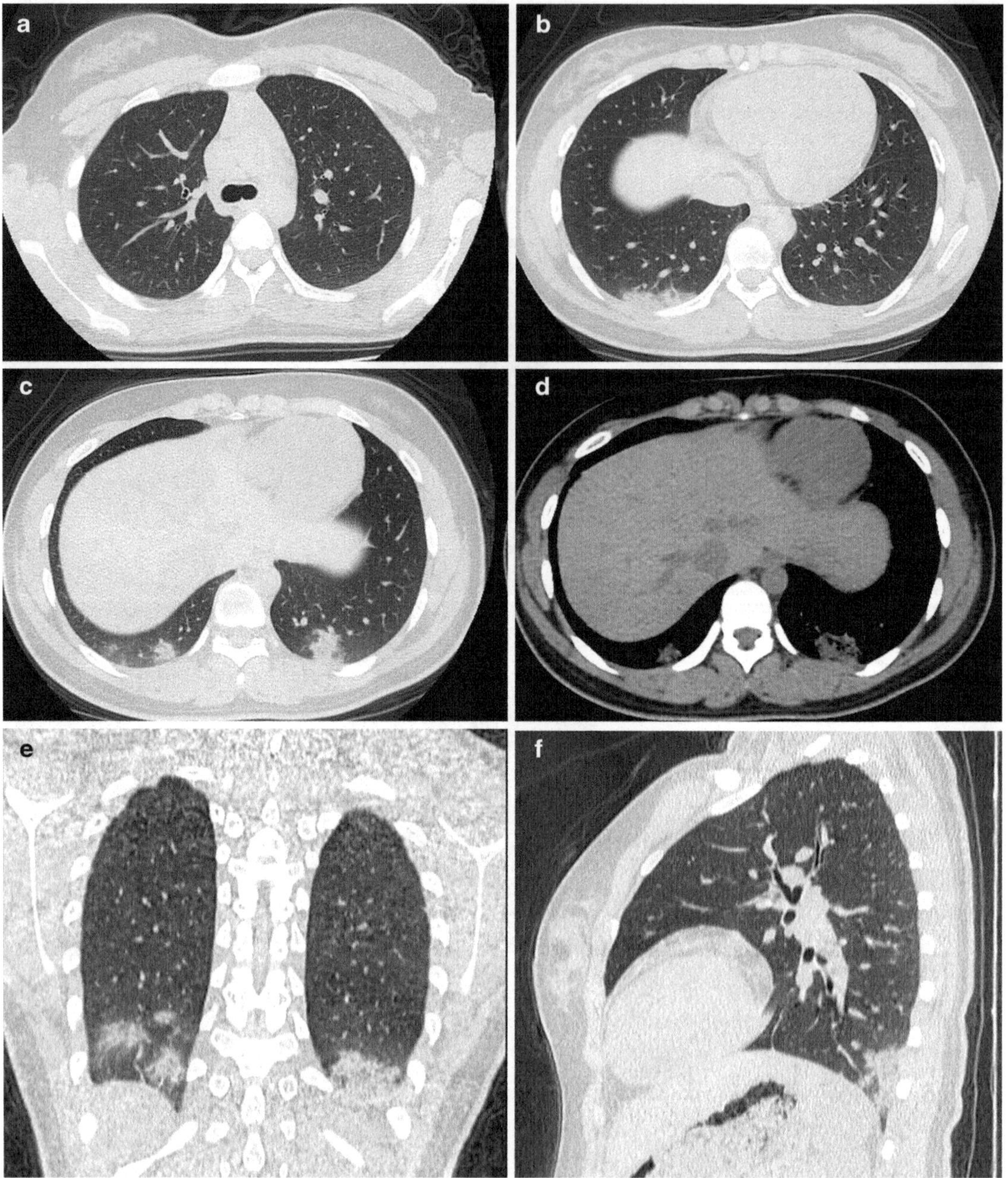

Fig. 7.7 Follow-up axial chest CT (**a**–**d**), reconstructed coronal (**e**) and sagittal (**f**) images 6 days after initial scan

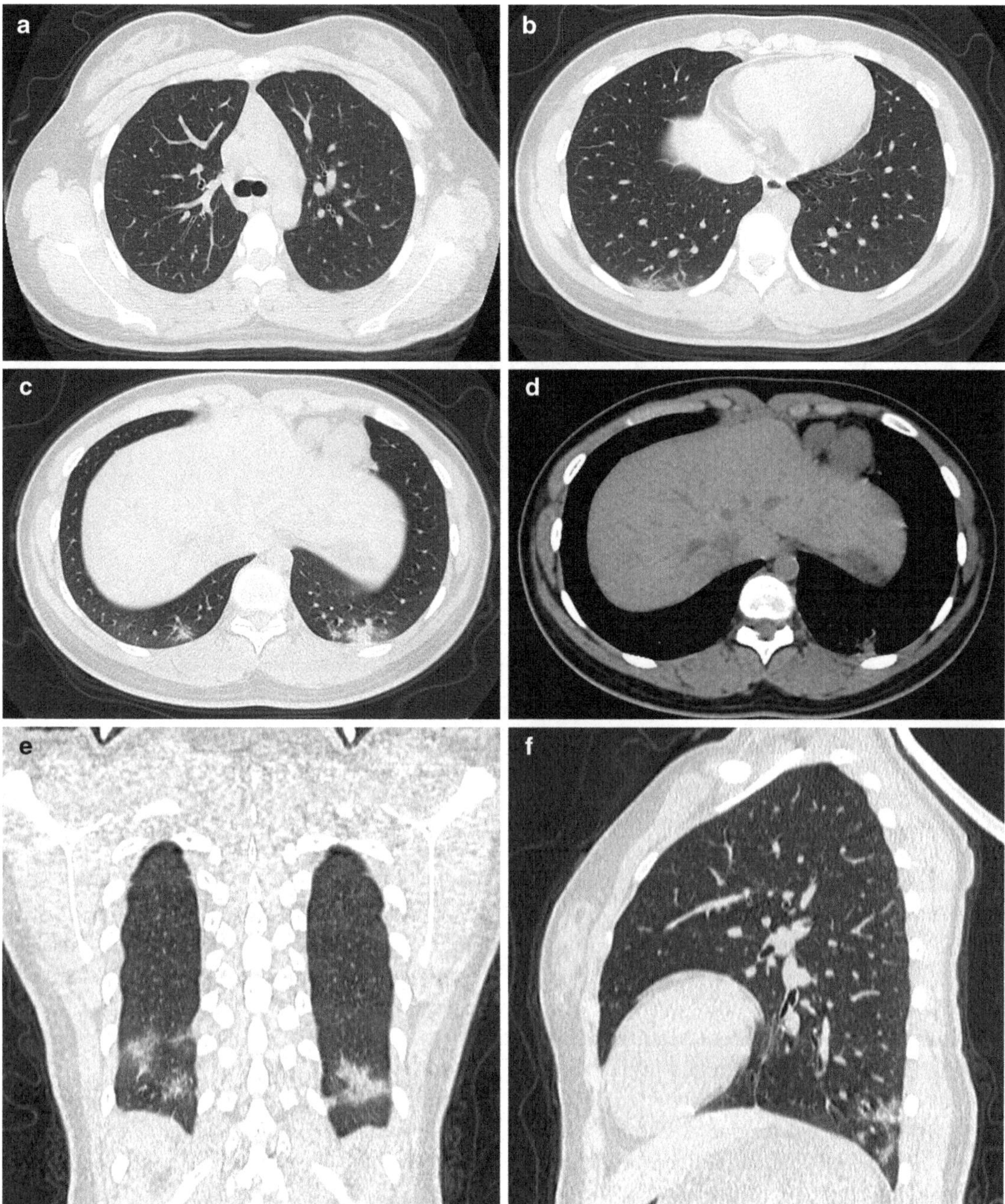

Fig. 7.8 Follow-up axial chest CT (**a**–**d**), reconstructed coronal (**e**) and sagittal (**f**) images 10 days after initial scan

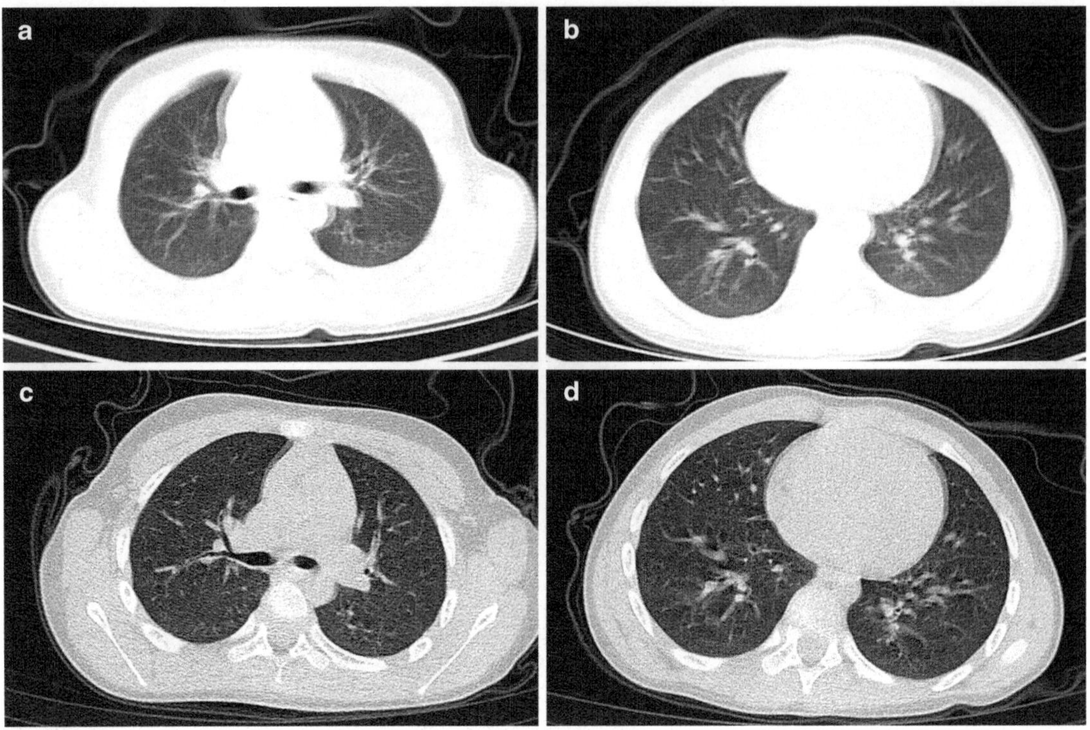

Fig. 7.9 Initial CT images and follow-up CT images 12 days after initial scan

second test for nucleic acid of the SARS-CoV-2. In the initial chest CT, patchy shadows were found in subpleural areas of the posterior basal segments of the lower lobes of the two lungs. Grid-like changes could be found in the lesions, so it is a relatively typical case of COVID-19 infection.

Case 3
Medical History and Clinical Manifestation

A 5-year-old girl was admitted in the hospital for 3 days with fever (highest body temperature: 38.3 °C), fatigue, and dizziness. Laboratory test results (at the outpatient department) indicated a normal white blood cell count of 6.9 × 10^9/L and a low level of lymphocytes (14.0%). The C-reactive protein is less than 0.499 mg/L and procalcitonin (PCT) is less than 0.25 ng/mL. The parents and grandmother of the child patient were all confirmed cases of COVID-19. She was tested positive for nucleic acid of the SARS-CoV-2 on the day of admission.

Imaging Features

Both initial chest CT (Fig. 7.9a, b) and 12 days later follow-up chest CT (Fig. 7.9c, d) showed normal finding.

Comments: Although the child was positive in nuclear acid of the SARS-CoV-2 test and had some systemic symptoms of infection, there was no evidence of COVID-19.

Case 4
Medical History and Clinical Manifestation

A 15-year-old girl was admitted in the hospital for 3 days with fever (highest body temperature: 38.1 °C) and chills. Laboratory test results indicated a low level of white blood cell count of 3.8 × 10^9/L. lymphocytes (32.9%) and lymphocytes (61.0%) are normal. CRP is 1.7 mg/L and PCT is less than 0.25 ng/mL. The parents and grandmother of the child patient are all confirmed cases of COVID-19. She was tested positive for nucleic acid of the SARS-CoV-2 on the day of admission.

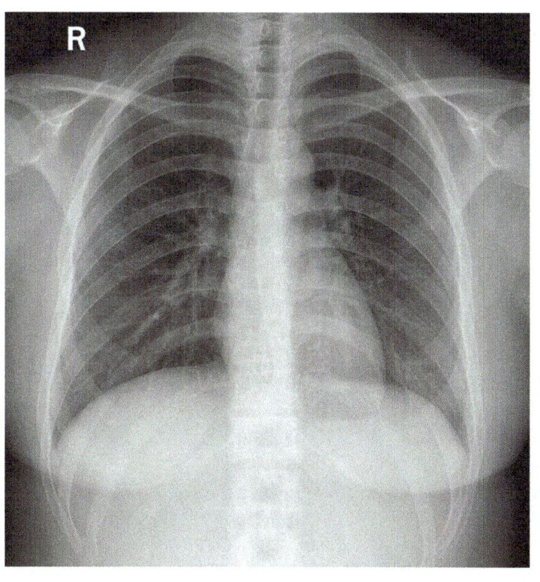

Fig. 7.10 Initial chest radiography image

Imaging Features

Initial chest radiography showed no abnormality (Fig. 7.10).

Chest CT showed small GGO (**c**, red arrow) in the subpleural area of the upper lobe of the left lung (Fig. 7.11).

Follow-up chest CT (4 days after Initial CT examination) showed CT indicates that the small ground-glass opacities had been absorbed (**c**, red arrow) (Fig. 7.12).

Comments: Children's COVID-19 has mild clinical symptoms and atypical imaging manifestations.

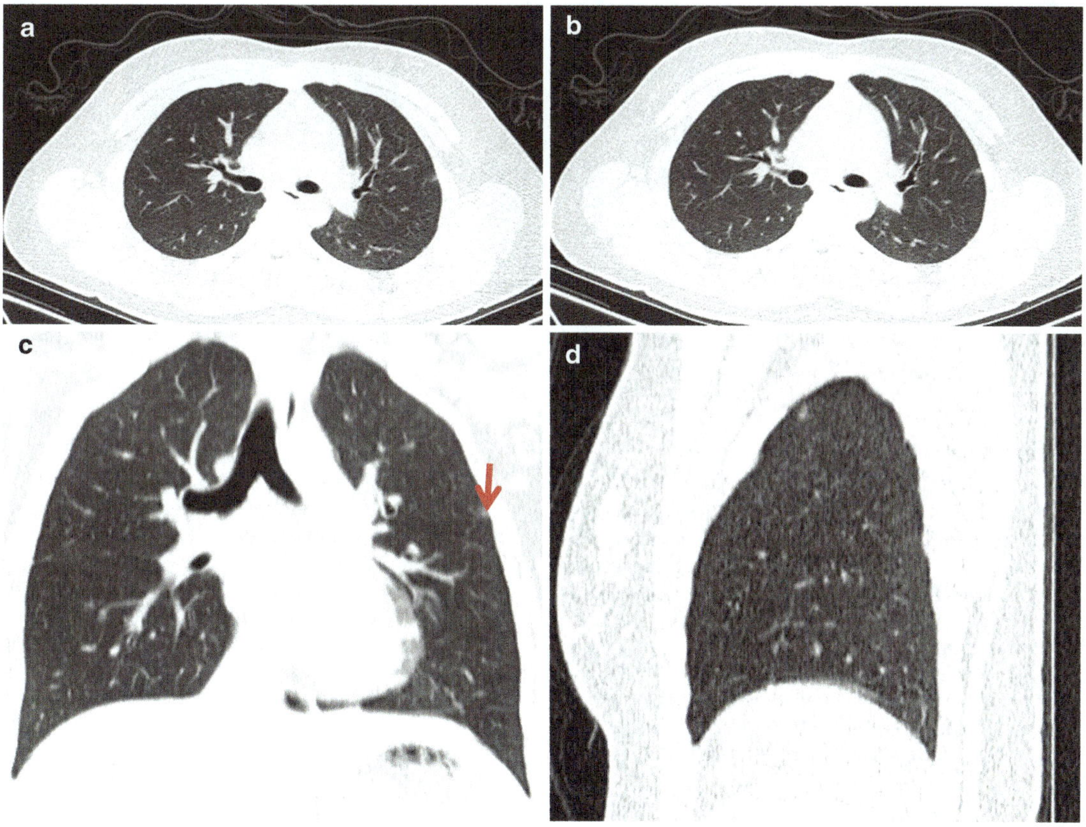

Fig. 7.11 Initial chest CT (**a**, **b**), reconstructed coronal (**c**) and sagittal (**d**) images of the patient

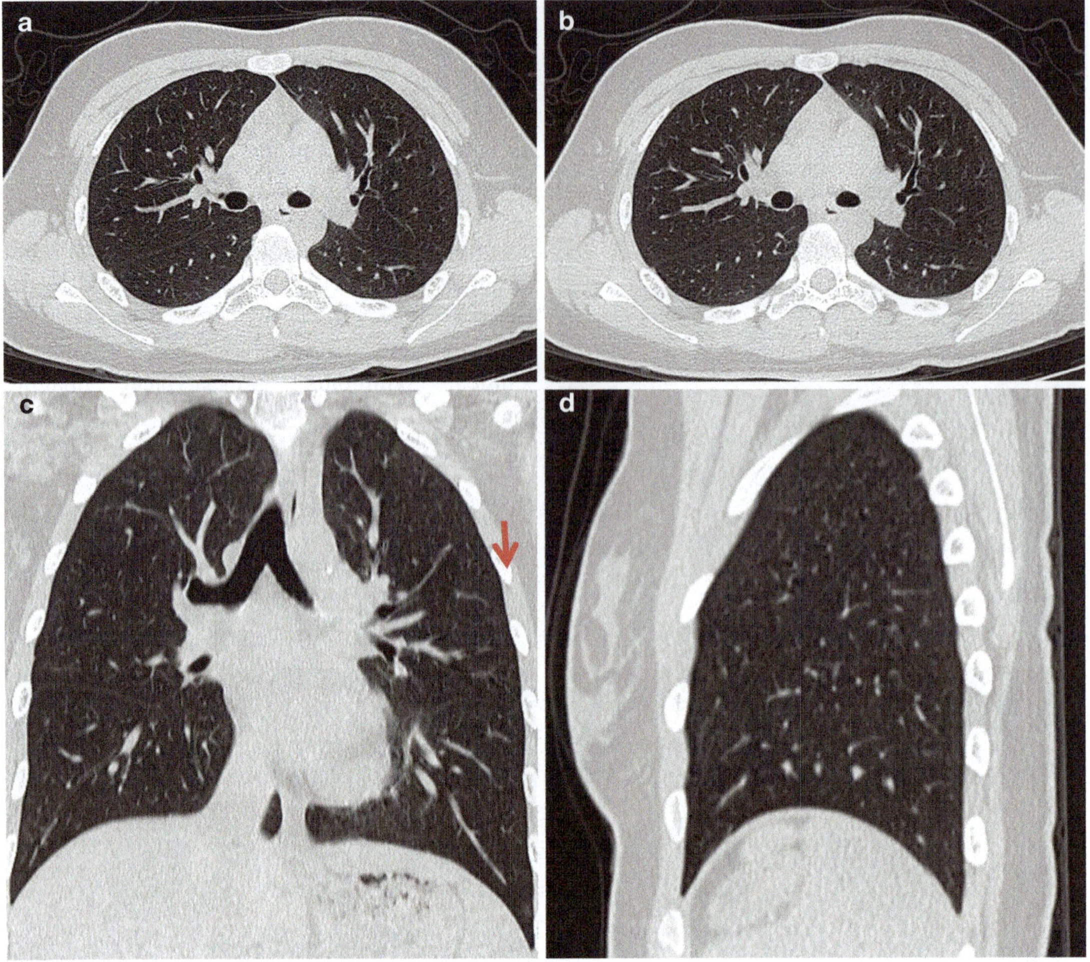

Fig. 7.12 Follow-up axial chest CT (**a**, **b**), reconstructed coronal (**c**) and sagittal (**d**) images 4 days after initial scan

References

1. The Society of Pediatrics, Chinese Medical Association, the Editorial Board, Chinese Journal of Pediatrics. Recommendations for the diagnosis, prevention and control of the 2019 novel coronavirus infection in children (first interim edition). Chin J Pediatr. 2020;58(3):169–74.
2. Long XR, Zhu J, Zhao RQ, et al. Epidemiology and clinical features of highly pathogenic human coronavirus infection in children. Zhonghua er ke za zhi = Chinese Journal of Pediatrics. 2020;58(5):E014.
3. Fang F, Luo X. Facing the pandemic of 2019 novel coronavirus infections: the pediatric perspectives. Chin J Pediatr. 2020;58(2):81–5.
4. Wei M, Yuan J, Liu Y, et al. Novel coronavirus infection in hospitalized infants under 1 year of age in China. JAMA. 2020;323(13):1313–4.
5. Chan JF, Yuan S, Kok KH, et al. A familial cluster of pneumonia associated with the 2019 novel coronavirus indicating person-to-person transmission: a study of a family cluster. Lancet. 2020;395(10223):514–23.
6. Dong Y, Mo X, Hu Y, et al. Epidemiology of COVID-19 among children in China. Pediatrics. 2020:145(6).

8 Differentiating COVID-19 CT Manifestations from Other Types of Pneumonia

Pingding Kuang, Xiaocheng Zhang, Bin Lin, Hui Mao, and Minming Zhang

In the early days of COVID-19 pandemic in China, the RT-PCR test reported only 59–71% positive cases among those tested [1, 2]. However, among the patients admitted to the hospitals, there were some patients with typical imaging features of viral pneumonia, but negative test results for RT-PCR tests, even after being tested for several times. The accuracy of nucleic acid RT-PCR test depends on the time of infection, samples and sampling method, quality of the reagent, and different interpretation standards. Thus, RT-PCR tests are often conducted repeatedly if patients have the typical imaging features of pneumonia. The CT manifestations of COVID-19 are mainly that of interstitial pneumonia. The distribution, shape, density, and bronchial and vascular manifestations of lesions are typical, but not specific to COVID-19. Therefore, it is necessary to make differential diagnosis to distinguish COVID-19 from other lung infections with similar CT manifestations, such as pneumonia caused by influenza A (H1N1), avian influenza (H7N9), influenza B, adenovirus, cytomegalovirus, and others (Table 8.1). The application of thoracic CT to COVID-19 diagnosis and imaging assessment of pulmonary infection and damage can add value to clinical management of patients with COVID-19.

P. Kuang · X. Zhang · B. Lin · M. Zhang (✉)
Department of Radiology, the Second Affiliated Hospital, Zhejiang University School of Medicine, Hangzhou, China
e-mail: zjdxlinbin@zju.edu.cn; zhangminming@zju.edu.cn

H. Mao
Department of Radiology and Imaging Sciences, Emory University School of Medicine, Atlanta, GA, USA
e-mail: hmao@emory.edu

8.1 Influenza A (H1N1) Virus Pneumonia

Typical Imaging Features

Distribution: Distributed in one or multiple lobes, mainly in the dorsal subpleural area of bilateral lower lobes, and usually symmetrical. The extent of the lesions increases and merges from periphery to the center if progressed. The lesions in severe patients are bilateral and have diffuse distribution.

Shape: Present as nodule, patch, or flake, the typical lesions are wedge-shaped or fan-shaped along the bronchovascular bundle or parallel to the pleura.

Density: Early lesions show ground glass density, smooth air bronchogram, thickened interlobular septum, and reticulation. Nodular or patchy consolidations can be seen in the progressed lesions or patients with bacterial infection [3–5].

M. Zhang, B. Lin (eds.), *Diagnostic Imaging of Novel Coronavirus Pneumonia*,
https://doi.org/10.1007/978-981-15-5992-1_8

Table 8.1 The CT manifestations of COVID-19 and other types of pneumonia

Types of pneumonia	Distribution	Shape	GGO	Consolidation	Paving stone sign	Thickened vessels	Pleural effusion
COVID-19	Subpleural of multiple lobes	Nodular, patchy, or large patchy	+++	+	+++	+++	–
H1N1 pneumonia	Subpleural of inferior lobes, symmetrically	Patchy or large patchy	++	++	++	++	++
H7N9 pneumonia	One or more whole lobes	Large patchy	++	++	++	++	+
Influenza B pneumonia	Random in multiple lobes	Nodular or patchy	+	+++	+	+	–
Adenovirus pneumonia	Random in one or more lobes	Nodular or large patchy	+	+++	+	–	+
Cytomegalovirus pneumonia	Diffuse in both lungs	Large patchy	–	++++	+	+	–
Cryptogenic organizing pneumonia	Subpleural or bronchovascular bundle	Nodular, patchy or large patchy	+	+++	+	+	–
Pneumocystis pneumonia	Diffuse in two lungs except subpleural	Nodular or large patchy	+++	+	+	+	+
Cryptococcal pneumonia	Random in one or more lobes	Nodular, patchy, or large patchy	+	+++	–	+	–
Lobar pneumonia	One whole lobe	Large patchy	–	++++	–	+	++
Acute allergic alveolitis	Diffuse in lobular center of both lungs	Nodular	+++	+	–	–	–
Aspiration pneumonia	Diffuse in the dorsal part of both lungs	Nodular or patchy	+++	+	–	–	+
Alveolar pulmonary edema	Around the two lung hilus symmetrically	Large patchy like the butterfly wing	+	+++	+	+	+++
Alveolar hemorrhage	The dorsal part of one or more lobes	Patchy	+++	+	–	–	–

Differentiate COVID-19 from Influenza A (H1N1) Virus Pneumonia

Influenza A (H1N1) virus pneumonia often occurs in elderly and middle-aged people with underlying diseases. In chest CT, both COVID-19 and H1N1 virus pneumonia present the features of ground glass opacities (GGOs) in bilateral dorsolateral subpleural or along the bronchovascular bundle. The thickened interlobular septal, the reticular pattern, and ground glass opacities with halo sign are common in the lesions. The features of the lesions in COVID-19 are mostly ground glass opacities, with thickened blood vessels, while the lesions in H1N1 virus pneumonia are mostly patchy consolidation, thickened blood vessels are rare. The pathology reports indicate the numbers of leukocytes and neutrophils in patients with H1N1 virus pneumonia are higher than that in patients with COVID-19. The lesions in COVID-19 absorb more slowly than those of H1N1 virus pneumonia and fibrosis lesions appear in the early stage. Pleural effusion in COVID-19 is rare, while it is common in H1N1virus pneumonia [6, 7].

Case 1 (Ordinary Type)

Medical History and Clinical Manifestations

A 50-year-old male was admitted in the hospital with an aversion to cold, fever (highest body temperature: 39.6 °C), cough, expectoration, and chest distress for 1 week. Laboratory test results indicated a normal white blood cell count of 6.5×10^9/L and decreased lymphocytes (16.5%). There were elevated blood levels for neutrophils (77.8%) and C-reactive protein (84.6 mg/L). The H1N1 nucleic acid was positive.

Imaging Features

Initial CT image showed multiple subpleural patches in bilateral lungs and was mostly on the back. The lesions were mainly ground glass opacities and the reticular pattern (thick red arrows) was visible. Few effusions were seen in the left chest cavity (Fig. 8.1).

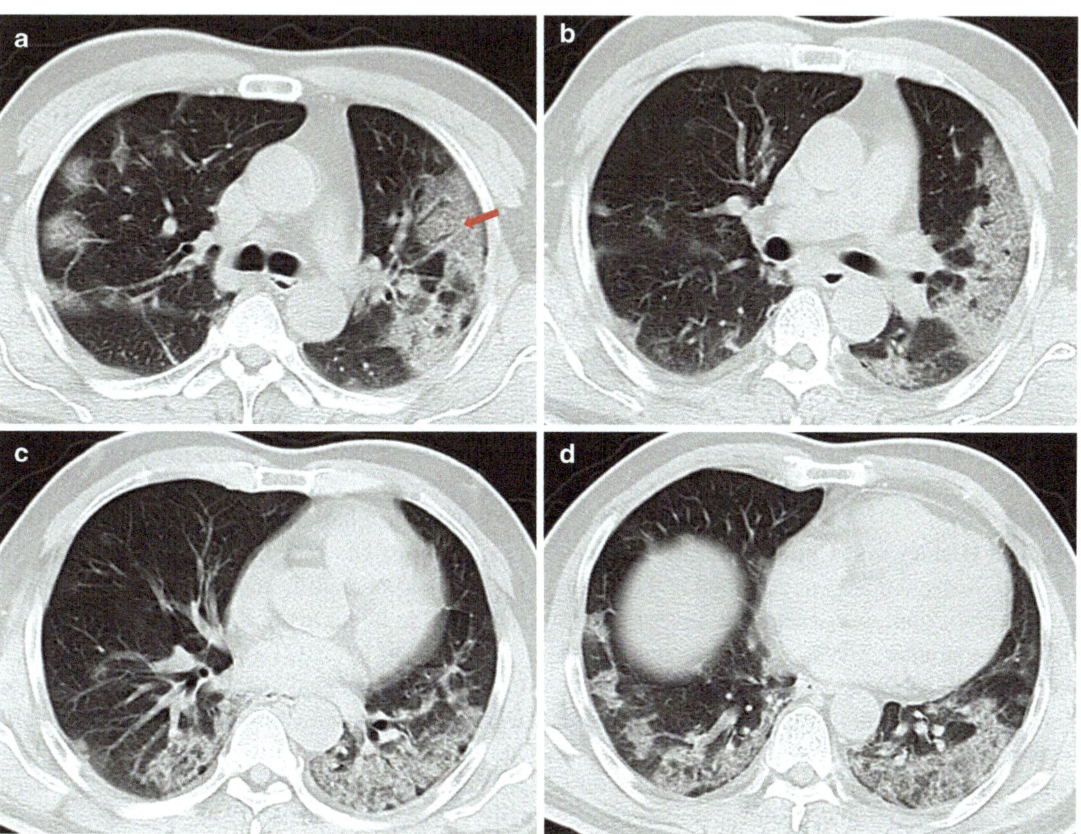

Fig. 8.1 Initial CT image

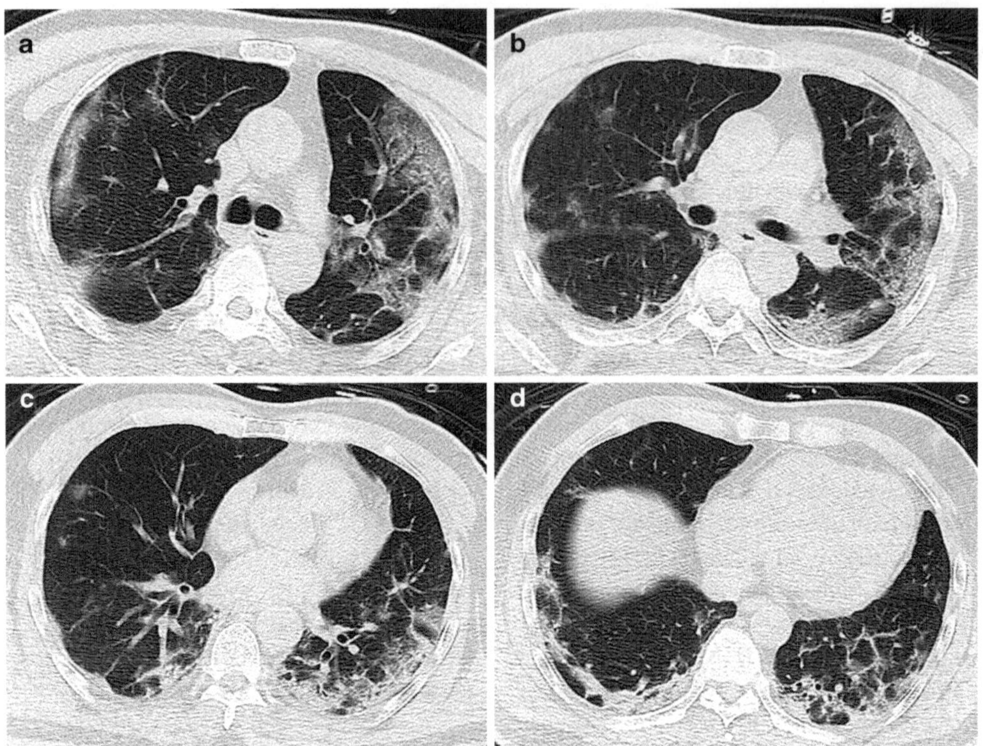

Fig. 8.2 Follow-up CT images 17 days after initial scan

Follow-up chest CT (7 days after Initial CT examination) showed the lesions were absorbed obviously after treatment (Fig. 8.2).

Comments: This case is an ordinary type of H1N1virus pneumonia, whose lung CT manifestations are similar to COVID-19. The relatively symmetrical lesions in both lungs accompanied with a few pleural effusions may indicate the diagnosis of H1N1 virus pneumonia.

Case 2

Medical History and Clinical Manifestations

A 30-year-old male was admitted in the hospital with the symptoms of repeated fever (highest body temperature: 39.0 °C) and cough for 1 week, chest distress and breathlessness for 1 day. Laboratory test results indicated decreased blood levels for white blood cell count (2.7×10^9/L), lymphocytes (11.0%), and arterial oxygen saturation (70–80%). There were elevated blood levels for neutrophils (87.5%) and C-reactive protein (129.5 mg/L). The H1N1 nucleic acid was positive.

Imaging Features

Initial CT image showed diffuse consolidations with a few ground glass opacities and mainly distributed in subpleural area or along the bronchovascular bundle. There were a small amount of pleural effusions in the bilateral chest cavity (Fig. 8.3).

Follow-up chest CT (1 day after Initial CT examination) showed the extent and density of the lesions increased, and the pleural effusions increased in bilateral chest cavity (Fig. 8.4).

Follow-up chest CT (5 days after Initial CT examination) showed the lesions in both lungs were resolved significantly and a small amount of fibrosis lesions (red arrow) were seen. The pleural effusions on both sides were reduced (Fig. 8.5).

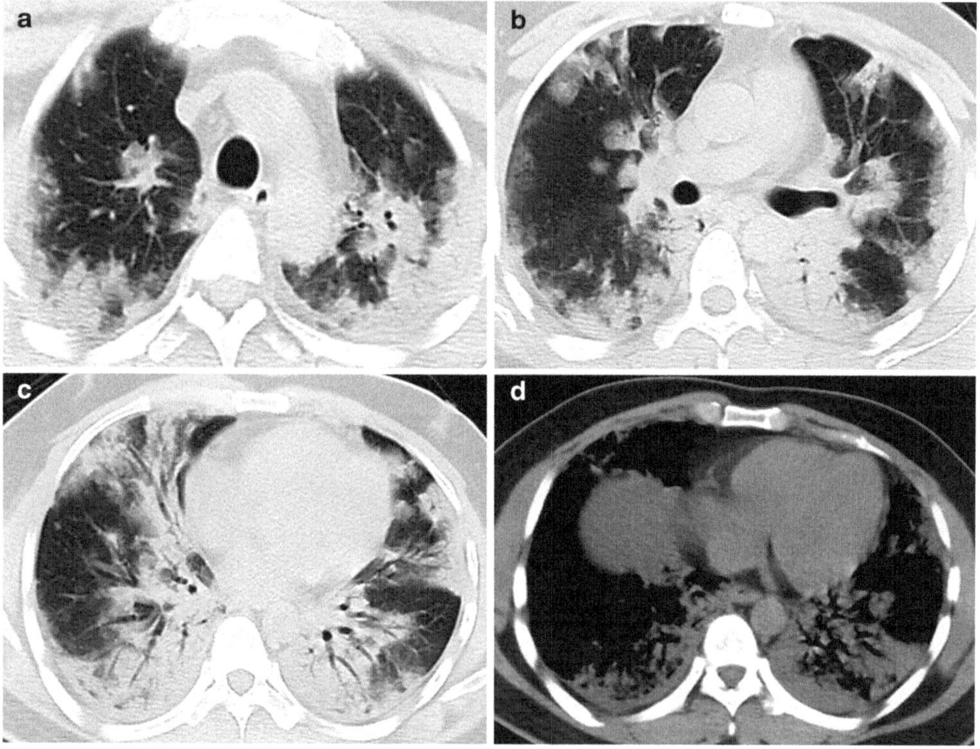

Fig. 8.3 Initial CT image

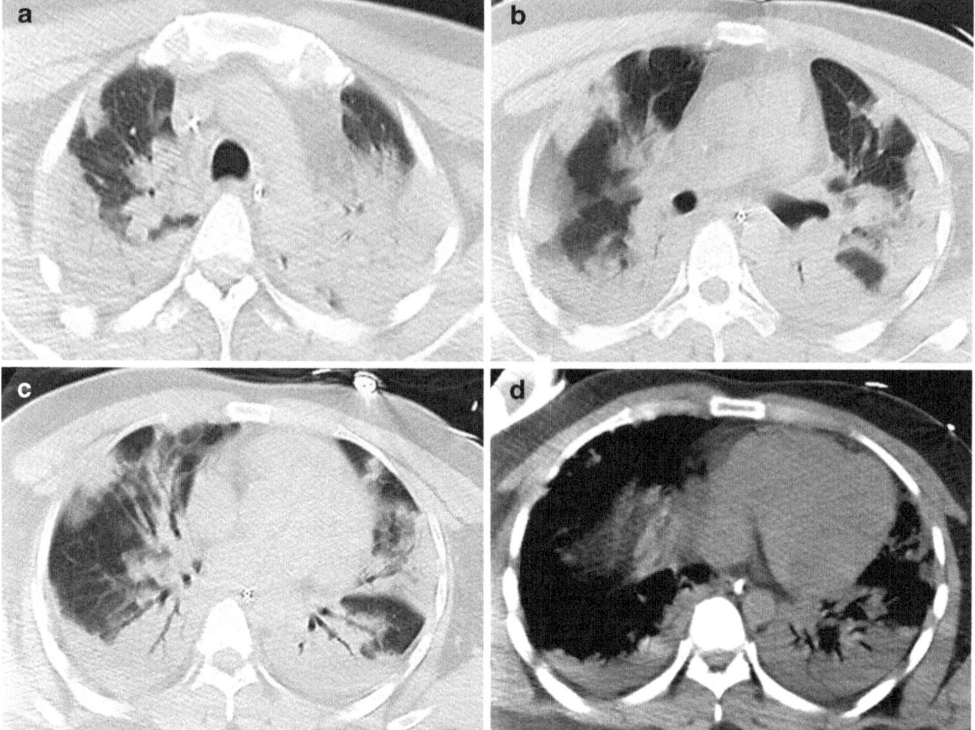

Fig. 8.4 Follow-up CT images 1 day after initial CT scan

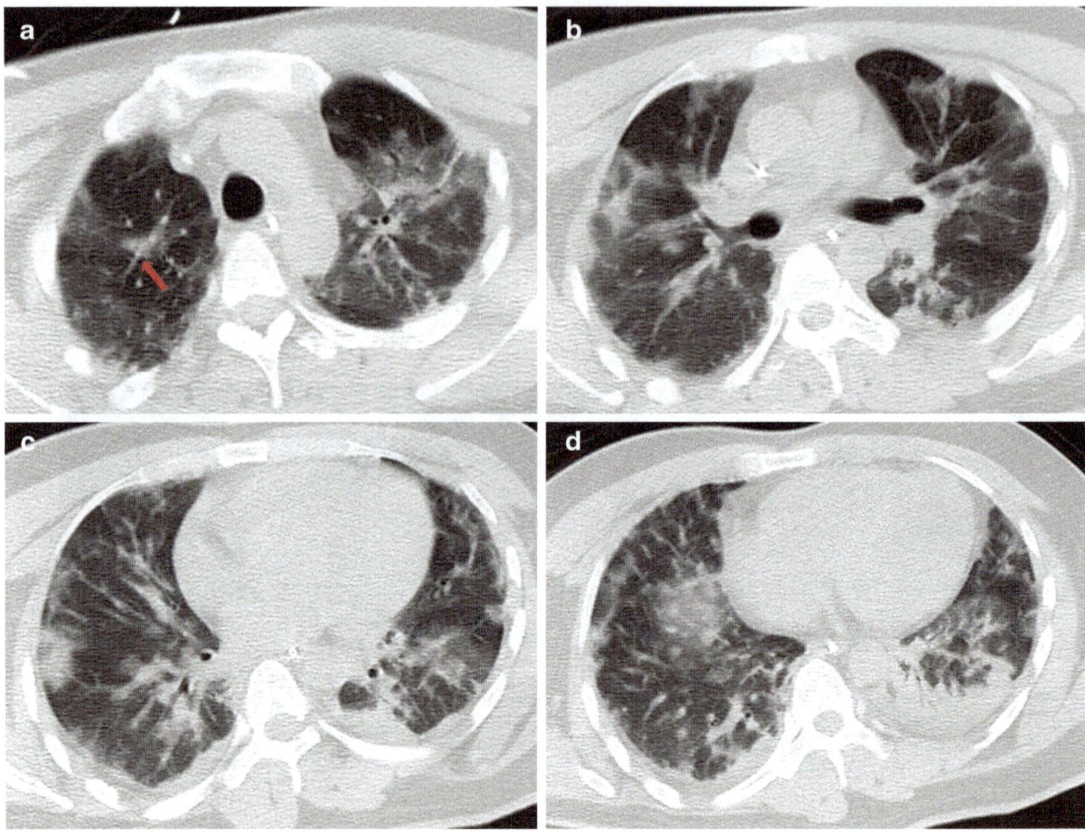

Fig. 8.5 Follow-up CT images 5 days after initial CT scan

Comments: This case is a severe type of H1N1 virus pneumonia. The lesions mainly located in the dorsal part of the lung lobes symmetrically and show higher density; pleural effusions are common in H1N1 virus pneumonia. These manifestations can help differentiating from COVID-19.

8.2 Avian Influenza (H7N9) Virus Pneumonia

Typical Imaging Features

Distribution: Often involve multiple lobes and there is no obvious distribution trend of prone lobes or segments. It is not limited in subpleural area or along the bronchovascular bundle and is often asymmetrically distributed.

Shape: Present as nodule, patch, or flake, mostly involve the whole lung lobe.

Density: Early stage lesions show ground glass density, reticular thickened interlobular septum, and most of the lesions progress rapidly with consolidations [8, 9].

Differentiate COVID-19 from Avian Influenza (H7N9) Virus Pneumonia

The CT imaging features of Avian influenza (H7N9) virus pneumonia are bilateral asymmetric patchy ground glass opacities with some consolidations. The lesions mostly involve the whole lung lobes. However, the lesions in COVID-19 mainly symmetrical distribute in subpleural area or along the bronchovascular bundle. It is helpful for differential diagnosis when combined with recent contact history of living birds.

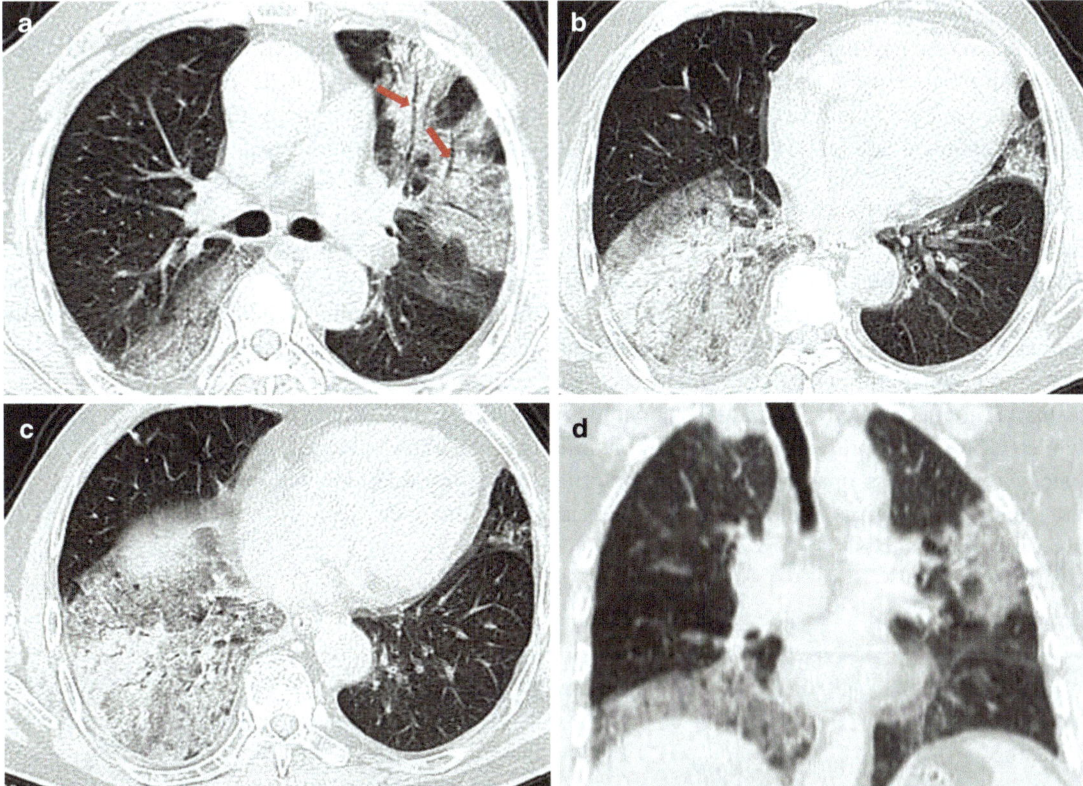

Fig. 8.6 Initial CT image

Case 3
Medical History and Clinical Manifestations

A 65-year-old male was admitted in the hospital with fever (highest body temperature: 39.5 °C), cough, expectoration, abdominal pain, and hypodynamia for 6 days. He had been to vegetable market to buy living birds prior to symptom onset. Laboratory test results indicated normal lymphocytes (20.0%) and decreased white blood cell count of 3.0×10^9/L. There were elevated blood levels for neutrophils (73.3%) and C-reactive protein (195.1 mg/L). The H7N9 nucleic acid was positive and he was transferred to a designated hospital for treatment.

Imaging Features

Initial CT image showed asymmetric large ground glass opacities with a few consolidations in left upper lobe and right lower lobe. The air bronchogram (thick red arrows) in left lung and no effusions were seen in the bilateral chest cavity (Fig. 8.6).

Comments: The CT manifestations of H7N9 virus pneumonia are mainly asymmetric large ground glass opacities in the two lungs with some consolidations and the lesions mostly involve the whole lung lobes. Combined with the recent contact history of living birds, it is helpful for differential diagnosis.

8.3 Influenza B Virus Pneumonia

Typical Imaging Features

Distribution: One or multiple lobes are involved and there is no obvious distribution trend of prone lobes or segments. It is not limited in subpleural area or along the bronchovascular bundle.

Shape: Present as nodule, patch, or flake, and most lesions are nodular and patchy.

Density: Most of the lesions are solid density with fuzzy margin, and reticular thickened interlobular septum is rare [10, 11].

Differentiate COVID-19 from Influenza B Virus Pneumonia

Most cases of influenza B virus pneumonia are sporadic or local epidemic. The CT features in influenza B virus pneumonia are mainly bilateral scattered nodular and patchy consolidations, and a small amount of patchy ground glass opacities, while COVID-19 presents as the subpleural patchy ground glass opacities, which is helpful for identification. Virus nucleic acid detection is necessary for diagnosis.

Case 4

Medical History and Clinical Manifestations

A 25-year-old female came to the hospital with fever (highest body temperature: 38.2 °C), cough, expectoration, and pharyngodynia for 2 days. Laboratory test results indicated a normal white blood cell count of 3.0×10^9/L and decreased lymphocytes (16.3%). There were elevated blood levels for neutrophils (73.9%) and C-reactive protein (128.9 mg/L). The nucleic acid of influenza B was positive.

Imaging Features

Initial CT image showed bilateral scattered ground glass opacities, multiple patchy, and nodular consolidations with obscurity boundary. No effusions were seen in the bilateral chest cavity (Fig. 8.7).

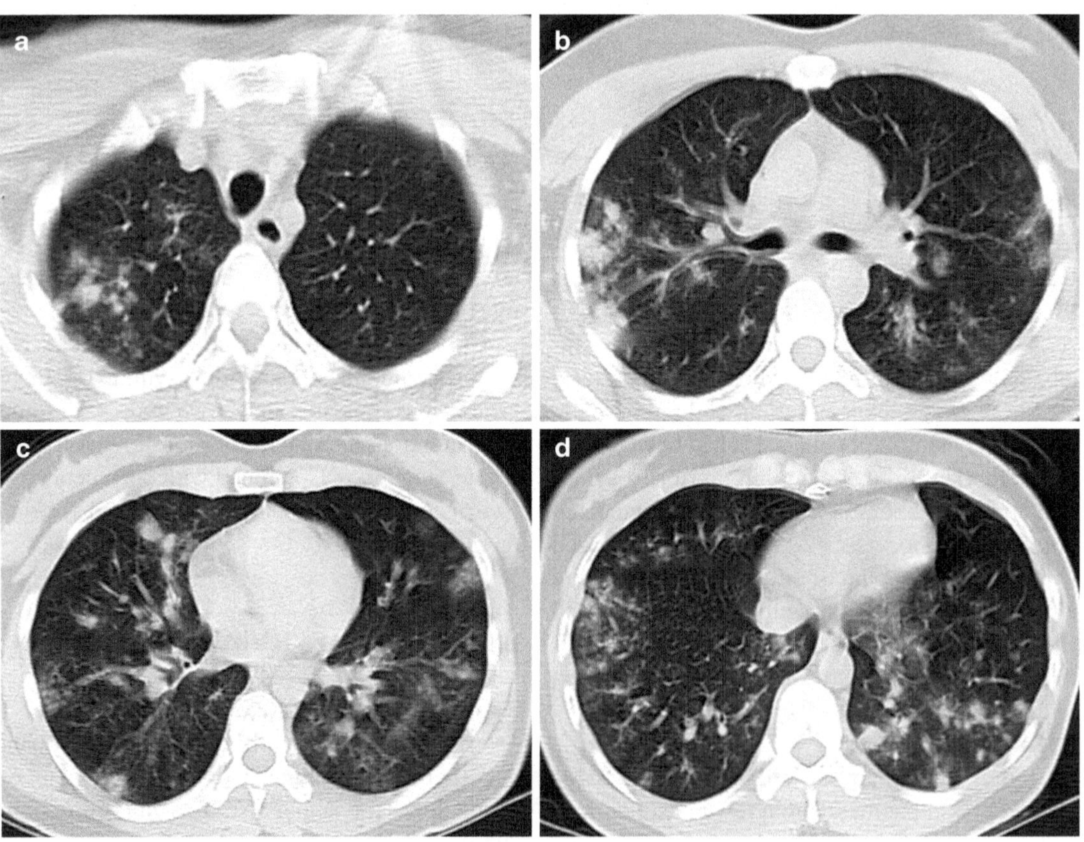

Fig. 8.7 Initial CT image

Comments: The CT manifestations of influenza B virus pneumonia show bilateral scattered multiple nodular ground glass opacities and patchy consolidations.

8.4 Adenovirus Pneumonia

Typical Imaging Features

Distribution: Often involve one or multiple lobes. There is no obvious distribution trend of prone lobes or segments.

Shape: The lesions are nodular, patchy, or flaky at the same time.

Density: Round and patchy consolidations accompanied by mottled ground glass opacities with fuzzy edges, and reticular thickened interlobular septa is rare [12].

Differentiate COVID-19 from Adenovirus Pneumonia

Adenovirus pneumonia often infects children and is rarely seen in adults. The CT imaging features are mainly flakey consolidations, accompanied by nodular patches with fuzzy edges. There is no obvious tendency of subpleural distribution and may be accompanied by a small amount of pleural effusions. These manifestations are helpful for the differentiation from COVID-19.

Case 5

Medical History and Clinical Manifestations

A 29-year-old male was admitted in the hospital with fever (highest body temperature: 39.4 °C), cough, and expectoration for 1 week. Laboratory test results indicated normal 67.5% neutrophils, 25.8% lymphocytes, and a decreased white blood cell count of 3.5×10^9/L. There were elevated blood levels for erythrocyte sedimentation rate (21 mm/h) and C-reactive protein (53.2 mg/L). The H1N1 and H7N9 nucleic acids were negative. Adenovirus was found in bronchoalveolar lavage fluid.

Imaging Features

Initial CT image showed consolidations in left upper lobe with air bronchogram (thick red arrow), multiple patches and nodules with halo sign (red arrow) in left upper and lower lobes, and there was a small amount of pleural effusion in the left chest cavity (Fig. 8.8).

Comments: The lesions of adenovirus pneumonia are mainly consolidations without obvious tendency of subpleural distribution.

8.5 Cytomegalovirus Pneumonia

Typical Imaging Features

Distribution: The lesions are bilateral and diffuse distribution and mainly in upper lobes. It is not limited in subpleural area or along the bronchovascular bundle.

Shape: Bilaterally symmetrical flaky lesions are common.

Density: Ground glass opacities with reticular thickened interlobular septum are common, and consolidations and pleural effusions are rare [13].

Differentiate COVID-19 from Cytomegalovirus Pneumonia

The CT manifestations of cytomegalovirus (CMV) pneumonia show diffuse and symmetrical patchy ground glass opacities with few consolidations in both lungs. The lesions are mainly in the upper lobes and the middle zones are affected obviously, but subpleural lesions are rare. Theses manifestations are different from COVID-19, which can be used for differentiation.

Case 6

Medical History and Clinical Manifestations

A 47-year-old male with a history of kidney transplantation 5 months ago was admitted in the hospital with fever (highest body temperature: 38.7 °C), cough, and shortness of breath for 3 days. Laboratory test results indicated a normal white blood cell count of 5.3×10^9/L and decreased lymphocytes (17.2%). There were elevated blood levels for neutrophils (75.3%), C-reactive protein (23.1 mg/L), and CMV-IgG (>500 μmol/L). The nucleic acids of influenza A/B and H7N9 were negative for three times.

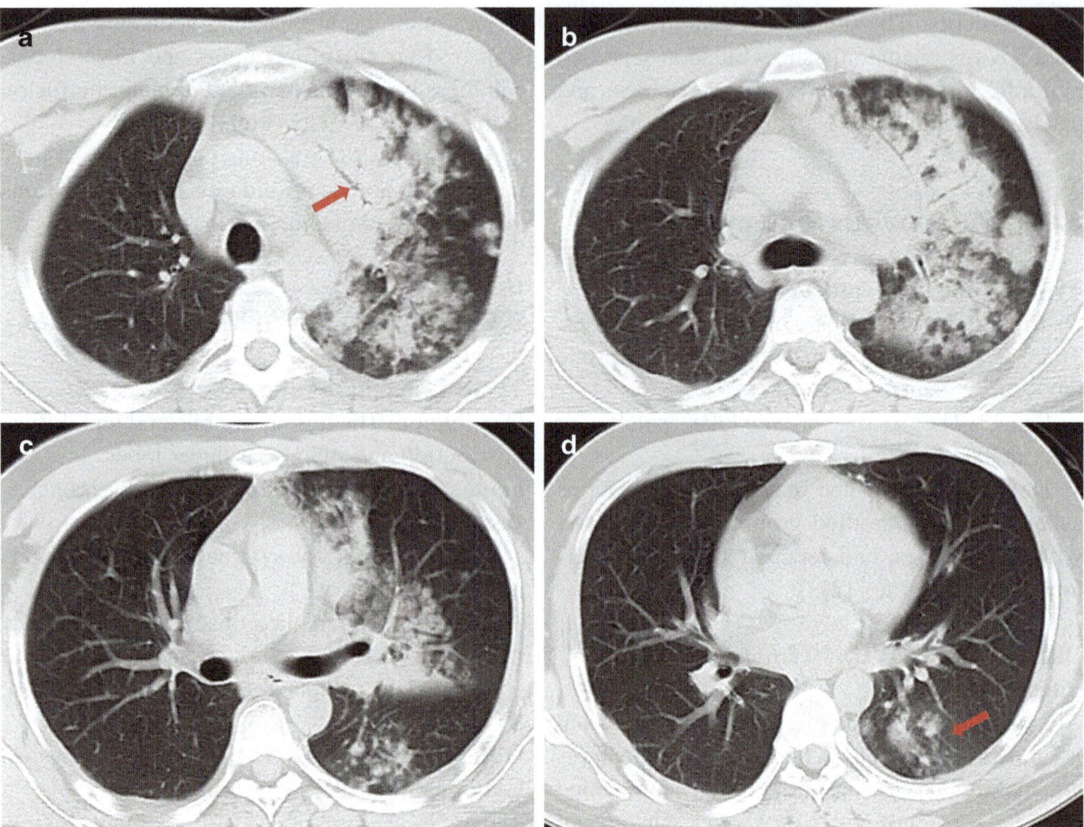

Fig. 8.8 Initial CT image

Imaging Features

Initial CT image showed diffused inhomogeneous patchy ground glass opacities and more lesions in upper lungs, and no pleural effusions were seen (Fig. 8.9).

Comments: The patient has a history of renal transplantation in an immunocompromised state; CT shows bilateral diffuse and flaky ground glass opacities, mainly in upper lobes, which is different from the COVID-19 that often occurs in the subpleural area.

8.6 Cryptogenic Organic Pneumonia

Typical Imaging Features

Distribution: The lesions are confine to one lung lobe or involve multiple lung lobes, and usually in subpleural area or along the bronchovascular bundle. There is no obvious distribution tendency of lung lobes and segments and the lesions are often asymmetrically.

Shape: The lesions are nodular, patchy, or flakey, the typical lesions are wedge-shaped or fan-shaped along the bronchovascular bundle or parallel to the pleura.

Density: Mixed ground glass opacities or consolidations are common and simple ground glass opacities are rare. Smooth air bronchogram is common but reticular pattern is rare [14, 15].

Differentiate COVID-19 from Cryptogenic Organic Pneumonia

Cryptogenic organic pneumonia is an acute or subacute interstitial pneumonia. The shape and distribution are similar to those of COVID-19. It is prone to occur under the pleura or along the bronchovascular bundle. The lesions can be ground glass opacities or consolidations with the

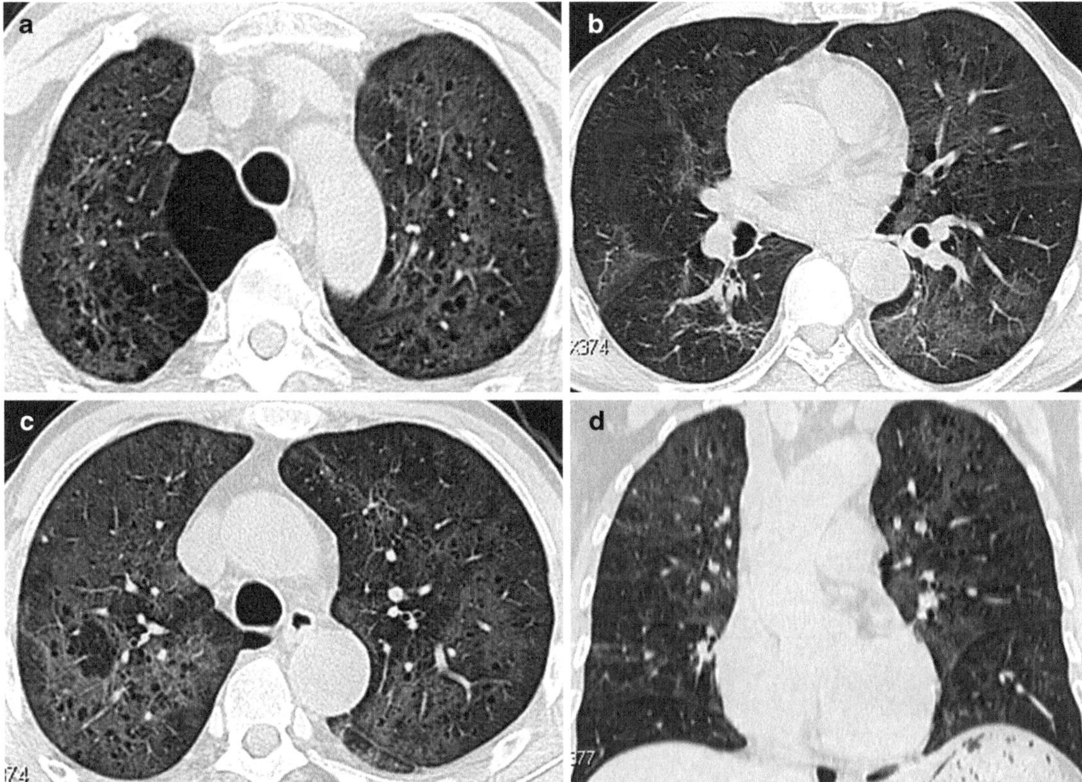

Fig. 8.9 Initial CT image

reverse halo sign, and reticular pattern is rare. COVID-19 is prone to occur in spring and winter. White blood cell count and neutrophils are usually normal or decreased. While cryptogenic organic pneumonia is not seasonal, and white blood cell count and neutrophils were decreased. These differences are helpful for differential diagnosis.

Case 7

Medical History and Clinical Manifestations

A 63-year-old female came to the hospital with fever (highest body temperature: 38.7 °C), cough, and shortness of breath for 2 months. Laboratory test results indicated decreased lymphocytes (10.5%). There were elevated blood levels for white blood cell count of 10.5×10^9/L, neutrophils (83.0%), and C-reactive protein (86.6 mg/L). The nucleic acids of influenza A/B and H7N9 were negative for three times. Lung biopsy guided by CT was performed and pathology reported chronic interstitial pneumonia.

Imaging Features

Initial CT image showed multiple wedge-shaped or strip-like consolidations in right upper lobe and two lower lobes. The lesions were along the bronchovascular bundle and air bronchograms were seen in right upper lobe (red arrow). Ring-shaped nodular consolidations (thick red arrow) were in left lower lobe, and there were micro pleural effusions in the left chest cavity (Fig. 8.10).

Follow-up chest CT (8 days after initial CT examination) showed the lesions increased slightly after anti-inflammatory treatment for 8 days (Fig. 8.11).

Follow-up chest CT (22 days after initial CT examination) showed the lesions were resolved obviously after 2 weeks of treatment with Methylprednisolone (Fig. 8.12).

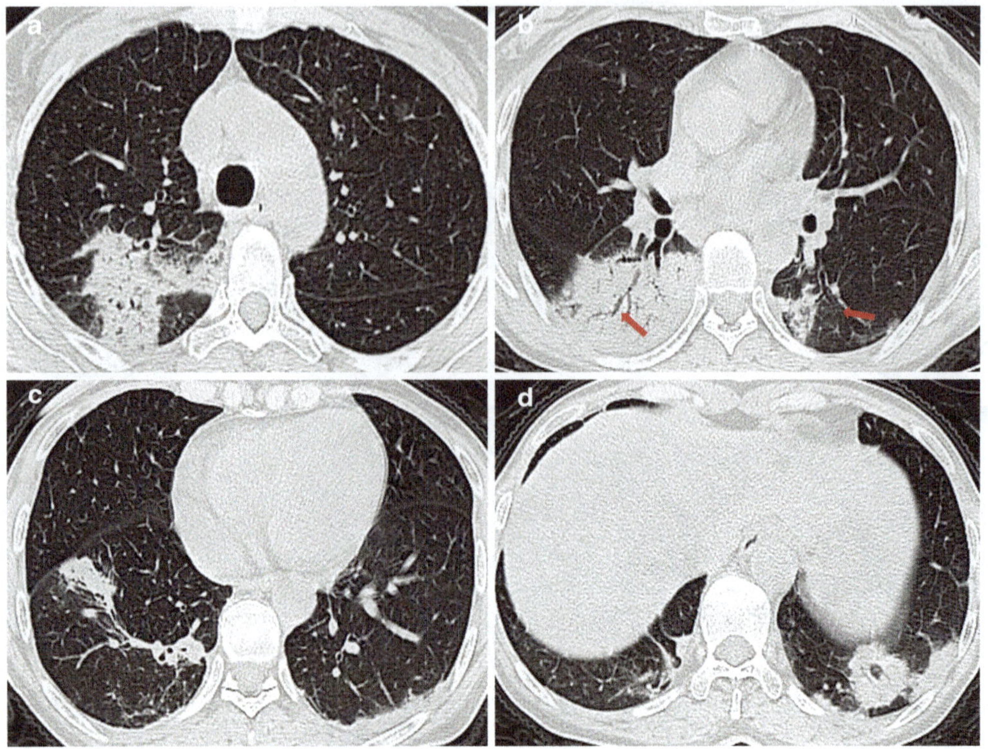

Fig. 8.10 Initial CT image

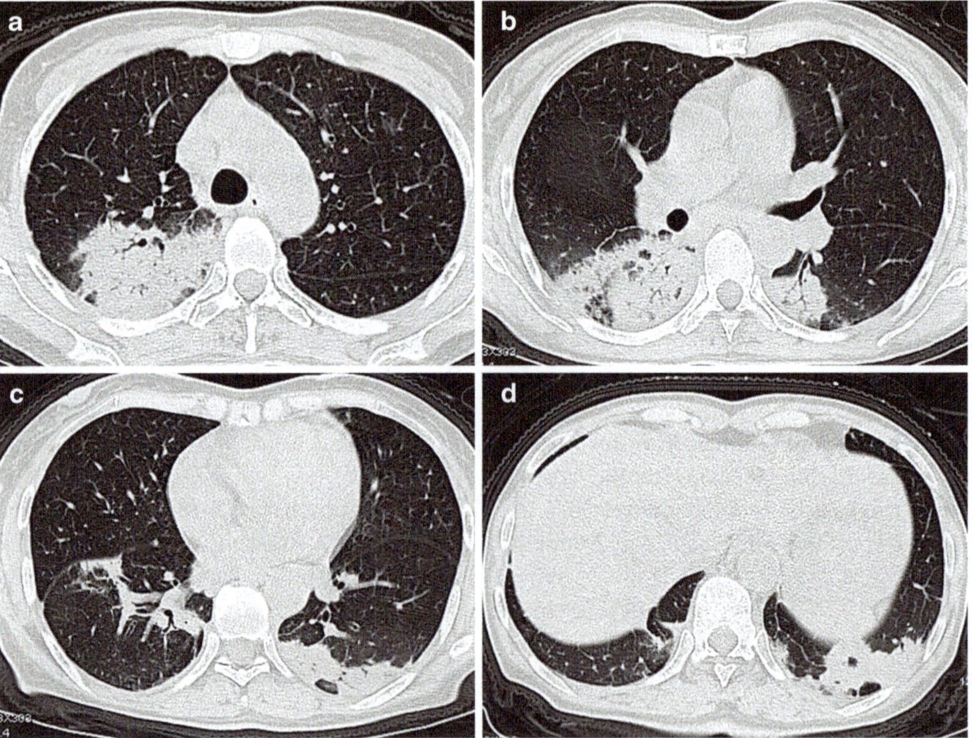

Fig. 8.11 Follow-up CT images 8 days after initial scan

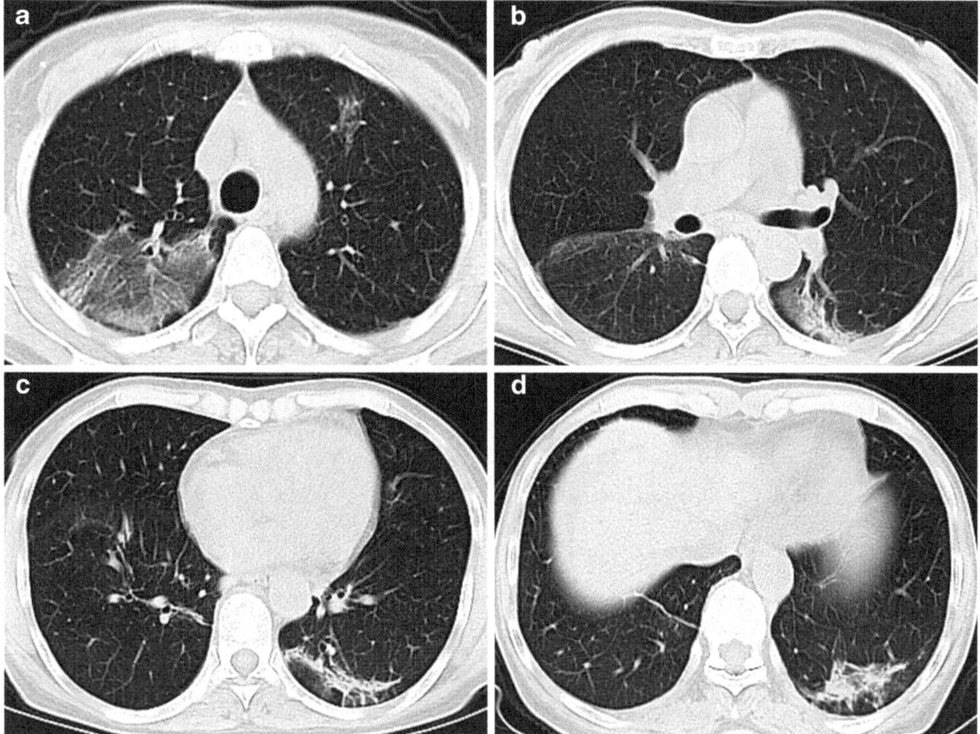

Fig. 8.12 Follow-up CT images 22 days after initial scan

Comments: This patient has elevated blood levels of leukocytes and neutrophils. The lesions are mainly consolidations with micro left pleural effusion, which may be different from COVID-19.

8.7 Pneumocystis Pneumonia

Typical Imaging Features

Distribution: The lesions are symmetrical centered in two lung hilum, rarely involve subpleural, two apex and costophrenic angle regions.

Shape: The lesions are flakey or strip like, ground glass opacities are fused into a piece, and nodular consolidations are seen inside.

Density: Ground glass or mixed ground glass opacities, with high peripheral density. Smooth air bronchogram is common and reticulated reticular pattern is rare [16].

Differentiate COVID-19 from Pneumocystis Pneumonia

Patients usually have a history of immune damage. The lesions present as large ground glass opacities or consolidations, with rare pleural effusions, which are similar to the COVID-19. However, the focus of Pneumocystis pneumoniae is located in the central axis of both lungs, and subpleural area involvement is rare, which can be differentiated from the COVID-19. Pneumocystis pneumonia can be further diagnosed when combine with significantly reduced CD4:CD8 and positive of HIV.

Case 8

Medical History and Clinical Manifestations

A 47-year-old male came to the hospital with fever (highest body temperature: 39.2 °C), cough, and shortness of breath for 3 days. Laboratory test results indicated a normal white blood cell

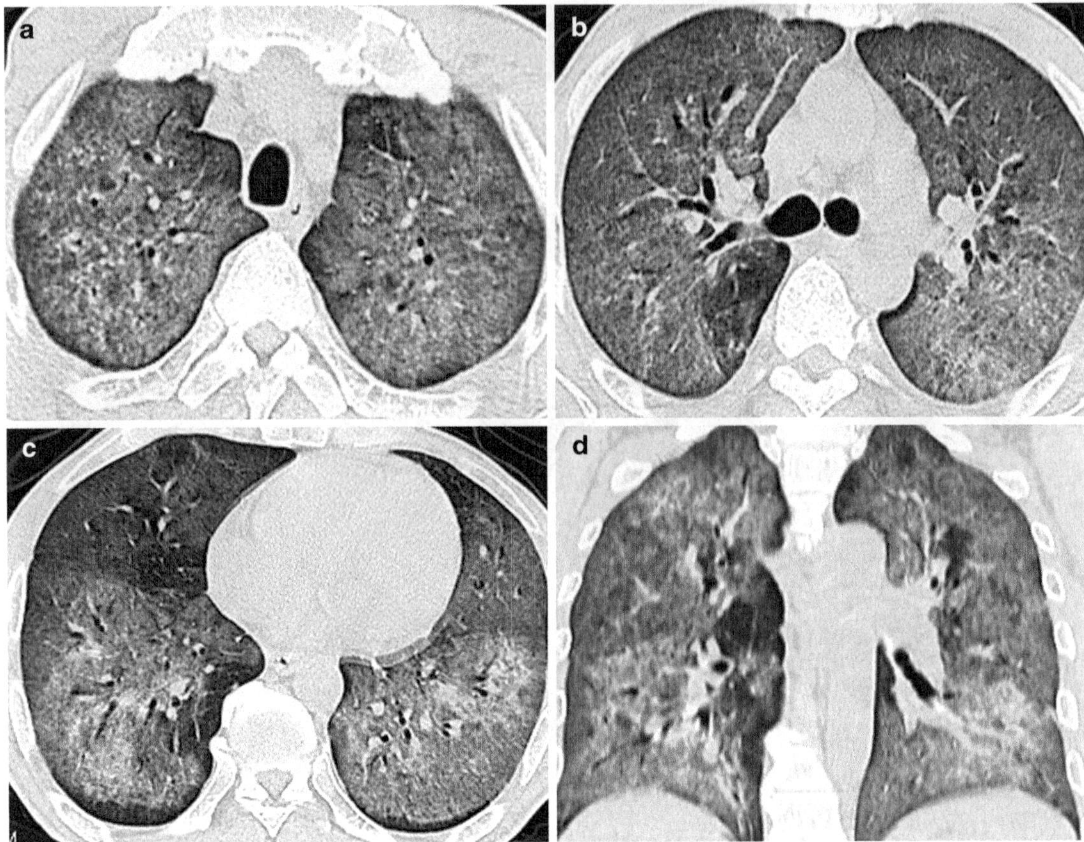

Fig. 8.13 Chest CT image

count of 7.3 × 10^9/L and decreased lymphocytes (15.1%). There were elevated blood levels for neutrophils (83.0%), erythrocyte sedimentation rate (21 mm/h), and C-reactive protein (35.2 mg/L). The nucleic acids of influenza A/B, H7N9 were negative twice and HIV was positive. Yersinia pneumonia was diagnosed by bronchoalveolar lavage, then the patient was transferred to a designated hospital for treatment.

Imaging Features

Chest CT image showed bilateral and diffused miliary lesions, patchy ground glass opacities, and consolidations. The lesions were distributed centered in the lung hilum. Subpleural area, costophrenic angle, and the apex of the two lungs were not involved. Air bronchogram was seen and there were no pleural effusions (Fig. 8.13).

Comments: The patient has a history of being HIV (+). The lesions diffused distribute around two lung hilum.

8.8 Cryptococcal Pneumonia

Typical Imaging Features

Distribution: The lesions are often subpleural distribution and there is no obvious tendency of lung lobes or segments.

Shape: Present as single, multiple nodule, or multiple patches and nodules, the edge is irregular, but there is no obvious burr and pleura traction.

Density: Most are solid and surrounded by ground glass opacities which are called "halo sign." There are smooth cavities in the solid lesions [17, 18].

Differentiate COVID-19 from Cryptococcal Pneumonia

Cryptococcal pneumonia occurs not only in patients with hypoimmunity, but also those with normal immunity. Generally, the clinical symptoms are mild and fever is rare. The imaging manifestations of cryptococcal pneumonia can be divided into single nodule, multiple nodule, or multiple patchy nodules types. Multiple patchy nodules type needs to be differentiated from COVID-19. Multiple patchy nodules type cryptococcus pneumonia is commonly distributed in subpleural area, but the density of the lesions is higher and halo signs are common, and thickened blood vessel or reticular pattern is rare. These are helpful to distinguish from COVID-19 when combined with the clinical manifestations.

Case 9

Medical History and Clinical Manifestations

A 44-years-old male was admitted in the hospital with cough and blood in sputum for 1 month. Laboratory test results indicated a normal white blood cell count of 5.7×10^9/L and 20.2% lymphocytes. There were elevated blood levels for neutrophils (72.3%), erythrocyte sedimentation rate (15.5 mm/h), and C-reactive protein (31.2 mg/L). The nucleic acids of influenza A/B and H7N9 were negative twice. Anti-inflammatory treatment was invalid. Pathology of lung biopsy in the left lower lobe reported "multiple granulomas, multiple fungal spores in the multinuclear giant cells; PAS(+), pasm(+), cryptococcal pneumonia was considered."

Imaging Features

Chest CT image showed subpleural multiple patchy and nodular opacities with halo sign (red arrow) in right middle lung and left lower lobe. The air bronchogram (thick red arrow) in left lower lobe, and no pleural effusions were seen in the bilateral chest cavity (Fig. 8.14).

Comments: The solid lesions with "halo sign" are the characteristic CT finding of cryptococcal pneumonia.

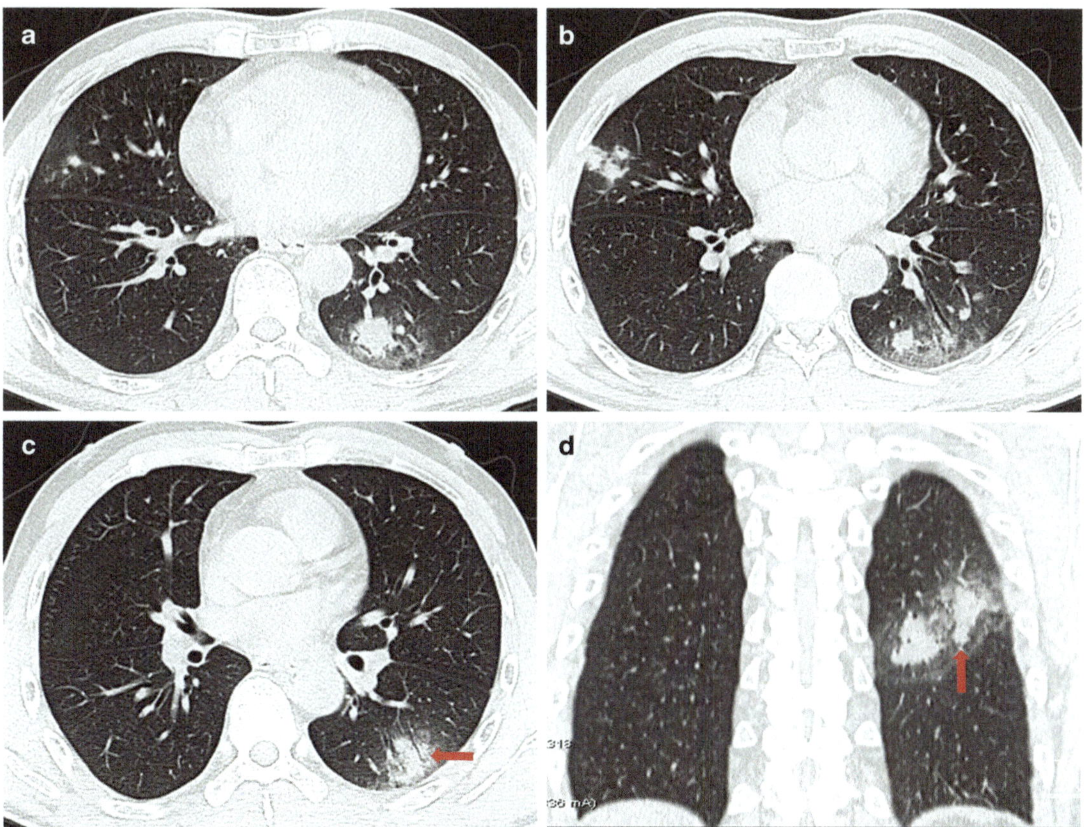

Fig. 8.14 Initial CT image

8.9 Lobar Pneumonia

Typical Imaging Features

Distribution: The lesions usually involve the whole lung lobe from hilum to subpleural area, but there is no obvious tendency of lung lobe distribution.

Shape: The lesions are large wedge-shaped or fan-shaped.

Density: Present as heterogeneous flakey consolidations with smooth air bronchogram.

Differentiate COVID-19 from Lobar Pneumonia

Lobar pneumonia is more common in young adults and the typical clinical manifestations are cough, rust, and sputum. It usually involves one lung lobe and presents large consolidations with air bronchogram, and without reticular pattern. Pleural effusions are common. Combined with the significant increase of white blood cell count and neutrophils, these features are helpful to distinguish from COVID-19 [19].

Case 10

Medical History and Clinical Manifestations

A 68-year-old female was admitted in the hospital with cough for 4 days and fever (highest body temperature: 39.3 °C) for 1 day. Laboratory test results indicated elevated blood levels for white blood cell count (19.5×10^9/L), neutrophils (83.1%), and C-reactive protein (182.6 mg/L). The nucleic acids of influenza A/B and H7N9 were negative for three times.

Imaging Features

Initial chest CT image showed large consolidation with a slightly fuzzy edge in right middle lobe. The smooth air bronchogram (thick red arrow) and a small amount of right pleural effusions were seen (Fig. 8.15).

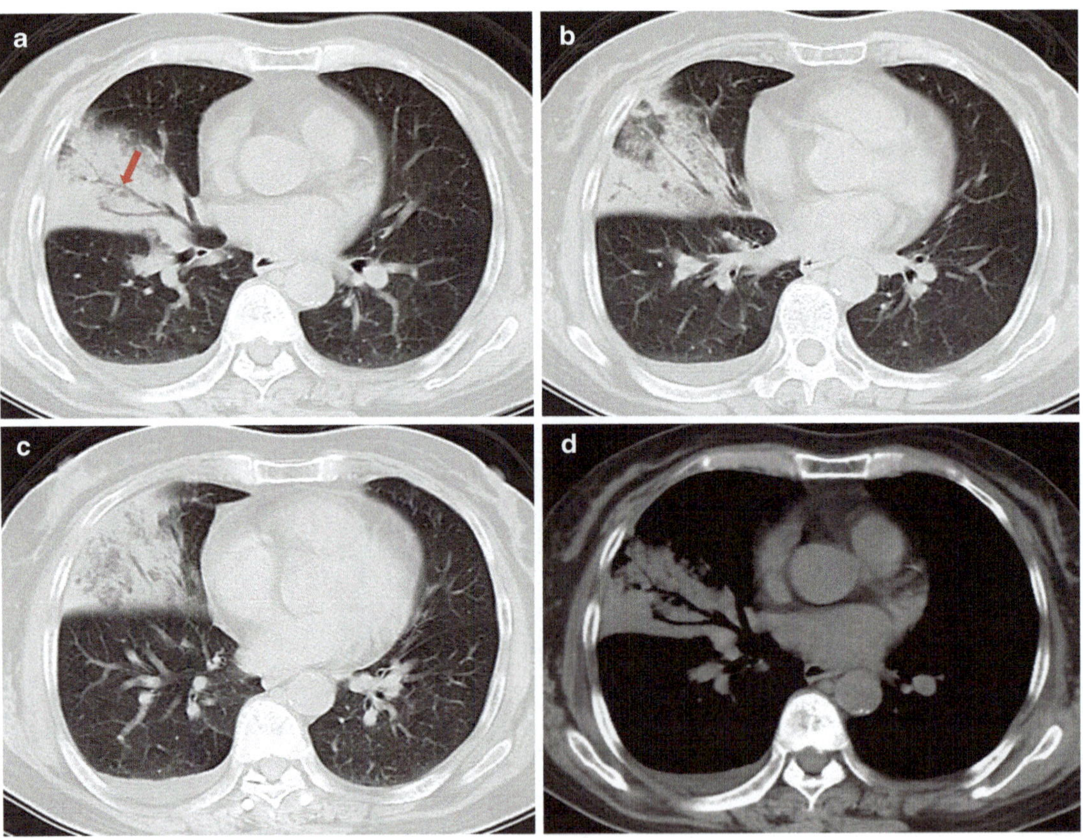

Fig. 8.15 Initial CT image

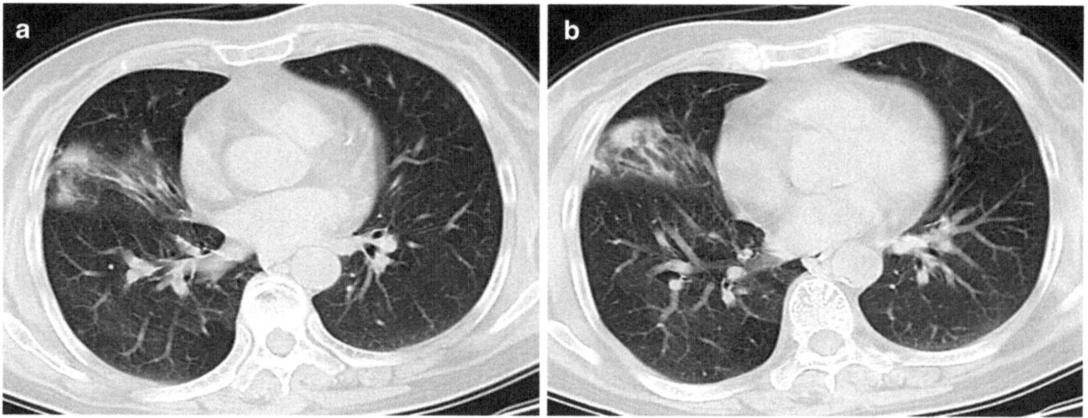

Fig. 8.16 Follow-up CT images 14 days after initial scan

Follow-up chest CT (14 days after Initial CT examination) showed the lesions in right middle lobe and right pleural effusions were resolved obviously after 14 days treatment of anti-inflammatory (Fig. 8.16).

Comments: Large consolidations in one lung lobe are the characteristic CT finding of lobar pneumonia. The blood routine leukocytes and neutrophils are significantly increased, which is helpful to distinguish from COVID-19.

8.10 Acute Allergic Alveolitis

Typical Imaging Features

Distribution: The lesions are diffused distribution from hilum to subpleural, most of them are centrilobular, the interlobular septum is not involved.

Shape: The lesions are small nodular, tree bud shaped or patchy.

Density: Present as ground glass opacities and some are consolidation [20].

Differentiate COVID-19 from Acute Allergic Alveolitis

The CT manifestations of acute allergic alveolitis are diffused multiple centrilobular ground glass nodules with tree bud sign and without thickened interlobular septum, while COVID-19 commonly presents ground glass opacities and reticular pattern. Combined with the patient's history, blood levels of eosinophils, and IgE, it can be distinguished from COVID-19.

Case 11

Medical History and Clinical Manifestations

A 40-year-old male was admitted in the hospital with cough for 2 months and chest tightness for 1 month, who had been engaged in carpentry over 10 years. Laboratory test results indicated a normal white blood cell count of 7.0×10^9/L and decreased lymphocytes (15.1%). There were elevated blood levels for neutrophils (70.2%), eosinophils (10.2%), erythrocyte sedimentation rate (18 mm/h), C-reactive protein (31.2 mg/L), and IgE (125.3 mg/L). The TSPOT was negative and the nucleic acids of influenza A/B and H7N9 were negative for three times. Acute allergic alveolitis was diagnosed on admission and the lesions absorbed obviously after treatment with methylprednisolone for 1 month.

Imaging Features

Initial CT image showed bilateral, diffuse, and multiple homogeneous centrilobular ground glass nodules. The tree bud sign was seen, and there was no pleural effusion in the bilateral chest cavity (Fig. 8.17).

Comments: The occupational history and imaging features of the patients are helpful for differential diagnosis.

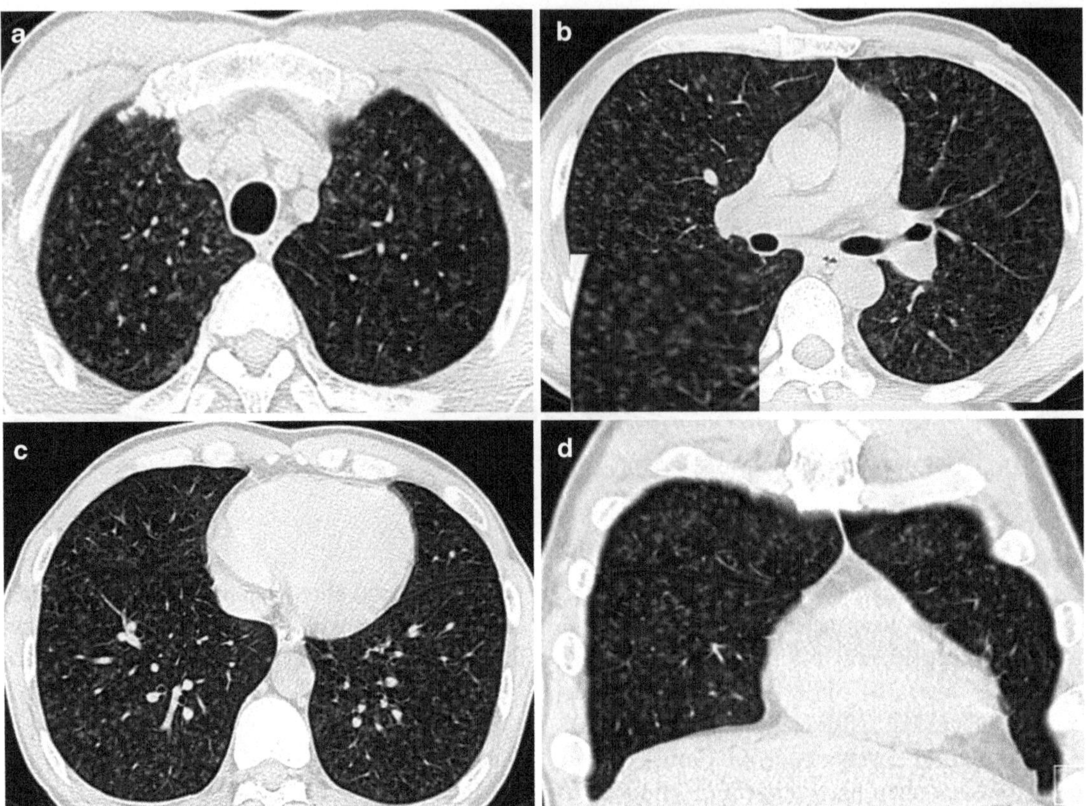

Fig. 8.17 Initial CT image

8.11 Aspiration Pneumonia

Typical Imaging Features

Distribution: The lesions are distributed unevenly in the center of the lobules and mainly in the dorsal side of the lower field of both lungs.

Shape: The lesions are nodular, tree bud shaped or patchy.

Density: Mixed ground glass and patchy opacities with solid nodules. The density of lesions close to the dorsal pleura is usually higher than that on the centripetal side, and the edge is fuzzy [21].

Differentiate COVID-19 from Aspiration Pneumonia

The history of inhalation and CT features of lobular distribution are helpful for differential diagnosis.

Case 12

Medical History and Clinical Manifestations

A 49-year-old male was admitted in the hospital with chest distress and shortness of breath for 13 h after inhaling nitrosylsulfuric acid. Laboratory test results indicated a normal white blood cell count of 6.3×10^9/L and 23.1% lymphocytes. There were elevated blood levels for erythrocyte sedimentation rate (18 mm/h) and C-reactive protein (25.2 mg/L). The nucleic acids of influenza A/B and H7N9 were negative twice.

Imaging Features

Initial CT image showed bilateral multiple patchy opacities and centrilobular nodules in different sizes. The tree bud sign (thick red arrow) was seen, and there were a small amount of pleural effusions (Fig. 8.18).

Comments: The CT manifestations of aspiration pneumonia are similar to viral pneumonia. The history of inhalation of nitrosylsulfuric acid is helpful for the diagnosis.

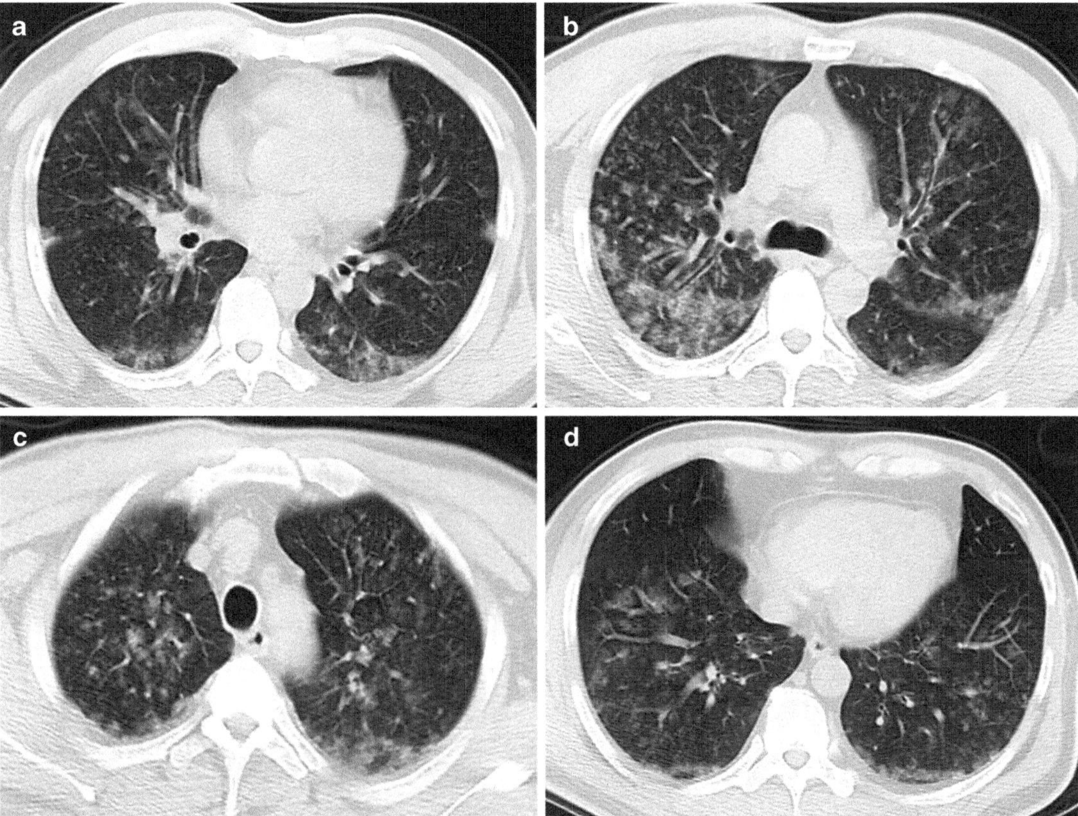

Fig. 8.18 Initial CT image

8.12 Alveolar Pulmonary Edema

Typical Imaging Features

Distribution: The lesions are bilateral symmetrical centered in two lung hilum and mainly in the dorsal lung.

Shape: Present as "butterfly wing."

Density: Mixed ground glass, patchy opacities with solid nodules. Mixed ground glass opacities, flakey ground glass nodular consolidations, and thickened interlobular septum and pleural effusion are common [22].

Differentiate COVID-19 from Pulmonary Alveolus Edema

The CT manifestations of pulmonary vesicular edema were "butterfly wing" ground glass opacity, thickening of interlobular septum, left heart enlargement, and pleural effusion. Typical CT features and clinical information such as cardiac insufficiency are helpful for differential diagnosis.

Case 13

Medical History and Clinical Manifestations

A 60-year-old male was admitted in the hospital with repeated chest distress and shortness of breath for more than 2 years, aggravated for 3 days. Laboratory test results indicated a normal white blood cell count of 8.3×10^9/L and decreased lymphocytes (19.1%). There were elevated blood levels for neutrophils (75.2%), erythrocyte sedimentation rate (17.5 mm/h), and C-reactive protein (34.2 mg/L). Echocardiography showed mitral valve prolapse with severe regurgitation and left ventricular enlargement. The nucleic acid of influenza A/B and H7N9 was negative twice. He was diagnosed as left ventricular insufficiency and pulmonary alveolar edema. After 1 week of treatment of cardiotonic diuresis

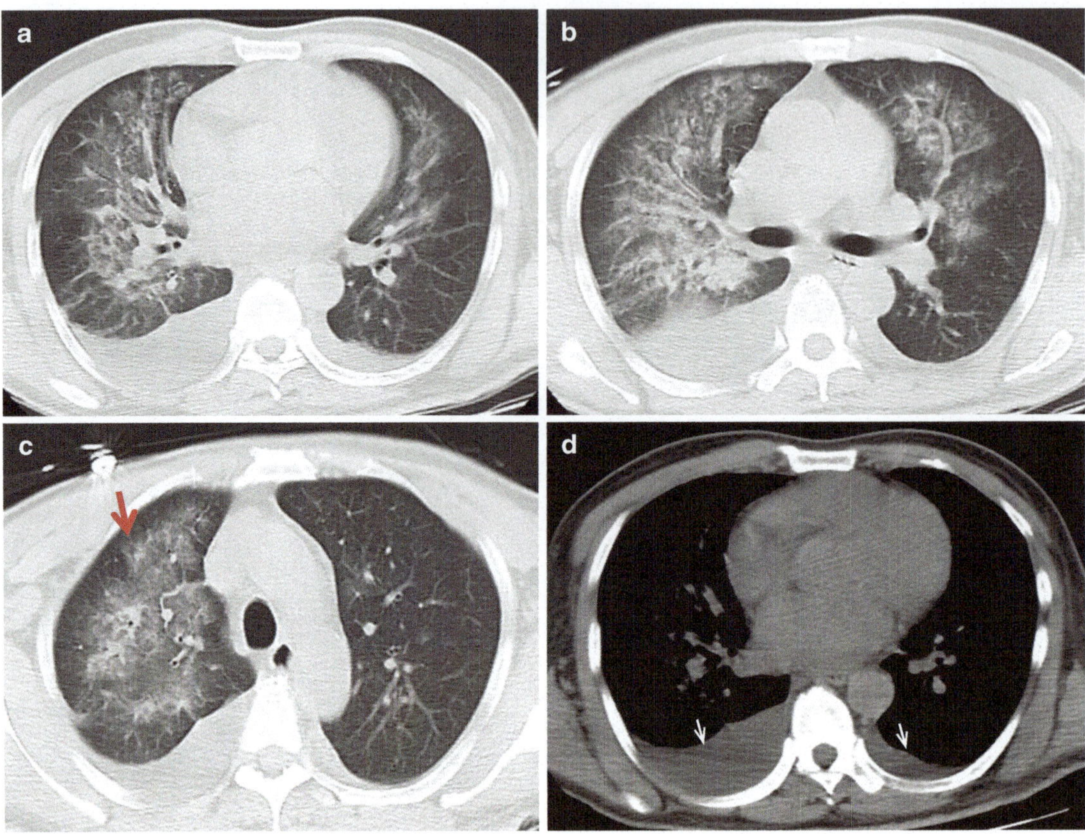

Fig. 8.19 Initial CT image

and anti-inflammatory, the bilateral lesions were obviously absorbed.

Imaging Features

Initial CT image showed left heart enlargement, multiple patchy ground glass opacities, and consolidations centered in two lung hilum. The interlobular septum was thickened (thick red arrow), and there were pleural effusions in the bilateral chest cavity (thick white arrow) (Fig. 8.19).

Comments: The patient has basic heart disease. CT shows butterfly-wing like ground glass opacities and consolidations centered to the lung hilum, thickened interlobular septum, left heart enlargement, and massive pleural effusion.

8.13 Alveolar Hematocele

Typical Imaging Features

Distribution: Most of the lesions are located in one side of the lung, mostly under the pleura and close to the pleura of oblique fissure. There is no obvious distribution tendency of lung lobes or segments.

Shape: Present as flakey or polygon with a straight back edge.

Density: The density of the dorsal side of the lesion is usually higher and the density of the thoracic side is lighter [23].

Differentiate COVID-19 from Alveolar Hematocele

Pulmonary alveolar hematocele has a history of hemoptysis and the lesions are mainly on one side. Chest CT scan shows patchy ground glass opacities with consolidations. The dorsolateral of the lesions has high density with a relatively straight edge and clear boundary. The chest side of the lesions has fuzzy boundary. These features are different from those of COVID-19 and can be distinguished by combining it with the history of hemoptysis.

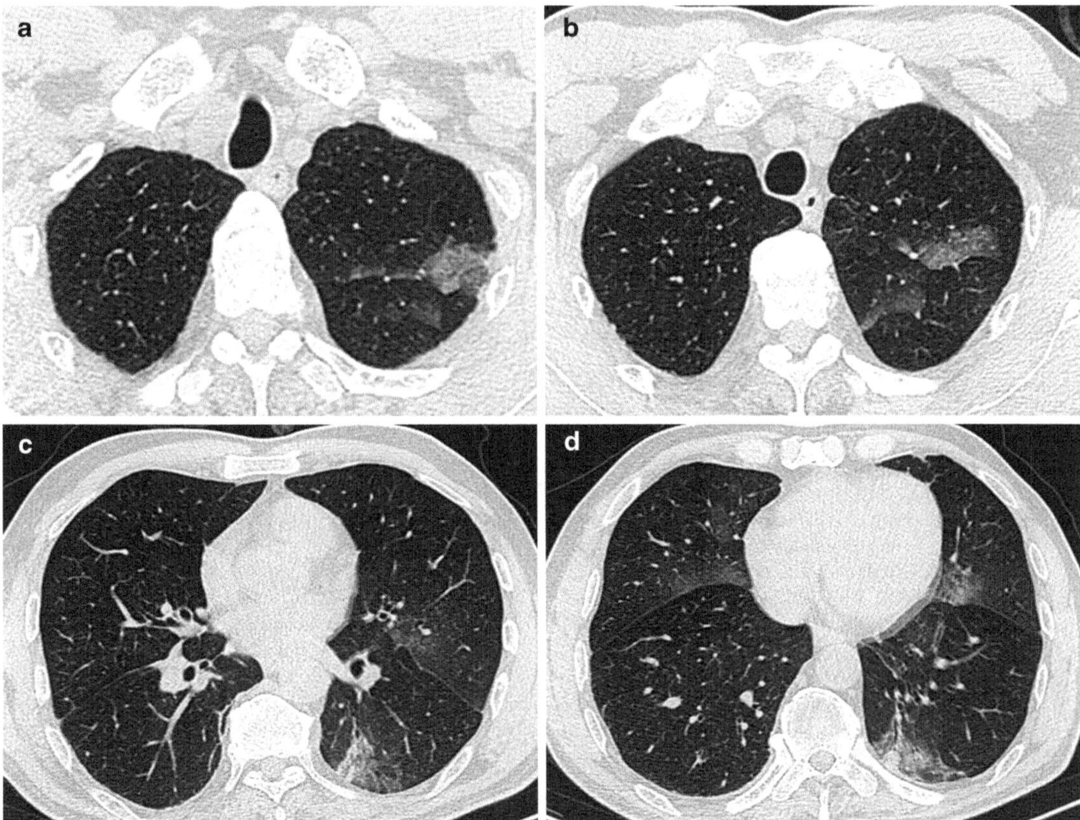

Fig. 8.20 Chest CT image

Case 14

Medical History and Clinical Manifestations

A 62-year-old male was admitted in the hospital and had hemoptysis for 3 days. Laboratory test results indicated a normal white blood cell count of 5.3 × 10^9/L, lymphocytes (23.1%) and erythrocyte sedimentation rate (15 mm/h). There were elevated blood levels for neutrophils (71.2%) and C-reactive protein (23.2 mg/L). The nucleic acid of influenza A/B and H7N9 was negative twice.

Imaging Features

Chest CT image showed multiple patchy ground glass opacities in left lung and right middle lobe. The lesions in left upper lobe mostly had straight edges and clear borders, and some lesions had fuzzy edges (Fig. 8.20).

Comments: The patient has a clear history of hemoptysis. The CT shows flake ground glass opacities with relatively straight edge and higher density on the dorsal side of the lesion, which is different from COVID-19.

References

1. Ai T, Yang Z, Hou H, et al. Correlation of chest CT and RT-PCR testing in coronavirus disease 2019 (COVID-19) in China: a report of 1014 cases. Radiology. 2020:200642. Online ahead of print.
2. Fang Y, Zhang H, Xie J, et al. Sensitivity of chest CT for COVID-19: comparison to RT-PCR. Radiology. 2020:200432. Online ahead of print.
3. Ajlan AM, Quiney B, Nicolaou S, et al. Swine-origin influenza A (H1N1) viral infection: radiographic and CT findings. AJR. 2009;193(6):1494–9.
4. Marchiori E, Zanetti G, D'Ippolito G, et al. Swine-origin influenza A (H1N1) viral infection: thoracic findings on CT. AJR. 2011;196(6):W723–8.
5. Li P, Su DJ, Zhang JF, et al. Pneumonia in novel swine-origin influenza A (H1N1) virus infection: high-resolution CT findings. Eur J Radiol. 2011;80(2):e146–52.

6. Tang X, Du R, Wang R, et al. Comparison of hospitalized patients with ARDS caused by COVID-19 and H1N1. Chest. 2020 Mar 26 [Epub ahead of print].
7. Yin Z, Kang Z, Yang D, et al. A comparison of clinical and chest CT findings in patients with Influenza A (H1N1) virus infection and coronavirus disease (COVID-19). AJR. 2020, May 26:1–7. [Epub ahead of print].
8. Lin ZQ, Xu XQ, Zhang KB, et al. Chest X-ray and CT findings of early H7N9 avian influenza cases. Acta Radiol. 2015;56(5):552–6.
9. Joob B, Wiwanitkit V. Chest X-ray and CT findings in H7N9 influenza. Acta Radiol. 2015;56(1):NP5.
10. Bai HX, Hsieh B, Xiong Z, et al. Performance of radiologists in differentiating COVID-19 from viral pneumonia on chest CT. Radiology. 2020, Mar 10:200823. [Epub ahead of print].
11. Wang H, Wei R, Rao G, et al. Characteristic CT findings distinguishing 2019 novel coronavirus disease (COVID-19) from influenza pneumonia. Eur Radiol. 2020, Apr 22. [Epub ahead of print].
12. Chong S, Lee KS, Kim TS, et al. Adenovirus pneumonia in adults: radiographic and high-resolution CT findings in five patients. AJR. 2006;186(5):1288–93.
13. Kunihiro Y, Tanaka N, Matsumoto T, et al. The usefulness of a diagnostic method combining high-resolution CT findings and serum markers for cytomegalovirus pneumonia and pneumocystis pneumonia in non-AIDS patients. Acta Radiol. 2015, Jul;56(7):806–13.
14. Chung MP, Nam BD, Lee KS, et al. Serial chest CT in cryptogenic organizing pneumonia: evolutional changes and prognostic determinants. Respirology. 2018;23(3):325–30.
15. Lee JW, Lee KS, Lee HY, et al. Cryptogenic organizing pneumonia: serial high-resolution CT findings in 22 patients. AJR. 2010;195(4):916–22.
16. Hidalgo A, Falcó V, Mauleón S, et al. Accuracy of high-resolution CT in distinguishing between *Pneumocystis carinii* pneumonia and non-*Pneumocystis carinii* pneumonia in AIDS patients. Eur Radiol. 2003;13(5):1179–84.
17. Sui X, Huang Y, Song W, et al. Clinical features of pulmonary cryptococcosis in thin-section CT in immunocompetent and non-AIDS immunocompromised patients. Radiol Med. 2020;125(1):31–8.
18. Xie LX, Chen YS, Liu SY, et al. Pulmonary cryptococcosis: comparison of CT findings in immunocompetent and immunocompromised patients. Acta Radiol. 2015;56(4):447–53.
19. Bai HX, Wang R, Xiong Z, et al. AI augmentation of radiologist performance in distinguishing COVID-19 from pneumonia of other etiology on chest CT. Radiology, 2020 Apr 27:201491. [Epub ahead of print].
20. Ban CJ, Dai HP, Zhang S, et al. Chest high resolution CT features of extrinsic allergic alveolitis and its diagnostic value. Zhonghua Yi Xue Za Zhi. 2010, Apr 27;90(16):1105–8.
21. Lee KH, Kim WS, Cheon JE, et al. Squalene aspiration pneumonia in children: radiographic and CT findings as the first clue to diagnosis. Pediatr Radiol. 2005;35(6):619–23.
22. Komiya K, Ishii H, Murakami J, et al. Comparison of chest computed tomography features in the acute phase of cardiogenic pulmonary edema and acute respiratory distress syndrome on arrival at the emergency department. J Thorac Imaging. 2013;28(5):322–8.
23. Kloth C, Thaiss WM, Beck R, et al. Potential role of CT-textural features for differentiation between viral interstitial pneumonias, *Pneumocystis jirovecii* pneumonia and diffuse alveolar hemorrhage in early stages of disease: a proof of principle. BMC Med Imaging. 2019;19(1):39.

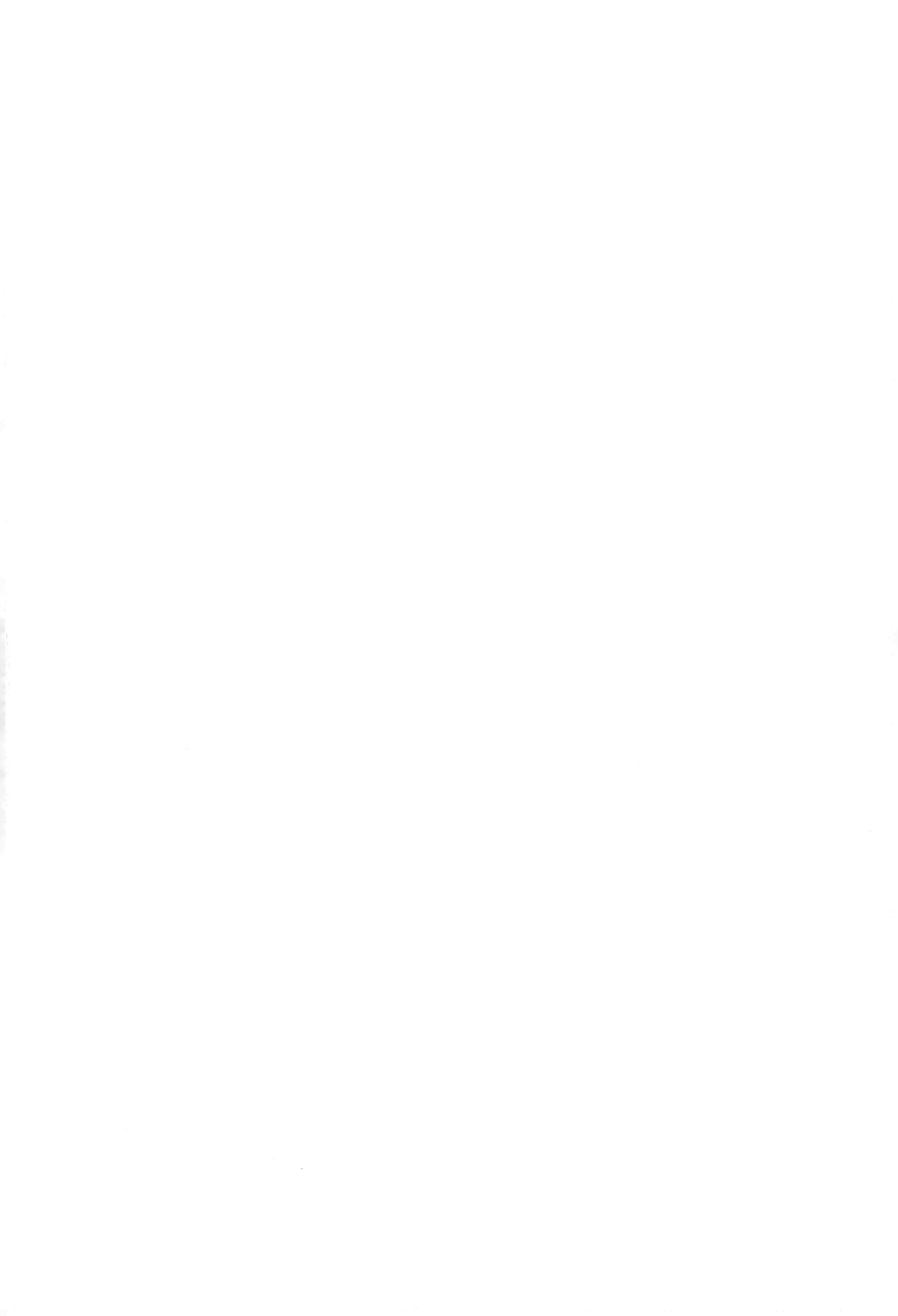

GPSR Compliance

The European Union's (EU) General Product Safety Regulation (GPSR) is a set of rules that requires consumer products to be safe and our obligations to ensure this.

If you have any concerns about our products, you can contact us on ProductSafety@springernature.com

In case Publisher is established outside the EU, the EU authorized representative is:

Springer Nature Customer Service Center GmbH
Europaplatz 3
69115 Heidelberg, Germany

Batch number: 10406427

Printed by Printforce, the Netherlands